ADVANCES IN ALLOGENEIC HEMATOPOIETIC STEM CELL TRANSPLANTATION

Cancer Treatment and Research

Steven T. Rosen, M.D., *Series Editor*

Sugarbaker, P.H. (ed): Management of Gastric Cancer. 1991. ISBN 0-7923-1102-7.

Pinedo H.M., Verweij J., Suit, H.D., (eds): Soft Tissue Sarcomas: New Developments in the Multidisciplinary Approach to Treatment. 1991. ISBN 0-7923-1139-6.

Ozols, R.F., (ed): Molecular and Clinical Advances in Anticancer Drug Resistance. 1991. ISBN 0-7923-1212-0.

Muggia, F.M. (ed): New Drugs, Concepts and Results in Cancer Chemotherapy 1991. ISBN 0-7923-1253-8.

Dickson, R.B., Lippman, M.E. (eds): Genes, Oncogenes and Hormones: Advances in Cellular and Molecular Biology of Breast Cancer. 1992. ISBN 0-7923-1748-3.

Humphrey, G. Bennett, Schraffordt Koops, H., Molenaar, W.M., Postma, A., (eds): Osteosarcoma in Adolescents and Young Adults: New Developments and Controversies. 1993. ISBN 0-7923-1905-2.

Benz, C. C., Liu, E. T. (eds): Oncogenes and Tumor Suppressor Genes in Human Malignancies. 1993. ISBN 0-7923-1960-5.

Freireich, E.J., Kantarjian, H., (eds): Leukemia: Advances in Research and Treatment. 1993. ISBN 0-7923-1967-2.

Dana, B. W., (ed): Malignant Lymphomas, Including Hodgkin's Disease: Diagnosis, Management, and Special Problems. 1993. ISBN 0-7923-2171-5.

Nathanson, L. (ed): Current Research and Clinical Management of Melanoma. 1993. ISBN 0-7923-2152-9.

Verweij, J., Pinedo, H. M., Suit, H. D. (eds): Multidisciplinary Treatment of Soft Tissue Sarcomas. 1993. ISBN 0-7923-2183-9.

Rosen, S. T., Kuzel, T. M. (eds): Immunoconjugate Therapy of Hematologic Malignancies. 1993. ISBN 0-7923-2270-3.

Sugarbaker, P. H. (ed): Hepatobiliary Cancer. 1994. ISBN 0-7923-2501-X. .

Rothenberg, M. L. (ed): Gynecologic Oncology: Controversies and New Developments. 1994. ISBN 0-7923-2634-2.

Dickson, R. B., Lippman, M. E. (eds.): Mammary Tumorigenesis and Malignant Progression. 1994. ISBN 0-7923-2647-4.

Hansen, H. H., (ed): Lung Cancer. Advances in Basic and Clinical Research. 1994. ISBN 0-7923-2835-3.

Goldstein, L.J., Ozols, R. F. (eds.): Anticancer Drug Resistance. Advances in Molecular and Clinical Research. 1994. ISBN 0-7923-2836-1.

Hong, W.K., Weber, R.S. (eds.): Head and Neck Cancer. Basic and Clinical Aspects. 1994. ISBN 0-7923-3015-3.

Thall, P.F. (ed): Recent Advances in Clinical Trial Design and Analysis. 1995. ISBN 0-7923-3235-0.

Buckner, C. D. (ed): Technical and Biological Components of Marrow Transplantation. 1995. ISBN 0-7923-3394-2.

Winter, J.N. (ed.): Blood Stem Cell Transplantation. 1997. ISBN 0-7923-4260-7.

Muggia, F.M. (ed): Concepts, Mechanisms, and New Targets for Chemotherapy. 1995. ISBN 0-7923-3525-2.

Klastersky, J. (ed): Infectious Complications of Cancer. 1995. ISBN 0-7923-3598-8.

Kurzrock, R., Talpaz, M. (eds): Cytokines: Interleukins and Their Receptors. 1995. ISBN 0-7923-3636-4.

Sugarbaker, P. (ed): Peritoneal Carcinomatosis: Drugs and Diseases. 1995. ISBN 0-7923-3726-3.

Sugarbaker, P. (ed): Peritoneal Carcinomatosis: Principles of Management. 1995. ISBN 0-7923-3727-1.

Dickson, R.B., Lippman, M.E. (eds.): Mammary Tumor Cell Cycle, Differentiation and Metastasis. 1995. ISBN 0-7923-3905-3.

Freireich, E.J, Kantarjian, H. (eds.): Molecular Genetics and Therapy of Leukemia. 1995. ISBN 0-7923-3912-6.

Cabanillas, F., Rodriguez, M.A. (eds.): Advances in Lymphoma Research. 1996. ISBN 0-7923-3929-0.

Miller, A.B. (ed.): Advances in Cancer Screening. 1996. ISBN 0-7923-4019-1.

Hait , W.N. (ed.): Drug Resistance. 1996. ISBN 0-7923-4022-1.

Pienta, K.J. (ed.): Diagnosis and Treatment of Genitourinary Malignancies. 1996. ISBN 0-7923-4164-3.

Arnold, A.J. (ed.): Endocrine Neoplasms. 1997. ISBN 0-7923-4354-9.

Pollock, R.E. (ed.): Surgical Oncology. 1997. ISBN 0-7923-9900-5.

Verweij, J., Pinedo, H.M., Suit, H.D. (eds.): Soft Tissue Sarcomas: Present Achievements and Future Prospects. 1997. ISBN 0-7923-9913-7.

Walterhouse, D.O., Cohn, S. L. (eds.): Diagnostic and Therapeutic Advances in Pediatric Oncology. 1997. ISBN 0-7923-9978-1.

Mittal, B.B., Purdy, J.A., Ang, K.K. (eds.): Radiation Therapy. 1998. ISBN 0-7923-9981-1.

Foon, K.A., Muss, H.B. (eds.): Biological and Hormonal Therapies of Cancer. 1998. ISBN 0-7923-9997-8.

Ozols, R.F. (ed.): Gynecologic Oncology. 1998. ISBN 0-7923-8070-3.

Noskin, G. A. (ed.): Management of Infectious Complications in Cancer Patients. 1998. ISBN 0-7923-8150-5

Bennett, C. L. (ed.): Cancer Policy. 1998. ISBN 0-7923-8203-X

Benson, A. B. (ed.): Gastrointestinal Oncology. 1998. ISBN 0-7923-8205-6

Tallman, M.S. , Gordon, L.I. (eds.): Diagnostic and Therapeutic Advances in Hematologic Malignancies. 1998. ISBN 0-7923-8206-4

von Gunten, C.F. (ed.): Palliative Care and Rehabilitation of Cancer Patients. 1999. ISBN 0-7923-8525-X

Burt, R.K., Brush, M.M. (eds): Advances in Allogeneic Hematopoietic Stem Cell Transplantation. 1999. ISBN 0-7923-7714-1

ADVANCES IN ALLOGENEIC HEMATOPOIETIC STEM CELL TRANSPLANTATION

edited by

Richard K. Burt
and
Mary M. Brush

Northwestern University Medical Center
Chicago, USA

KLUWER ACADEMIC PUBLISHERS
Boston / Dordrecht / London

Distributors for North, Central and South America:
Kluwer Academic Publishers
101 Philip Drive
Assinippi Park
Norwell, Massachusetts 02061 USA

Distributors for all other countries:
Kluwer Academic Publishers Group
Distribution Centre
Post Office Box 322
3300 AH Dordrecht, THE NETHERLANDS

Library of Congress Cataloging-in-Publication Data

Printed on acid-free paper.

Printed in the United States of America

TABLE OF CONTENTS

CONTRIBUTORS

Rodolfo Alejandro, Diabetes Research Institute, Departments of Medicine and Surgery, University of Miami School of Medicine and Miami VA Medical Center, Miami, FL, USA

Claudio Anasetti, MD, Fred Hutchinson Cancer Research Center, Seattle, WA

J. Christian Barrett, MD, University of Alabama-Birmingham, Birmingham, AL

Bruce Blazar, MD, University of Minnesota, Minneapolis, MN 55455

William H. Burns, MD, Medical College of Wisconsin, Milwaukee, WI 53226

Richard K. Burt, MD, Northwestern University Medical Center, 250 E. Superior Street, Wesley 162, Chicago, IL 60611

Richard Champlin, University of Texas, M.D. Anderson Cancer Center, Houston, TX 77030

C.L. Chastang, Hôpital Saint Louis, 1 Ave Claude Vellefaux, 75475 Paris Cedex 10, France

Maria Chatzipetrou, Diabetes Research Institute, Departments of Medicine and Surgery, University of Miami School of Medicine and Miami VA Medical Center, Miami, FL, USA

G. J. Clark, Mater Medical Research Institute, South Brisbane 4101, Queensland, Australia

Patricia D. Conrad, MD, University of Pennsylvania School of Medicine, Philadelphia, PA 19104

William R. Drobyski, Department of Medicine and the Bone Marrow Transplant Program, Medical College of Wisconsin, Milwaukee, WI 53226

Stephen G. Emerson, MD, PhD, University of Pennsylvania School of Medicine, Philadelphia, PA 19104

James L.M. Ferrara, MD, University of Michigan Cancer Center, Ann Arbor, MI 48109

Sergio Giralt, MD, University of Texas, M.D. Anderson Cancer Center, Houston, TX 77030

Rocha E. Gluckman, Hôpital Saint Louis, 1 Ave Claude Vellefaux, 75475 Paris Cedex 10, France

John A. Hansen, Fred Hutchinson Cancer Research Center, Seattle, WA

D.N.J. Hart, Mater Medical Research Institute, South Brisbane 4101, Queensland, Australia

P. Jean Henslee-Downey, MD, South Carolina Cancer Center, University of South Carolina and Palmetto Richland Memorial Hospital Center for Cancer Treatment and Research, Columbia, South Carolina, USA

Ernst Holler, MD, Regensberg University Hospital, Regensburg, Germany D93042

Gabriel N. Hortobagyi, Department of Blood and Marrow Transplantation, University of Texas, M.D. Anderson Cancer Center, Houston, TX 77030

Norma S. Kenyon, Diabetes Research Institute, Departments of Medicine and Surgery, University of Miami School of Medicine and Miami VA Medical Center, Miami, FL, USA

Issa Khouri, MD, University of Texas, M.D. Anderson Cancer Center, Houston, TX 77030

Martin Körbling, University of Texas, M.D. Anderson Cancer Center, Houston, TX 77030

Charles J. Link, Jr., MD, Human Gene Therapy Research Institute, Des Moines, IA 50309

Kenneth G. Lucas, MD, University of Alabama-Birmingham, Birmingham, AL

Paul J. Martin, MD, Fred Hutchinson Cancer Research Center, Seattle, WA

Ian K. McNiece, PhD, Bone Marrow Transplant Unit, University of Colorado Health Sciences Center, Denver, CO 80262

Joshua Miller, Diabetes Research Institute, Departments of Medicine and Surgery, University of Miami School of Medicine and Miami VA Medical Center, Miami, FL, USA

Stephen J. Noga, MD, PhD, The Johns Hopkins Oncology Center, Room 804, 550 N. Broadway Avenue, Baltimore, MD 21205

Effie W. Petersdorf, MD, Fred Hutchinson Cancer Research Center, Seattle, WA

Camillo Ricordi, Diabetes Research Institute, Departments of Medicine and Surgery, University of Miami School of Medicine and Miami VA Medical Center, Miami, FL, USA

V. Rocha, Hôpital Saint Louis, 1 Ave Claude Vellefaux, 75475 Paris Cedex 10, France

Jean E. Sanders, MD, Fred Hutchinson Cancer Research Center, Seattle, WA

Tatiana Seregina, PhD, Human Gene Therapy Research Institute, Des Moines, IA 50309

Alan M. Ship, MD, CM, Emory University School of Medicine, Atlanta, GA 30322

Ann Traynor, MD, Northwestern University Medical Center, 250 E. Superior Street, Wesley 162, Chicago, IL 60611

Andreas Tzakis, Diabetes Research Institute, Departments of Medicine and Surgery, University of Miami School of Medicine and Miami VA Medical Center, Miami, FL, USA

Naoto T. Ueno, Department of Blood and Marrow Transplantation, University of Texas, M.D. Anderson Cancer Center, Houston, TX

Alan M. Ship, MD, CM, Emory University School of Medicine, Atlanta, GA 30322

Edmund K. Waller, MD, PhD, FACP, Emory University School of Medicine, Atlanta, GA 30322

Ann E. Woolfrey, MD, Fred Hutchinson Cancer Research Program, Seattle, WA

PREFACE

The field of hematopoietic stem cell transplantation is rapidly evolving. Realization that hematopoietic stem cells give rise to the immune compartment has resulted in clinical trials of hematopoietic stem cell transplantation for patients with autoimmune diseases. Allogeneic hematopoietic transplants are a form of adoptive immunotherapy resulting in beneficial graft versus tumor effects. Large numbers of hematopoietic cells can be collected with ease. Therefore, a renewable source of cells for *ex vivo* genetic manipulations is readily available. Multiple trials combining hematopoietic transplants and gene therapy are in progress. One such application is the infusion of allogeneic lymphocytes containing a suicide gene to abort graft versus host disease.

Hematopoietic stem cell transplantation is in reality the clinical and practical application of cellular therapy. Hematopoietic transplant physicians are by design or by practical application evolving into cell and gene therapy specialists. The excitement and enthusiasm in hematopoietic transplantation is that it offers a door to the future. A future not of drugs or titrating poisonous chemotherapy but rather of cellular and gene therapy.

1

ALLOGENEIC PERIPHERAL BLOOD STEM CELL TRANSPLANTATION FOR HEMATOLOGIC DISEASES

Martin Körbling

University of Texas M.D.Anderson Cancer Center, Houston, Texas 77030

INTRODUCTION

Circulating hematopoietic stem cells have emerged as an alternative to bone marrow (BM) stem cells for allografting. For many years the reconstitutive potential of circulating stem cells was questioned; peripheral blood stem cells (PBSC) were even characterized a waste product (1). The preclinical experience with allogeneic, sex-mismatched PBSC transplantations in canine littermates, has clearly shown that blood-derived stem cells reconstitute hematopoiesis completely and permanently (2,3) including long-lasting evidence of donor chimerism (4). The first reported case of allogeneic PBSC transplantation in a patient with acute lymphoblastic leukemia was published in 1989 by Kessinger et al. (5) showing clear evidence of trilineage engraftment. This was followed in 1994 and 1995, by various reports of successful allogeneic PBSC transplantations using PBSC from rhG-CSF mobilized donors (6-9).

STEADY-STATE CIRCULATING HEMATOPOIETIC STEM CELLS

In the unperturbed peripheral blood (PB) from normal subjects the percentage of $CD34^+$ cells among circulating nucleated cells is on the average 0.06% (10) (Table 1). The absolute number of circulating $CD34^+$ cells in normal individuals has been reported to be 3.8 (± 0.8 standard deviation) x 10^6/L (n=14) (10) or 3.8 (± 3.2 standard deviation) x 10^6/L (n=10) (11). The more primitive circulating $CD34^+$ subsets such as $CD34^+$ Thy-1^{dim} and $CD34^+$ Thy-1^{dim} $CD38^-$ encompass 30% and 2.5%, respectively, of the unperturbed circulating $CD34^+$ cell pool (10) (Table 1).

Table 1. CD34$^+$ cell and subset concentrations in the donor's peripheral blood at steady state and prior to apheresis at day 4 of rhG-CSF treatment in normal donors.

		CD34$^+$ cells	CD34$^+$ Thy-1^{dim} cells	CD34$^+$ Thy-1^{dim} CD38$^-$ cells
at steady-state	cell concentration x 10^6/L	3.8	1.1	0.095
	% of TNC	0.06	0.018	0.0015
	% of CD34$^+$ cells		30	2.5
prior to apheresis at day 4 of rhG-CSF treatment	cell concentration x 10^6/L	61.9	26.6	2.2
	% of TNC	0.9	0.4	0.033
	% of CD34$^+$ cells		43.1	3.5
fold increase preapheresis over precytokine cell concentration values		16.3	24.2	23.2

[modified: Körbling et al. Blood 86: 2842-2848, 1995]

MOBILIZATION OF HEMATOPOIETIC STEM CELLS

For complete and sustained hematopoietic engraftment after myeloablative chemo- or chemo/radiotherapy, patients must receive a sufficient number of pluripotent hematopoietic stem cells with indefinite self-renewal potential. The stem cell concentration in steady-state peripheral blood is insufficient to provide CD34$^+$ cell engraftment by single or multiple apheresis in a reasonable time period. A temporary peripheralization of CD34$^+$ cells and subsets into the circulating blood is therefore a necessity to increase significantly the yield of blood stem cells, thus minimizing the number of aphereses needed to achieve sufficient CD34$^+$ cells for engraftment. As shown by Molineux et al. (12) in a sex-mismatched mouse model, the transplantation of 10 µl rhG-CSF treated PB was equivalent to 3,000 µl unperturbed PB in rescuing 98% of lethally irradiated mice.

For obvious ethical reasons, mobilization of stem cells from normal donors for allogeneic transplantation cannot rely on chemotherapy combined with cytokine treatment as used in autologous setting. Cytokine priming alone, however, has emerged as an acceptable and efficient treatment alternative in normal, patient-related donors for stem cell mobilization. PBSC donation by unrelated donors listed in the North American National Marrow Donor Program (NMDP) or other Western European Registries and undergoing cytokine mobilization treatment is presently being discussed or has already been performed in a limited number of cases.

The optimal cytokine for stem cell mobilization in normal donors
RhG-CSF has emerged as the preferred cytokine for stem cell mobilization in normal donors partly based on the positive experience and toxicity profile reported with its administration to granulocyte donors (13,14). The mechanism(s) underlying the release of stem cells into circulation are not well understood. Prosper and Verfaillie (15) suggested that downregulated α_4 integrin expression and/or function on rhG-CSF mobilized PB 34^+ colony-forming cells may be responsible for the aberrant circulation of mobilized PBSC.

Flt3 ligand, a new cytokine is currently being tested in phase I/II clinical trials in combination with rhG-CSF or rhGM-CSF. It is believed to have biologic activities similar to stem cell factor (SCF) on the hematopoietic system. In a recently published randomized study on healthy volunteers using Flt3 ligand at escalating doses, the following mobilization characteristics were observed (16): The WBC, especially the monocyte fraction was elevated after Flt3 ligand administration,
-	Flt3 ligand treated subjects exhibited sustained blood levels following subcutaneous administration,
-	Flt3 ligand produced sustained mobilization of progenitor cells with elevated circulating levels persisting for up to a week after the last dose of Flt3 ligand,
-	circulating dendritic cells were increased up to 30-fold following Flt3 ligand administration.

Since Flt3 ligand primarily acts through lymphoid proliferation as compared with the mast cell degranulation effect of SCF, Flt3 ligand might also have a different toxicity profile. Flt3 ligand was well tolerated by healthy volunteers without the need for premedication. Injection site reactions and enlarged lymph nodes seem to be the only adverse events related to Flt3 ligand administration.

Combined rhG-CSF and rhGM-CSF treatment has been reported to result in a significantly reduced number of circulating and collected $CD3^+$ cells, $CD4^+$ cells and $CD8^+$ cells as compared to rhG-CSF treatment alone (17). This could potentially result in the development of less graft-vs-host disease (GVHD) although clinical data are not available yet.

Effect of rhG-CSF treatment on the peripheral blood concentrations of white blood cells (WBC), polymorphonuclear (PMN) cells, lymphocytes, and CD34+ cells and subsets in normal subjects

To assess the effects of rhG-CSF (12 μg/kg/day) on the peripheralization of hematopoietic stem cells and lymphoid subsets, we studied a cohort of 41 normal blood stem cell donors. After 3 days of rhG-CSF treatment, the WBC, PMN, and lymphocyte concentrations in the donor's PB exceeded baseline by 6.4, 8.0 and 2.2-fold, respectively (10). A similar increase of T-lymphocytes by day 3 of 16 μg/kg/day rhG-CSF has been reported by Weaver et al. (18), namely 1.5 to 2.0 times over baseline. On the other hand, PB CD34+ cells and primitive subsets such as CD34+ Thy-1^{dim}, and CD34+ Thy-1^{dim} CD38- cells increased by 16.3-fold, 24.2-fold and 23.2-fold, respectively, suggesting a selective peripheralization effect of rhG-CSF on hematopoietic progenitor cells and, in particular, on their more primitive stem cell subsets (10,19) (Table 1). The percentage of CD34+ cells among total nucleated cells (TNC) increases up to almost 1% at the 4th day of rhG-CSF treatment (Table 1).

The clonogenic potential of rhG-CSF mobilized PBSC is also reported to be significantly higher. In a study on PBSC obtained from G-CSF treated normal individuals, the replating capacity of primary colonies from 5-week-old long-term culture (LTC) systems was found to be significantly higher than the 5-week-old LTC initiated in a steady state (20). In normal donors, a 5-day course of G-CSF increased the frequency of LTC-initiating cells among CD34+ cells by 9-fold over baseline (19).

The course of peripheral blood CD34+ cell and subset concentrations under rhG-CSF mobilization treatment

The kinetics of WBC and progenitor cell subsets under rhG-CSF treatment is quite uniform in an unperturbed, normal hematopoietic system (11,21,22). When monitored over 6 days on a daily basis under rhG-CSF treatment (12 μg/kg/day), the kinetics of circulating CD34+ cells and subsets paralleled each other reaching a plateau from day 4 on (day 1 = first day of cytokine treatment) (Figure 1). Based on those data and data reported by others (11,21,22,23,24), the most favorable day for stem cell collection (15- to 35-fold increase of circulating CD34+ cells at peak level over baseline values) would appear to be day 4 or day 5 of cytokine treatment. Continuation of rhG-CSF administration beyond a 5-day course leads to a progressive decline in the mobilization efficiency of CD34+ progenitors (22,25).

RhG-CSF dose-dependent mobilization of CD34$^+$ progenitor cells
It has been shown that, at least for rhG-CSF doses between 5 and 10 µg/kg/day, a dose-response relationship exists for the degree of mobilization of CD34$^+$ progenitor cells (25,26,27). Although rhG-CSF doses up to 24 µg/kg/d have been employed (8,28), experience with such a dose range remains limited. RhG-CSF given to normal donors at a dose of 10 - 12 µg/kg twice daily resulted in a higher yield of CD34$^+$ cells as compared with 10 µg/kg given once a day (28). Nevertheless, bone pain and headache were more severe in the high-dose rhG-CSF donor cohort but still tolerable.

Donor age and mobilization of CD34$^+$ progenitor cells
In an effort to elucidate factors affecting mobilization in normal donors and stem cell yield by apheresis, the CD34$^+$ cell yield from the first day of apheresis in 119 donors who underwent apheresis on days 4-6 of rhG-CSF treatment (12 µg/kg/day) was analyzed. The CD34$^+$ cell yield was significantly lower in donors >55 years of age, or who underwent apheresis on day 4 of rhG-CSF treatment. There was also a correlation between CD34$^+$ cell yield and baseline WBC, pre-apheresis WBC and pre-apheresis mononuclear cell (MNC) count. Twenty-one (18%) donors were considered "poor mobilizers" yielding less than 20 x 10^6 CD34$^+$ cells/L donor blood processed. In the multivariate analysis, the only significant risk factor for inferior mobilization was age > 55 years, which conferred a 3.8-fold increased risk (p=0.04). As poor mobilizers occurred in all age groups, the predictive value (and clinical usefulness) of the model was limited (29).

Side effects of rhG-CSF treatment for stem cell mobilization in normal donors and safety considerations
There are now sufficient data on the short-term safety profile of rhG-CSF in normal apheresis donors (30). The most commonly reported adverse effects, which are partly dose-related, include bone pain, headache, fatigue and nausea. They ordinarily resolve within a few days of rhG-CSF discontinuation and can be managed successfully in most cases with minor analgesics. Severe adverse events requiring rhG-CSF discontinuation have been rare. RhG-CSF-induced laboratory abnormalities include transient increases (about 2- to 3-fold) of alkaline phosphatase and lactate dehydrogenase, and less commonly decreases in serum potassium and magnesium. These are seemingly related to the expanding myeloid cell mass (31). One case of splenic rupture 4 days following a 6 day course of rhG-CSF treatment for stem cell mobilization has been reported although the etiology of this event was probably multifactorial (32).

Although the short-term rhG-CSF safety profile seems acceptable (30), experience remains limited and the optimal dose and schedule have not been defined. Only limited data exist regarding long-term safety (i.e. the development of myelodysplasia or myeloid leukemia), primarily derived from experience in patients with chronic neutropenia (33). Available data are largely limited to isolated case reports (34). It has been estimated, for instance, that to detect a 10-fold increase in the leukemia risk (a substantial risk increase), more than 2000 normal donors would need to be followed for up to 10 years or longer, and the detection of a smaller risk increase would require the follow-up of a comparably larger donor pool (35). This can conceivably be accomplished only by international registries and will require an intensive cooperative effort with individual transplant teams and centers. The data available on the long-term effects of rhG-CSF in patients with severe congenital neutropenia and aplastic anemia do not answer these questions, as these diseases have been shown to carry a predisposition to the development of acute leukemia even regardless of rhG-CSF therapy (36,37).

Partly related to the long-term effects issue is the issue of PBSC collections from unrelated, HLA-matched donors. Only a very limited number of PBSC allografts from matched unrelated donors has been performed worldwide (38). Until now, in the United States the NMDP has endorsed PBSC collections only for second transplants (i.e. for treatment of relapse following marrow transplantation). Currently many national registries are gradually becoming more open to the idea of administering rhG-CSF to unrelated HLA-matched donors, although some logistical issues and safety concerns still remain. PBSC collection seems to be gaining increasing acceptance in the blood banking community as well (39). A more user-friendly and possibly safer collection procedure may allow a substantial expansion of the stem cell unrelated donor pool in national and international registries, particularly among minorities and older individuals (40).

The consensus reached (41) regarding safety issues related to rhG-CSF administration to normal donors is as follows:

1) rhG-CSF has an acceptable short-term safety profile.
2) rhG-CSF doses up to 12 µg/kg/day show a consistent dose-response relationship with the mobilization and collection of CD34$^+$ cells.
3) transient cytopenias following cytokine treatment and apheresis are generally asymptomatic and self-limited (see below).
4) donors should meet the eligibility criteria which apply to platelet apheresis donors with the exception of multiple donations on consecutive days and the donor's age.
5) the creation of an International PBSC Donor Registry is desirable to assess long-term effects of cytokine treatment for stem cell mobilization.

STEM CELL COLLECTION BY APHERESIS

Donor eligibility for stem cell apheresis

Adult stem cell donors meet similar apheresis eligibility criteria as known for platelet donation. Guidelines for stem cell donation by apheresis are provided by the American Association of Blood Banks (AABB) (42) and by the Foundation for the Accreditation of Hematopoietic Cell Therapy (FAHCT) (43). In normal PBSC donors it is common practice not to place a central line but rather use the peripheral vein needle approach to avoid the risk(s) involved with central venous catheter placement. In some cases, however, (approximately 3%-5% at our institution) peripheral venous access is insufficient, and placement of a central line after appropriate consent or, alternatively, BM harvesting is required. According to our institutional guidelines, the donor's hemoglobin prior to cytokine mobilization treatment and prior to apheresis should be ≥ 11.0 g/dl. Because of an expected significant drop in the PB platelet count due to apheresis, the baseline platelet concentration should be $\geq 150,000/\mu l$, prior to apheresis. The difference in platelet concentration requirements is explained by the fact that rhG-CSF treatment may cause a decrease in platelet concentration due to increased intravascular volume (dilution effect) or by other mechanisms (44). Hepatitis, HIV, and Rapid Plasma Reagin (RPR) screening of all stem cell donors within 30 days of the collection procedure as well as strict compliance with the donor deferral policy are obligatory requirements for donor acceptance. The eligibility criteria for subsequent stem cell donations are hemoglobin ≥ 10 g/dl and a platelet concentration $\geq 70,000/\mu l$. Contrary to unrelated platelet donation, patient-related stem cell donation is not restricted by the donor's age. In our experience, stem cell donors as young as 4 years and as old as 79 years have been eligible for stem cell apheresis.

Eligibility criteria for unrelated stem cell donors are currently being discussed under the guidance of the NMDP.

Continuous-flow stem cell apheresis

PBSCs are collected by single or multiple continuous-flow apheresis. The total blood volume processed per run is usually 2 - 3 times the donor's total blood volume. Large volume stem cell apheresis processing more than three times the donor's total blood volume or more than 15 liters of blood, up to 46 liters has been reported (45-48). Typically, 3 - 5 x 10^8 MNC per kg patient body weight are collected per run with MNC encompassing between 70% and 90% of total nucleated cells (TNC) collected. In case of cryopreserving the apheresis product, the cell collection volume per apheresis procedure should not exceed 200 ml to minimize storage volume and dimethyl sulfoxide (DMSO) exposure to the recipient. The hematocrit of the collected cell suspension should be less than 5%.

Table 2. Cell yield by apheresis

# aphereses	
1	66 donors
2	35 donors
3	8 donors
4	3 donors
median blood volume processed per apheresis [liters]	13.6 [4.4-27.7] (n=112)
median cell number collected per donor	
TNC x 10^8/kg$_{recipient}$ [range]	10.3 [1.47 - 33.0] (n=112)
CD3$^+$ cells x 10^6/kg$_{recipient}$ [range]	294 [48 - 1376] (n=111)
CD4$^+$ cells x 10^6/kg$_{recipient}$ [range]	187 [53 - 874] (n=111)
CD8$^+$ cells x 10^6/kg$_{recipient}$ [range]	104 [7 - 421] (n=111)
CD19$^+$ cells x 10^6/kg$_{recipient}$ [range]	60 [10 - 225] (n=111)
CD3$^-$ 56$^+$ 16$^+$ cells x 10^6/kg$_{recipient}$ [range]	34 [5 - 196] (n=111)
CD34$^+$ cells x 10^6/kg$_{recipient}$ [range]	7.58 [2.05 - 27.96] (n=112)
median cell number transfused per patient	
TNC x 10^8/kg$_{recipient}$ [range]	7.93 [2.31 - 26.45] (n=112)
CD34$^+$ cells x 10^6/kg$_{recipient}$ [range]	5.87 [1.81 - 40.10] (n=70)

TNC: total nucleated cells

Cell yield by stem cell apheresis
The CD34$^+$ cell yield data from 112 normal individuals evaluated for stem cell donation by apheresis, are listed in Table 2. The median number of CD34$^+$ cells collected was 7.58 x 10^6 /kg of recipient body weight. After cryopreservation the median number of CD34$^+$ cells was reduced by 23 % to 5.87 x 10^6/kg of recipient body weight. The collection data of CD3, CD4, CD8, CD 19 and CD3$^-$ 56$^+$ 16$^+$ lymphoid subsets are listed as well. It is noteworthy that in 66 of 112 donors only one single apheresis was needed to collect an engraftment dose CD34$^+$ cells (49).

Second stem cell collections from the same donor
Second stem cell collections in normal apheresis donors have been performed even as early as one month after the first. The donor's pre-apheresis leukocyte concentration under rhG-CSF treatment was not significantly different nor was the CD34$^+$ cell yield (50). These data support the concept that mobilization efficiency in normal donors remains mostly unchanged over time and is not significantly altered by previous rhG-CSF exposure.

TRANSIENT CYTOPENIAS FOLLOWING STEM CELL APHERESIS IN NORMAL DONORS

Stem cell apheresis, especially large-volume stem cell apheresis, has been reported to cause a transient decrease in the donor's platelet count (45,48). Clinically asymptomatic, transient drops in PB lymphocyte and granulocyte concentrations below baseline occasionally resulting in lymphocytopenia and/or granulocytopenia have been reported following rhG-CSF mobilization and stem cell collection (44,51,52). CD34$^+$ cells and subsets as well as lymphoid subsets (CD3, CD4, CD8, CD3-16$^+$56$^+$, CD 19) bottom by day 7 to regain baseline values by day 30 to 100 (51). A reactive lymphocytopenia by day 7 was also reported by Martinez et al. regaining baseline values by 30 - 90 days(52). There is no evidence as yet of a possible clinical relevance of these findings.

TARGET PROGENITOR CELL DOSE FOR SUCCESSFUL ALLOENGRAFTMENT

The indicators for hematopoietic progenitor cells with reconstitutive potential contained in the apheresis products are clonogenic short-/long-term culture assays or their immunophenotype including the CD34 surface antigen. Since clonogenic assays are time consuming and difficult to standardize, the immunophenotyping of progenitor cells has widely replaced culture assays.

The minimal CD34$^+$ cell dose required in the *autologous* transplant situation for complete three lineage engraftment is not well defined, but may be in the range of 0.5 and 1 x 10^6/kg (53). Successful allogeneic BMT among HLA-matched siblings has been reported with CD34$^+$ cell doses as low as 0.7 x 10^6/kg patient body weight (54). The same study also showed that patients receiving more than 2 x 10^6 CD34$^+$ cells/kg recovered their hematopoietic system earlier, and treatment related mortality was significantly less. A similar threshold CD34 dose range might apply for blood-derived stem cell allografts although comparative data on minimal CD34 dose requirements between BM and PBSC allografts are not available. For complete and sustained *allogeneic* engraftment among HLA matched siblings, we propose the transfusion of 3 to 4 x 10^6 or more CD34$^+$ cells per kg of recipient body weight. At our institution this target CD34$^+$ cell dose is reached with one leukapheresis in approximately 75% of the donors and with two in the majority of the others. A similar target dose (2 to 3 x 10^6 CD34$^+$ cells per kg) has recently been recommended by the EBMT (38).

PBSC MOBILIZATION IN PEDIATRIC DONORS

Given the promising data reported with clinical trials on allogeneic PBSC transplantation in adults and the potential advantage to the donor over a BM harvest under general anesthesia, collection of PBSCs in normal children is an appealing approach.

In the autologous transplant setting, rhG-CSF treatment at a dose ranging from 5 to 10 µg/kg/day, combined with chemopriming for transient stem cell peripheralization and collection, is well tolerated in small children (55,56). This appears to be true for normal pediatric donors as well at a dose of 12 µg/kg/day rhG-CSF. In a series of five allogeneic blood stem cell transplantations (57) using normal pediatric donors age 4 to 13 years, we processed a median of 2.2 times the donor's total blood volume (TBV) per apheresis, which provided a sufficient CD34$^+$ cell yield in an acceptable time period (2-3 hours). The mean CD34$^+$ cell yield per kg of donor body weight and per liter of donor blood processed was 128×10^4 in these five children, as compared to 63×10^4 for adult donors (10). One apheresis using rhG-CSF mobilization treatment was sufficient to collect 4×10^6 CD34$^+$ cells from an 8-year old boy for successful engraftment of his leukemic father despite the substantial body weight discrepancy between donor (27 kg) and recipient (93 kg) (57).

Venous access in small children providing sufficient blood flow is the major limiting factor for apheresis. To ensure an adequate and consistent blood flow rate of 20 ml/min during apheresis, Takaue et al. (56) successfully used a temporary radial artery catheter for blood withdrawal and return through a peripheral vein. Inserting a femoral catheter is in our experience an efficient and low risk approach to achieve a sufficient flow rate.

Based on preliminary clinical data, pediatric blood stem cell collection from normal donors is feasible and safe with adequate CD34$^+$ cell doses, even for adult recipients. Engraftment characteristics and clinical outcome appear comparable to those achieved with adult PBSC allotransplantation. Unrelated cord blood transplantation offers an alternative option in the pediatric transplant setting. Related allogeneic PBSC transplantation combines the advantages of higher stem cell availability, even for adult recipients, with rapid cell recovery; the incidence of developing GVHD is, however, expected to be higher after PBSC allotransplantation.

IMMUNOPHENOTYPIC CHARACTERIZATION OF MOBILIZED PB- AS COMPARED TO BM-DERIVED STEM CELLS AND LYMPHOID SUBSETS

We performed flow cytometric analyses on rhG-CSF mobilized PBSC collections from 41 normal donors and compared it with BM harvests from 43 normal donors. The $CD34^+$ cell yield of PBSC collections exceeded that of BM harvests by 3.7-fold and that of lymphoid subsets by 16.1-fold ($CD3^+$), 13.3-fold ($CD4^+$), 27.4-fold ($CD8^+$), 11.0-fold ($CD19^+$), and 19.4-fold ($CD56^+ CD3^-$) (10). The percentage of $CD34^+$ cells is approximately 1% of the nucleated cells in harvested BM, which is not significantly different from the $CD34^+$ cell percentage in rhG-CSF mobilized apheresis products (Table 1). When compared to the $CD34^+$ progenitor cell profile in the BM, rhG-CSF mobilization treatment of normal individuals causes a substantial increase in the percentage of circulating $CD34^+CD13^+$ and $CD34^+CD33^+$ cells (myeloid precursors) and a decrease in the percentage of circulating $CD34^+CD10^+$and $CD34^+CD19^+$ cells (B lymphocyte precursors) (21).

EX VIVO MANIPULATION OF THE APHERESIS PRODUCT

As is widely used for BM allografts, ex vivo manipulation including T-cell depletion and CD34 selection can also be used for PBSC allografts. However, as outlined in the previous paragraph, the total cell numbers significantly differ between BM- and PBSC collections, with apheresis-derived PBSC harvests containing a 5-fold higher total number of nucleated cells (10). Use of density gradient separation methods that reduce the total cell number by roughly 1 log are now being tested in phase I/II clinical trials (58). Alternatively, counterflow elutriation (59) has been proposed as a first step $CD34^+$ cell selection procedure but with considerable loss of progenitor cells.

T-cell depletion and $CD34^+$ cell selection methods to prevent GVHD include the biotin-avidin immunoadsorption and the immunomagnetobead separation technologies. However, the 4-times higher $CD34^+$ cell yield of apheresis products has, among others, the advantage of compensating for the significant loss of progenitor cells as a result of such ex vivo depletion or selection procedures. On a more experimental basis, preparative fluorescence activated cell sorting (60) have gained interest as the latest technology to generate purified $CD34^+ Lin^- Thy^+$ progenitor cells and lymphoid subsets that might, after transplantation, mediate a graft facilitating (61) and/or graft-versus-leukemia (GVL) effect without inducing severe GVHD.

Ex vivo transduction of apheresis-derived donor lymphocytes with the herpes simplex virus thymidine kinase (HSV-TK) suicide gene has recently gained much interest (62).

11

In a first clinical trial, it was shown that by treating the recipient with ganciclovir after lymphocyte infusion GVHD development potentially can be controlled.

ENGRAFTMENT CHARACTERISTICS FOLLOWING ALLOGENEIC PBSC TRANSPLANTATION

As first reported by Przepiorka et al (63), when comparing consecutive patient cohorts after BMT with those after PBSC transplantation, the time to neutrophils >0.5 x 10^9/L was similar (9 and 10 days, respectively), whereas the time to platelets >20 x 10^9/L was significantly shorter following allogeneic PBSC transplantation (19 and 14 days, respectively). In a retrospective comparison of patients receiving PBSC for transplantation with those receiving BM, the time to reach >0.5 x 10^9/L neutrophils was 14 days versus 16 days after BMT. On the other hand, the time to reach >20 x 10^9/L platelets without transfusions occurred on days 11 and 15, respectively (64). An evaluation of 112 consecutive patients receiving HLA identical PBSC transplants in our institution revealed a neutrophil recovery of 10 days and 10.5 days to reach 0.5 x 10^9/L and 1.0 x 10^9/L, respectively, and a platelet recovery of 13 days to reach 20 x 10^9/L without platelet support (65).

From those and other reported data, the recovery of granulocytes seems to be at least comparable, if not somewhat faster. As known from autologous PBSC transplantation and confirmed by most investigators, platelet recovery after allogeneic PBSC transplantation is faster (63,64,66,67) compared to control patients receiving steady-state BM allografts.

In view of the fast myeloid engraftment after allogeneic PBSC transplantation, it is unclear whether post-infusion cytokines (i.e. rhG-CSF) are actually beneficial or cost-effective (66).

IMMUNOLOGIC RECONSTITUTION AFTER ALLOGENEIC PBSC TRANSPLANTATION

The number of T and NK cells contained in the apheresis product exceeds the BM allograft by 10 to 20-fold (10). Apart from GVHD, this would also be expected to impact the speed of immunologic reconstitution after PBSC allografting. Ottinger et al. (68) reported an improved immune reconstitution after allogeneic PBSC transplantation as compared to BM allotransplantation. Naive (CD4$^+$ CD45RA$^+$) and memory (CD4$^+$ CD45RO$^+$) helper T-cells were found to be significantly elevated in patients receiving an allogeneic PBSC transplant, and proliferative responses to phytohemaglutinin, pokeweed mitogen, tetanus toxoid and candida were found to be more pronounced as well. In another report (69) the recovery of $CD3^+$ cells was similar in allogeneic PBSC recipients and concurrent marrow transplant recipients. On the other hand, the recovery of $CD4^+$ and, to a lesser extent, $CD8^+$ cells was significantly faster in the former group, resulting in a more rapid increase in the CD4/8 ratio as well. Whether this more rapid immunologic reconstitution will decrease morbidity and mortality from infectious complications (e.g. cytomegalovirus, fungal infections) remains to be determined.

ALLOGENEIC PBSC TRANSPLANTATION: TREATMENT-RELATED TOXICITY

Regimen-related toxicity and early morbidity/mortality

The impact of PBSC allografting on regimen-related toxicity and infectious or bleeding complications has not been fully evaluated. We analyzed early treatment-related morbidity and mortality after HLA-matched allogeneic transplantation of rhG-CSF mobilized PBSC as compared to BM allografted recipients. Three cohorts of patients were analyzed: cohort I (n = 30) received a BM allograft and was treated with cyclosporine + methotrexate for GVHD prophylaxis, cohort II (n = 19) received a BM allograft as well, but was prophylactically treated with cyclosporine + methylprednisolone, and cohort III (n = 25) received a PBSC allograft with the same GVHD prophylaxis as cohort II. RhG-CSF (5 µg/kg/day) was given to all patients after transplant to enhance hematopoietic reconstitution. Grade 2 - 4 maximum regimen-related toxicity (70) (especially stomatitis) was significantly less in PBSC transplant recipients, and this was not accounted for by a shorter duration of neutropenia. PBSC recipients (cohort III) were discharged from the hospital on the average 4 days earlier than their BM counterparts (cohort II). The 180 day survival was significantly higher in the allogeneic PBSC transplant group (cohort III) with 68%, as compared to 53% in cohort I and 32% in cohort II (63). Those data are confirmed by Azevedo et al. describing significantly shorter hospital stays, as well as fewer days on antibiotic and antifungal agents in PBSC recipients (9), and by Russell et al. (67) reporting shorter hospitalization stays and fewer platelet transfusions for PBSC allograft recipients. According to a retrospective comparison by Bensinger et al. (64) the estimated risks of transplant-related mortality at 200 days post-transplant were 27% after HLA-identical allogeneic PBSC transplantation versus 45% after BM allotransplantation.

Incidence of acute and chronic GVHD

Whereas, compared with a BM allograft, the average number of $CD34^+$ cells collected by apheresis and transplanted is four times higher, the number of T- and natural killer (NK) cells in the apheresis product exceeds the BM allograft by 10 - 20-fold (10) raising concern that PBSC allotransplants could induce more severe GVHD.

The great majority of available data suggests that the incidence and severity of acute GVHD following PBSC allografting is similar (or possibly even lower) to that encountered after BM allografting. (63, 64,67), although these have employed historical or nonrandomized controls. As reported by our institution (63) the rate of grades 2 - 4 and grades 3 - 4 acute GVHD was 42% and 22%, respectively, and not significantly different from patients undergoing allogeneic BMT. Similar data were reported by Bensinger et al. showing a 37% estimated risk of developing grades 2 to 4 acute GVHD as compared with 56% for the BM group, while the estimated risks of grades 3 to 4 acute GVHD were 14% for the PBSC allotransplant group and 33% for the BM group.

It is well known from studies employing T-cell depletion of the stem cell allograft, that below a lower threshold dose of about 10^5 $CD3^+$ cells/kg the development of acute GVHD is significantly reduced (71). On the other hand, it is conceivable that, after reaching a critical upper threshold number of transplanted lymphoid cells, the infusion of additional lymphocytes does not necessarily translate into the development of more frequent or severe acute GVHD given the genetic disparity between donor and recipient. Other, and even more likely mechanisms may also be responsible for this finding such as cytokine induced shifting of T-cells toward $CD4^+$ Th-2 (type-2) cells (72, 73) leading to prevention of GVHD, or generation of natural suppressor cells ($CD4^-$ $CD8^-$ $TCR_{\alpha\beta}^+$) which have been shown to inhibit GVHD (73, 74).

The incidence of chronic GVHD following PBSC allografting has varied among reports due to the small sample size and the short follow-up of most studies to date. It is well known that the addition of buffy-coat cells to allogeneic BM infusion leads to a higher incidence of chronic GVHD (75). We have studied a group of 47 consecutive allogeneic PBSC transplant recipients (HLA-matched, siblings) surviving at least 100 days after transplant at a median follow-up of 27 months. When compared with a matched, historical control population undergoing allogeneic BM transplantation, the actuarial rate of chronic, mainly extensive GVHD, at 2 years was as high as 80% after PBSC transplantation versus 59% after BM transplantation (76). Based on a retrospective comparison reported by Bensinger et al (64), clinically extensive or limited chronic GVHD developed in 41% evaluable patients receiving PBSCs as compared with 26% receiving BM allografts. An updated report on the same patient cohorts revealed a 2.22 increased relative risk of developing chronic GVHD (clinical limited and extensive) by 2 years post-transplant among the PBSC recipients compared with BM recipients (77). The absolute higher incidence of chronic GVHD seen in our patient cohort (73% probability) could be related to either the use of more methylprednisolone-containing GVHD prophylaxis rather than methotrexate containing-regimens and/or to a longer median patient follow-up.

14

TRANSPLANTATION OF PBSC ALLOGRAFTS FROM MATCHED UNRELATED DONORS

Matched unrelated donor transplantations using PBSCs are still scarce, mainly due to the fact that regulatory issues regarding mobilized stem cell collections from unrelated donors are still missing or being prepared. Six high-risk patients receiving unrelated donor PBSC transplants have been recently reported by Ringden (78). Trilineage engraftment was similar to matched sibling PBSC transplantations. Acute GVHD did not seem to be a major risk in those patients.

ALLOGENEIC PBSC TRANSPLANTATION COMBINED WITH A POTENTIALLY ENHANCED GRAFT VERSUS LEUKEMIA EFFECT

It has been speculated that allogeneic PBSC transplantation might coincide with a more pronounced GVL effect. This assumption is based on the fact that mobilized PBSC allografts contain more than 1 log higher total number of lymphocytes (10) which have been shown in patients with relapsed chronic myelogenous leukemia after allogeneic BMT to induce long lasting remissions (79). Our retrospective analysis comparing patients undergoing allogeneic PBSC transplantation with those after allogeneic BMT, revealed a higher incidence of chronic GVHD. This, however, did not result in a higher mortality because of a significantly lower incidence of relapse in PBSC transplant recipients. This lower relapse rate would be consistent with an enhanced GVL effect (76).

Since GVHD targets liver and skin, among other organs, it may be possible to deliver a graft-versus-malignancy effect in patients with selected solid tumors by purposely inducing GVHD. Based on such considerations and preliminary reports by Tricot et al. (80) for multiple myeloma and Eibl et al. (81) for advanced stage breast cancer, phase I/II allogeneic PBSC transplantation trials have been initiated in our institution and elsewhere for patients primarily with advanced stage and metastasized breast cancer (82).

CD34 SELECTION OF PBSC ALLOGRAFTS

There is an increasing number of studies reported using $CD34^+$ cell selected PBSC allografts to prevent severe GVHD. Since the larger number of $CD34^+$ cells collected by PBSC apheresis (10) allows for some selective loss of progenitor cells, ex vivo selection procedures with consecutive partial T-cell depletion seems to be an attractive and easy approach. Link et al. (83) have described the clinical outcome after transplantation of HLA-identical, CD34 selected PBSC allografts. The total $CD3^+$ cells contained in the allograft were reduced by 2.1 to 3.4 log. The recovery of CD34$^+$ cells was, on the other hand, 50%. Engraftment was comparable to unmanipulated PBSC allotransplantation. Despite GVHD prophylaxis with cyclosporine, severe acute GVHD (grade III-IV) developed in 4 of the first 5 patients. In another study, 16 patients with advanced hematologic malignancies received HLA-identical PBSC allografts that were selected for CD34$^+$ cells (84). The median CD34$^+$ cell yield after the avidin-biotin immunoadsorption approach was reported to be 53% with a median purity of 62%; the median log reduction in T-cells was 2.8. The early (up to day 100) transplant-related mortality reached 44% (median patient age: 48 years). Surprisingly, the development of acute grade 2-4 GVHD was as high as 86%, and 43% for grade 3-4 acute GVHD. Six of 8 evaluable patients developed clinical chronic GVHD. Although the sample sizes of both studies are small, one might speculate about the high incidence of GVHD being a result of selecting CD34$^+$ cells in the allograft by eliminating GVHD suppressing T-cell subsets. Employing the same ex vivo CD34 selection approach for reducing contaminating T-cells, Urbano-Ispizua et al (85) reported a study involving 20 patients undergoing PBSC allotransplantation. However, in their study, virtually no significant acute or chronic GVHD was observed at a median follow-up of 7.5 months.

The therapeutic benefit of the CD34 selection techniques to reduce the incidence and severity of GVHD by partly depleting PBSC allografts of T-cells remains to be shown in prospective, randomized trials.

CONCLUSIONS

Clinical data on stem cell collection from normal, healthy donors and their allotransplantation are accumulating rapidly. Donor short- and long-term safety is of imperative importance that needs to be openly addressed in form of national and international data registries. Finally (and most importantly), measurable benefits of PBSC over BM allotransplantation in terms of clinical outcome need to be further demonstrated. This should include variables such as patient transfusion requirement and hospitalization duration, reduction of treatment-related mortality and improvement of survival and/or disease-free survival.

Present and future aspects of allogeneic PBSC transplantation are focusing on
- more effective stem cell mobilization regimens with less side effects,
- induction of a more pronounced GVL effect,
- cell component allotransplantation including highly purified CD34 and lymphoid subsets that
- guarantee engraftment even across major histocompatibility barriers,

- mediate anti-tumor effect, and avoid major GVHD,
- induction of donor-specific tolerance for organ allografting (86), and
- transduction of suicide genes into GVHD inducing T-cells by maintaining the allograft specific GVL effect (62)

Based on clinical data available so far, one might anticipate PBSC replacing, at least in part, BM as the preferred source of hematopoietic stem cells for transplantation, as is already the case for autologous transplantation.

REFERENCES

1. Micklem HS, Anderson N, Ross E. Limited potential of circulating haemopoietic stem cells. Nature 1975; 256:41-43.
2. Epstein RB, Graham TC, Buckner CD et al. Allogeneic marrow engraftment by cross circulation in lethally irradiated dogs. Blood 1966;28: 692-707.
3. Körbling M, Fliedner TM, Calvo W, Ross WM, Nothdurft W, Steinbach I. Albumin density gradient purification of canine hemopoietic blood stem cells (HBSC): Long-term allogeneic engraftment without GVH-reaction. Exp Hemat 1979;7: 277-288.
4. Carbonell F, Calvo W, Fliedner TM, et al. Cytogenetic studies in dogs after total body irradiation and allogeneic transfusion with cryopreserved blood mononuclear cells: Observations in long-term chimeras. International Journal of Cell Cloning 1984;2: 81-88.
5. Kessinger A, Smith DM, Strandjord SE, Landmark JD, Dooley DC, Law P, Coccia PF, Warkentin PI, Weisenburger DD, Armitage JO. Allogeneic transplantation of blood-derived, T cell-depleted hemopoietic stem cells after myeloablative treatment in a patient with acute lymphoblastic leukemia. Bone Marrow Transplant 1989;4: 643-646.
6. Körbling M, Przepiorka D, Huh YO, et al. Allogeneic blood stem cell transplantation for refractory leukemia and lymphoma: Potential advantage of blood over marrow allografts. Blood 1995;85: 1659-1665.
7. Schmitz N, Dreger P, Suttorp M, et al. Primary transplantation of allogeneic peripheral blood progenitor cells mobilized by filgrastim ;granulocyte colony-stimulating factor). Blood 1995;85: 1666-1672.
8. Bensinger WI, Weaver CH, Appelbaum FR, et al. Transplantation of allogeneic peripheral blood stem cells mobilized by recombinant human granulocyte colony-stimulating factor. Blood 1995;85: 1655-1658.
9. Azevedo WM, Aranha FJP, Gouvea JV, et al. Allogeneic transplantation with blood stem cells mobilized by rhG-CSF for hematological malignancies. Bone Marrow Transplant 1995;16: 647-653.

10. Körbling M, Huh YO, Durett A, et al. Allogeneic blood stem cell transplantation: Peripheralization and yield of donor-derived primitive hematopoietic progenitor cells (CD34+ Thy-1dim) and lymphoid subsets, and possible predictors of engraftment and GVHD. Blood 1995;86: 2842-2848.

11. Link H, Arseniev L, Bähre O, et al. Combined transplantation of allogeneic bone marrow and CD34+ blood cells. Blood 1995;86: 2500-2508.

12. Molineux G, Pojda Z, Hampson IN, Lord BI, Dexter TM. Transplantation potential of peripheral blood stem cells induced by granulocyte colony-stimulating factor. Blood 1990; 76: 2153-2158.

13. Bensinger WI, Price TH, Dale DC, et al. The effects of daily recombinant human granulocyte colony-stimulating factor administration on normal granulocyte donors undergoing leukapheresis. Blood 1993; 81: 1883-1888.

14. Caspar CB, Seger RA, Burger J, Gmur J. Effective stimulation of donors for granulocyte transfusions with recombinant methionyl granulocyte colony-stimulating factor. Blood 1993;81: 2866-2871.

15. Prosper F, Verfaillie CM. Mobilization and homing of peripheral blood progenitors is related to reversible down regulation of a4b1 integrin expression and function. Journal of Clinical Investigation 1998; 101:2456-2467.

16. Lebsack ME, McKenna HJ, Hoek JA, Hanna R, Feng A, Marashovsky E, Hayes FA. Safety of FLT3 ligand in healthy volunteers. Blood 1997; 90: (Suppl.1) 170a.

17. Ali SM, Brown RA, Adkins DR, Todd G, Haug JS, Goodnough LT, DiPersio JF. Analysis of lymphocyte subsets and peripheral blood progenitor cells in apheresis products from normal donors mobilized with either G-CSF or concurrent G-CSF and GM-CSF. Blood 1997; 90: (Suppl.1) 564a.

18. Weaver CH, Longin K, Buckner CD, Bensinger W. Lymphocyte content in peripheral blood mononuclear cells collected after administration of recombinant human granulocyte colony-stimulating factor. Bone Marrow Transplant 1994; 13: 411-415.

19. Prosper F, Stroncek D, Verfaillie CM. Mobilization of LTC-IC in normal donors treated with G-CSF: phenotypic analysis of mobilized PBSC. Blood 1995; 86: (Suppl.1): 464a.

20. Fujisaki T, Otsuka T, Harada M, Ohno Y, Niho Y. Granulocyte colony-stimulating factor mobilizes primitive hematopoietic stem cells in normal individuals. Bone Marrow Transplant 1995; 16: 57-62.

21. Tjønnfjord GE, Steen R, Evensen SA, Thorsby E, Egeland T. Characterization of CD34+ peripheral blood cells from healthy adults mobilized by recombinant human granulocyte-stimulating factor. Blood 1994; 84: 2795-2801.

22. Grigg AP,Roberts A.W, Raunow H, et al. Optimizing dose and scheduling of filgrastim (granulocyte colony-stimulating factor) for mobilization and collection of peripheral blood progenitor cells in normal volunteers. Blood 1995; 86: 4437-4445.

23. Tanaka R, Matsudaira T, Tanaka I, et al. Kinetics and characteristics of peripheral blood progenitor cells mobilized by G-CSF in normal healthy volunteers. Blood 1994; 84: (Suppl.1) 541a.
24. Dreger P, Haferlach T, Eckstein V, et al. Filgrastim-mobilized peripheral blood progenitor cells for allogeneic transplantation: Safety, kinetics and mobilization, and composition of the graft. British Journal of Haematology 1994; 87: 609.
25. Stroncek D, Clay M, Jaszcz W, Mills B, Oldham F, McCullough J. Longer than 5 days of G-CSF mobilization of normal individuals results in lower CD34+ cell counts. Blood 1994; 84: (Suppl.1): 541a.
26. Höglund M, Smedmyr B, Simonsson B, Tötterman T, Bengtsson M. Dose-dependent mobilisation of haematopoietic progenitor cells in healthy volunteers receiving glycosylated rHuG-CSF. Bone Marrow Transplant 1996; 18: 19-27.
27. Stroncek D, Clay M, Lennon S, Smith J, McCullough J. Collection of two blood progenitor cell components from healthy donors. Blood 1996; 88: (Suppl.1): 396a.
28. Waller CF, Bertz H, Wenger MK, et al. Mobilization of peripheral blood progenitor cells for allogeneic transplantation : efficacy and toxicity of a high-dose rhG-CSF regimen. Bone Marrow Transplant 1996; 18: 279-283.
29. Anderlini P, Przepiorka D, Seong D, et al. Factors affecting mobilization of CD34+ cells in normal donors treated with filgrastim. Transfusion 1997;37: 507-512.
30. Anderlini P, Przepiorka D, Champlin R, Körbling M . Biologic and clinical effects of granulocyte colony-stimulating factor in normal individuals. Blood 1996; 88: 2819-2825.
31. Anderlini P, Przepiorka D, Seong D, et al. Clinical toxicity and laboratory effects of granulocyte-colony-stimulating factor (filgrastim) mobilization and blood stem cell apheresis from normal donors, and analysis of charges for the procedures. Transfusion 1996; 36: 590-595.
32. Becker PS, Wagle M, Matous S, et al. Spontaneous splenic rupture following administration of granulocyte colony-stimulating factor (G-CSF): occurrence in an allogeneic donor of peripheral blood stem cells. Biology of Blood and Marrow Transplantation 1997; 3: 45-49.
33. Bonilla MA, Dale D, Zeidler C, et al. Long-term safety of treatment with recombinant human granulocyte colony-stimulating factor (r-metHuG-CSF) in patients with severe congenital neutropenias. British Journal of Haematology 1994; 88: 723-730.
34. Sakamaki S, Matsunaga T, Hirayama Y, Kuga T, Niitsu Y. Haematological study of healthy volunteers 5 years after G-CSF. Lancet 1995;346: 1432-1433 (letter).
35. Hasenclever D, Sextro M. Safety of alloPBSCT donors: biometrical considerations on monitoring long term risks. Bone Marrow Transplant 1996; 17: (Suppl 2) S28-S30.
36. Gilman P, Jackson D, Guild H. Congenital agranulocytosis: prolonged survival and terminal acute leukemia. Blood 1970; 36: 576-585.

37. de Planque MM, Bacigalupo A, Würsch A, et al. Long-term follow-up of severe aplastic anemia patients treated with antithymocyte globulin. British Journal of Haematology 1989; 73: 121-126.
38. Russell N, Gratwohl A, Schmitz N . The place of blood stem cells in allogeneic transplantation. British Journal of Haematology 1996; 93: 747-753.
39. Lane T. Allogeneic marrow reconstitution using peripheral blood stem cells : the dawn of a new era. Transfusion 1996; 36: 585-589.
40. Körbling M, Przepiorka D, Gajewski J, Champlin RE, Chan KW. With first successful allogeneic transplantations of apheresis-derived hematopoietic progenitor cells reported, can the recruitment of volunteer matched, unrelated stem cell donors be expanded substantially? Blood 1995;86: 1235 (letter).
41. Anderlini P, Körbling M, Dale D, et al. Allogeneic blood stem cell transplantation: considerations for donors. Blood 1997; 90: 903-908.
42. Standards for Blood Banks and Transfusion Services (18th Edition), 1997; edited by J.E.Menitove, American Association of Blood Banks Publications, Bethesda, MD.
43. Standards for Hematopoietic Progenitor Cell Collection, Processing & Transplantation. Foundation for the Accreditation of Hematopoietic Cell Therapy (FAHCT). 1996 First Edition - North America.
44. Stroncek D, Clay M, Lennon S, Smith J, Jaszcz W, McCullough J. Neutropenia following the collection of granulocyte colony-stimulating factor mobilized blood progenitor cell components is due to the collection of progenitor cells. Blood 1996; 88: (Suppl.1) 396a.
45. Malachowski ME, Comenzo RL, Hillyer CD, Tiegerman KO, Berkman EM. Large-volume leukapheresis for peripheral blood stem cell collection in patients with hematologic malignancies. Transfusion 1992; 32: 732-735.
46. Comenzo RI, Malachowski ME, Miller KB, et al. Engraftment with peripheral blood stem cells collected by large-volume leukapheresis for patients with lymphoma. Transfusion 1992; 32: 729-731.
47. Passos-Coelho JL, Braine HG, Wright SK, et al. Large volume leukapheresis using regional citrate anticoagulation to collect peripheral blood progenitor cells. Journal of Hematotherapy 1995; 4: 11-19.
48. Hillyer CD, Tiegerman KO, Berkman EM. Increase in circulating colony-forming units-granulocyte-macrophage during large-volume leukapheresis : evaluation of a new cell separator. Transfusion 1991; 31: 327-332.
49. Körbling M, Mirza N, Fischer H, Gee A, Giralt S. Circulating blood as a source of hematopoietic stem cells for allogeneic transplantation in 112 HLA-identical patients with advanced hematologic malignancies and solid tumors. Transfusion (submitted for publication).
50. Anderlini P, Lauppe J, Przepiorka D, Seong D, Champlin R, Körbling M. Peripheral blood stem cell apheresis in normal donors : feasibility and yield of second collections. British Journal of Haematology 1997; 96(2): 415-417.

51. Körbling M, Anderlini P, Durett A, et al. Delayed effects of rhG-CSF mobilization treatment and apheresis on circulating CD34+ and CD34+Thy-1dim CD38- progenitor cells, and lymphoid subsets in normal stem cell donors for allogeneic transplantation. Bone Marrow Transplant 1996; 18(6): 1073-1079.

52. Martinez C, Urbano-Ispizua A, Rozman C, et al. Effects of G-CSF administration and peripheral blood progenitor cell collection in 20 healthy donors. Ann Hematol 1996; 72: 269-272.

53. Shpall EJ, Jones RB, Bearman SI, et al. Transplantation of enriched CD34-positive autologous marrow into breast cancer patients following high-dose chemotherapy: Influence of CD34-positive peripheral-blood progenitors and growth factors on engraftment. Journal Clin Oncol 1994 ;12:28-36.

54. Mavroudis D, Read E, Cottler-Fox M, et al. CD34+ cell dose predicts survival, posttransplant morbidity, and rate of hematologic recovery after allogeneic marrow transplants for hematologic malignancies. Blood 1996;88:3223-3229.

55. Kanold J, Rapatel C, Berger M, et al. Use of G-CSF alone to mobilize peripheral blood stem cells for collection from children. Br J Haematology 1994;88:633-635.

56. Takaue Y, Kawano Y, Abe T, et al. Collection and transplantation of peripheral blood stem cells in very small children weighing 20 kg or less. Blood 1995;86: 372-380.

57. Körbling M, Chan KW, Anderlini P, et al. Allogeneic peripheral blood stem cell transplantation using normal patient-related pediatric donors. Bone Marrow Transplantation 1996;18:885-890.

58. Przepiorka D, Van Vlasselaer P, Huynh L, et al. Rapid debulking and CD34 enrichment of filgrastim-mobilized peripheral blood stem cells by semiautomated density gradient centrifugation in a closed system. Journal of Hematotherapy 1996;5: 497-502.

59. Wagner JE, Donnenberg AD, Noga SJ, et al. Bone marrow graft engineering by counter-flow centrifugal elutriation: results of a phase I-II clinical trial. Blood 1990;75:1370-1377.

60. Sasaki DT, Tichenor EH, Lopez F, et al. Development of a clinically acceptable high-speed flow cytometer for the isolation of transplantable human hematopoietic stem cells. Journal of Hematotherapy 1995;4:503-514.

61. Kaufman CL, Colson YL, Wren SM, Watkins S, Simmons RL, Ildstad ST. Phenotypic characterization of a novel bone marrow-derived cell that facilitates engraftment of allogeneic bone marrow stem cells. Blood 1994;84:2436-2446.

62. Bonini C, Ferrari G, Verzeletti S, et al. HSV-TK gene transfer into donor lymphocytes for control of allogeneic graft-versus-leukemia. Science 1997;276:1719-1724.

63. Przepiorka D, Anderlini P, Ippoliti C, et al. Allogeneic blood stem cell transplantation in advanced hematologic cancers. Bone Marrow Transplant 1997;19:455-460.

64. Bensinger WI, Clift R, Martin P, et al. Allogeneic peripheral blood stem cell transplantation in patients with advanced hematologic malignancies: a retrospective comparison with marrow transplantation. Blood1996;88:2794-2800.

65. Körbling M, Mirza N, Przepiorka D, Anderlini P, Chan KW, Champlin R. Clinical outcome in 112 patients following HLA-identical allogeneic peripheral blood stem cell (PBSC) transplantation. Blood 1997;90:(Suppl.1)224a-225a.

66. Rosenfeld C, Collins R, Piñeiro L, Agura E, Nemunaitis J. Allogeneic blood cell transplantation without posttransplant colony-stimulating factors in patients with hematopoietic neoplasm: a phase II study. J Clin Oncol ;14: 1314-1319, 1996.

67. Russell JA, Brown C, Brown T, et al. Allogeneic blood cell transplants for haematological malignancy : preliminary comparison of outcomes with bone marrow transplantation. Bone Marrow Transplant 1996;17:703-708.

68. Ottinger HD, Beelen DW, Scheulen B, Schaefer UW, Grosse-Wilde H. Improved immune reconstitution after allotransplantation of peripheral blood stem cells instead of bone marrow. Blood 1996;88:2775-2779.

69. Bacigalupo A, Van Lint MT, Valbonesi M, et al. Thiotepa cyclophosphamide followed by granulocye colony-stimulating factor mobilized allogeneic peripheral blood cells in adults with advanced leukemia. Blood 1996;88:353-357.

70. Bearman SI, Appelbaum FR, Buckner CD et al. Regimen related toxicity in patients undergoing bone marrow transplantation. J Clin Oncol 1988;6:1562-1568.

71. Verdonck LF, Dekker AW, de Gast GC, van Kempen ML, Lokhorst HM, Nieuwenhuis HK. Allogeneic bone marrow transplantation with a fixed low number of T-cells in the marrow graft. Blood 1994;83:3090-3096.

72. Pan L, Delmonte J Jr, Jalonen CK, Ferrara JLM. Pretreatment of donor mice with granulocyte colony-stimulating factor polarizes donor T lymphocytes toward type-2 cytokine production and reduces severity of experimental graft versus host disease. Blood 1995;86:4422-4429.

73. Zeng D, Dejbakhsh-Jones S, Strober S. Granulocyte colony-stimulating factor reduces the capacity of blood mononuclear cells to induce graft-versus-host disease: impact on blood progenitor cell transplantation. Blood 1997;90:453-463.

74. Kusnierz-Glaz CR, Still BJ, Amano M, et al. Granulocyte colony-stimulating factor-induced comobilization of CD4- CD8- T-cells and hematopoietic progenitor cells (CD34+) in the blood of normal donors. Blood 1997;89:2586-2595.

75. Storb R, Prentice RL, Sullivan KM, et al. Predictive factors in chronic graft-versus-host disease in patients with aplastic anemia treated by marrow transplantation from HLA-identical siblings. Ann Intern Med 1983;98:461-466.

76. Anderlini P, Przepiorka D, Khouri I, et al. Chronic graft-versus-host disease after allogeneic marrow or blood stem cell transplantation. Blood 1995;86:(Suppl.1)109a.

77. Storek J, Gooley T, Siadak M, et al. Allogeneic peripheral blood stem cell transplantation may be associated with a high risk of chronic graft-versus-host disease. Blood 1997;90:4705-4709.
78. Ringden O. Allogeneic peripheral blood stem cells from unrelated donors for transplantation. Bone Marrow Transplant 1997;19(Suppl.1): S72.
79. Kolb HJ, Schattenberg A, Goldman JM, et al. Graft-versus-leukemia effect of donor lymphocyte transfusions in marrow grafted patients. European Group for Blood and Marrow Transplantation Working Party Chronic Leukemia. Blood 1995;86:2041-2050.
80. Tricot G, Vesole DH, Jagannath S, Hilton J, Munshi N, Barlogie B. Graft-versus-myeloma effect: proof of principle. Blood 1996;87:1196-1198.
81. Eibl B, Schwaighofer H, Nachbaur D, et al. Evidence for a graft-versus-tumor effect in a patient treated with marrow ablative chemotherapy and allogeneic bone marrow transplantation for breast cancer. Blood 1996;88:1501-1508.
82. Ueno NT, Rondon G, Mirza NQ, et al. Allogeneic peripheral blood progenitor cell transplantation for poor-risk patients with metastatic breast cancer. J Clin Oncol 1998;16:986-993.
83. Link H, Arseniev L, Bähre O, Kadar JG, Diedrich H, Poliwoda H. Transplantation of allogeneic CD34+ cells. Blood 1996;87:4903-4909.
84. Bensinger WI, Buckner CD, Shannon-Dorcy K, et al. Transplantation of allogeneic CD34+ peripheral blood stem cells in patients with advanced hematologic malignancy. Blood 1996; 88(11): 4132-4138.
85. Urbano-Ispizua A, Rozman C, Martinez C, et al. Rapid engraftment without significant graft-versus-host disease after allogeneic transplantation of CD34+ selected cells from peripheral blood. Blood 1997;89:3967-3973.
86. Sykes M, Szot GL, Swenson KA, Pearson DA. Induction of high levels of allogeneic hematopoietic reconstitution and donor-specific tolerance without myelosuppressive conditioning. Nature Medicine 1997;3:783-787.

2

UNRELATED DONOR MARROW TRANSPLANTATION FOR TREATMENT OF CHILDHOOD HEMATOLOGIC MALIGNANCIES-EFFECT OF HLA DISPARITY AND CELL DOSE

Ann E. Woolfrey, MD, Claudio Anasetti, MD, Effie W. Petersdorf, MD, Paul J. Martin, MD, Jean E. Sanders, MD and John A. Hansen

Fred Hutchinson Cancer Research Center, Seattle, WA

Marrow and hematopoietic cell transplants provide the possibility of a cure for patients with high risk and therapy-resistant leukemia. However the minority of patients are fortunate enough to have an HLA identical sibling. Transplants from HLA matched unrelated donors were of only theoretical interest given the very high degree of polymorphism among HLA antigens throughout the human population and the lack of organized groups of HLA-typed volunteer donors. Demonstration in the early 1980's that unrelated marrow transplants were medically feasible gave great impetus to the creation of publicly supported donor registries (1-3). In the U.S., a national registry was authorized by congressional legislation in 1984, and in 1986 a federal contract initially administered by the Office of Naval Research was awarded to a consortium of investigators and centers headed by Dr. Jeffrey McCullough of the University of Minnesota (4). This consortium grew to become a comprehensive network of donor recruitment groups, donor centers, marrow and stem cell collection centers, and transplant centers known as the National Marrow Donor Program (NMDP). The NMDP currently consists of 96 donor centers and 127 transplant centers, including 8 donor centers located in countries outside the United States. National registries also exist in several other countries. Worldwide there are more than 4 million volunteers typed for at least HLA-A and B who are potentially available to donate stem cells for anyone in need. A preliminary search of potential matches worldwide can be performed through Internet access of Bone Marrow Donors Worldwide (BMDW) (http:// bmdw.leidenuniv.nl/), a service presented by the Europdonor Foundation located in Leiden, the Netherlands (5).

The NMDP Donor Registry currently contains more than 3.2 million donors typed for HLA-A and B, and more than 1.4 million donors typed for HLA-A, B, and DR. Patient diversity of the Registry is an important feature necessary to assure that patients of different racial origin will have an equitable chance of finding a match. The majority of donors in the NMDP Registry are Caucasian, but 252,773 (7%) are African American, 187,776 (5%) Asian-Pacific Islanders, 234,367 (7%) Hispanic and 43,027 (1%) are Native American. Approximately 470,000 new donors will be recruited to NMDP in the coming year, including 140,000 minority donors. In the last year, 85% of Caucasian patients found at least one potential HLA-A, B, and DR match at their initial search, whereas 58% of African Americans, 60% of Asian-Pacific Islanders and 78% Hispanics found at least one match at their initial search. This disparity has lead to new initiatives aimed at increasing the rate of minority donor recruitment.

Unrelated donor transplant activity has increased along with the very significant growth in donor registries. In 1997, NMDP received 6,256 preliminary and 3,532 formal donor search requests. The latter occurs with the request for a blood sample from a potentially matched donor for confirmatory and high-resolution HLA typing. Approximately 48% of formal searches result in transplants. The number of unrelated donor transplants facilitated by NMDP in 1998 is projected to total 1200. Over the last 3 years, the annual growth rate has averaged approximately 10-15%. The most common diagnosis of transplanted patients has been chronic myelogenous leukemia (CML) (34%), followed by acute myelogenous leukemia (AML) (20%) and acute lymphoblastic leukemia (ALL) (20%). The average age of transplanted patients is 27 years with a range from 2 months to 66 years. Since 1987, more than 2300 children less than 18 years of age had transplants facilitated through NMDP. Currently, more than 400 transplants per year are performed for children, accounting for one third of transplants facilitated through the NMDP. The majority of pediatric patients have received transplants for treatment of malignancies (74%), the most common diagnosis has been ALL (35%), followed by AML (17%), CML (14%) and MDS syndromes (8%).

UNRELATED MARROW TRANSPLANTATION FOR TREATMENT OF HEMATOLOGIC MALIGNANCIES

Elimination of hematologic malignancy using allogeneic marrow transplantation relies on three important therapeutic components: 1) delivery of myeloablative chemotherapy to eradicate the hematologic malignancy; 2) replacement of the diseased marrow with normal hematopoietic stem cells; and 3) control of residual leukemic clones by an anti-leukemic immune response. The use of unrelated donor grafts does not alter the essential therapeutic elements of marrow transplantation, but genetic disparities associated with unrelated donor grafts increase the immunologic barriers that must be overcome to ensure engraftment and achieve tolerance. The alloimmune reactions that form primary and opposing barriers to successful transplantation of unrelated marrow grafts include the graft-vs.-host (GVH) and host-vs.-graft (HVG) responses. While these immune mediated reactions must be controlled for successful outcome, they are associated with an important graft-vs.-leukemia (GVL) response that forms the third component of anti-leukemic therapy. The GVL reaction appears to be more significant in unrelated donor grafts, such that negative effects resulting from strengthened GVH and HVG reactions are counterbalanced by this favorable allogeneic response.

ENGRAFTMENT

Differences in histocompatibility antigens associated with unrelated donor grafts, including HLA as well as minor histocompatibility antigen (mHAg) disparities, promote a stronger HVG response, thereby increasing the risk of graft rejection. Studies that include matched and partially HLA-mismatched unrelated donors have shown graft rejection to occur in 4-7% of recipients, either as failure of primary engraftment or as secondary graft loss. (6-9).

In these studies, several specific factors have been shown to be important in determining the risk of graft failure, including the degree of donor-recipient HLA compatibility, pretransplant diagnosis, intensity of the conditioning regimen, and the number of marrow cells and T cells in the graft (6-8). Intensity of the conditioning regimen and pretransplant diagnosis, which may reflect extent of previous chemotherapy and subsequent host immunity, are important factors that determine magnitude of residual host T or NK cells capable of causing graft rejection (10,11). Because donor T cells play a primary role in preventing rejection, T depleted grafts are associated with an increased risk for graft failure (7). High marrow cell dose also appears to have a favorable affect on engraftment (8).

While it is not surprising that HLA disparity is associated with a higher incidence of graft rejection, the incidence of graft failure is also higher in recipients of HLA-A,-B,-DRB1 matched unrelated donor grafts compared to HLA-identical sibling grafts (1-3). This observation suggests that undetected class I HLA polymorphisms or non-A,B,DRB1 antigens also contribute to the host alloimmune response. When serologically HLA-matched unrelated donor-recipient pairs have been studied by using molecular typing techniques, approximately 30% of pairs have DNA sequence mismatches (12-14). To determine whether these molecular disparities contribute to graft failure, Petersdorf, et al analyzed extent of class I locus sequence mismatch in 21 unrelated donor patients with graft failure. Molecular typing of donor-recipient pairs detected a statistically significant increase in allelic disparity for HLA-C alone, or in combination with HLA-A or -B disparities, compared to case-matched unrelated marrow controls without graft failure (13). These results have recently have been confirmed in a larger group of unrelated donor patients. An increased risk of graft failure was associated with mismatching for two or more class I alleles, but not with mismatching for class II DRB1 or DQB1 alleles (14). Routine implementation of advanced typing technology for identification of class I HLA sequence-level donor-recipient mismatches should result in improvements in donor selection that will lead to a reduction in graft failure.

For patients with graft failure a second marrow transplantation has, until recently, had limited success (15). In our experience, 14 patients who rejected an unrelated donor graft were given a second unrelated donor graft, either from a different (n=2) or the original (n=11) donor. Twelve of these patient were conditioned with an anti-CD3 monoclonal antibody (mAb) (16-17). Seven of the 14 patients are alive at a median of 674 days after transplantation, 1 with autologous reconstitution.

Figure 1.

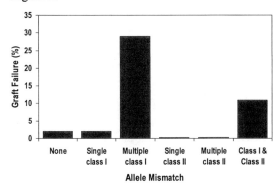

28

GRAFT VS. HOST DISEASE

The probability of developing acute graft vs. host disease (GVHD) is higher for recipients of unrelated donor grafts, compared to matched sibling grafts, presumably due to differences in major or minor histocompatibility antigens. Grade II-IV acute GVHD occurs in 49-83% of recipients of unmanipulated ABDRB1 matched donors and 67-98% of patients with mismatched donors (Table 1) (6, 18). Severe GVHD (grade III-IV) occurs in approximately 25% of matched and 35% of mismatched recipients, respectively. Significant factors associated with the development of acute GVH include HLA disparity (6), female donor (19) and older patient age (7), while T-cell depletion significantly decreases the risk for acute GVHD (7). Compared to recipients of HLA-identical related grafts, patients with an unrelated donor have a higher probability of developing extensive chronic GVHD (Table 1) (6, 7, 20). Furthermore, the duration of GVHD and length of treatment is significantly prolonged (median 3.2 years) (21). Significant factors associated with the development of chronic GVHD include HLA disparity, female donor for a male recipient, and patient age (19, 22). While prolonged therapy for chronic GVHD may affect quality of life, studies have demonstrated that quality of life for patients who survive two years after transplantation is not significantly different for unrelated donor patients compared to other groups of long-term survivors.

Our understanding of the relationship between HLA disparity and the risk for severe acute GVHD has evolved, corresponding with advances in tissue typing technologies. Initial studies of unrelated transplant recipients demonstrated an adverse effect on survival associated with serologic HLA-A or B incompatibility, at least in part due to increased incidence of GVHD, although this adverse effect was not observed for younger patients (18). Advances in DNA typing technologies have led to improved definitions of HLA compatibility, and prove particularly important when the donor and recipient are serologically HLA-identical. Results of initial studies using molecular typing to discriminate class II HLA alleles suggested that recipients of grafts that were serologically matched at HLA-A and –B had increased survival if there was molecular identity at DRB1 (23), while DRB1 or DQB1 disparity increased the risk for grades III-IV GVHD (24). However, these studies must now be reinterpreted given emerging information regarding the high incidence of molecular polymorphisms within serologically defined class I antigens. When donor-recipient pairs have been analyzed by using molecular techniques that identify allele disparities at class I (HLA-A, B, C) and class II (DRB1, DQB1) loci, the relative risk for grades III-IV GVHD previously associated with a single class II allelic disparity has become less significant (RR: 1.8, 95% CI:1.0-3.4; p=0.06) (Figure 2) (14). The risk for grades III-IV GVHD was significantly greater when allelic disparity at class II was found in combination with allelic disparity at one or more class I loci. Mortality was significantly higher when donors and recipients were disparate either for class II plus class I alleles (RR: 3.0, 95% CI: 1.8-5.0; p<0.001), or for multiple class I alleles (RR: 3.5, 95% CI: 2.1-5.9; p<0.001) (Figure 3), but a single allelic disparity for class I or class II was not associated with a significant increase in mortality. Results of this study and others (25) indicate that comprehensive matching of HLA class I and class II alleles should improve outcome for recipients of unrelated marrow grafts.

Figure 2.

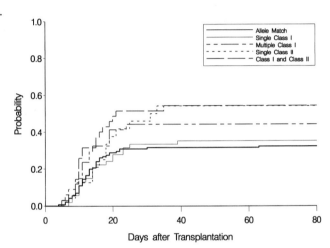

Figure 3.

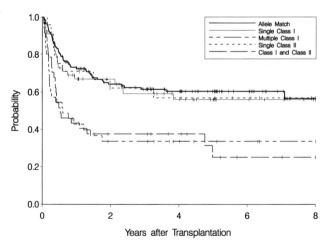

Relapse and Graft-vs.- Leukemia

The capacity of donor immune cells to generate anti-leukemic reactivity appears to be increased in unrelated marrow grafts, presumably induced by disparities in histocompatibility antigens. Enhancement of the GVL effect is supported by observations that recipients of unrelated marrow have a lower risk of relapse compared to recipients of genetically HLA-identical marrow (8, 19). Patients who receive HLA-mismatched unrelated grafts (6, 8) or those who develop GVHD (26-27) also have a lower risk of relapse. It remains to be established whether the GVL reaction is directed primarily toward disparate histocompatibility antigens, as a manifestation of the global GVH response, or whether leukemic-specific antigens may be identified, allowing separation of GVL from GVH responses.

MARROW TRANSPLANTATION FOR ACUTE LEUKEMIA

Despite the observations that unrelated marrow transplantation is associated with increased risk for rejection, GVHD, and transplant-related mortality, the use of unrelated donors as source of stem cells for children with acute leukemia does not appear to compromise outcome. While risk for graft rejection, acute and chronic GVHD are higher in unrelated marrow recipients, including children, risk for relapse is lower, and event-free survival (EFS) is not significantly different (6, 28). In patients with acute leukemia, primary engraftment occurs in 96-99% of patients who receive unmanipulated marrow grafts, although the incidence of late graft failure is 6-8%. Neutrophil recovery occurs at a median of 21 days, 50% of patients achieve platelet counts >50,000 by day 100, and 50% of patients no longer require platelet transfusions after day 25 (6, 8). Factors that are significantly associated with improved neutrophil and platelet engraftment include a high marrow cell dose (>3.6 x 10^8 cells/kg) and transplantation in complete remission. Acute GVHD grades II-IV occurs in 82% and severe (grade III-IV) GVHD occurs in 47% of patients who receive unmanipulated marrow (8). Higher marrow cell dose is significantly associated with a lower incidence of severe GVHD, as is younger patient age and T cell depletion (7, 29). Chronic GVHD occurs in 52% of surviving patients who receive unmanipulated marrow and occurs more frequently in recipients of HLA-disparate grafts, those with an antecedent history of severe acute GVHD, and in older patients, (8) and less frequently in patients with T cell depleted grafts (7, 29).

Phase of leukemia at time of transplant is highly predictive for the risks of leukemic relapse and death from non-relapse causes. In particular, patients transplanted in relapse with > 30% circulating blasts have very poor survival following unrelated transplantation (8). Overall, non-relapse death occurs in approximately 40% of unrelated marrow recipients, and most deaths occur within the first 100 days. One significant factor associated with non-relapse mortality is marrow cell dose, presumably due to more rapid engraftment and lower incidence of fatal infections in those receiving high cell doses, in addition to the association with lower risk for GVHD. In several studies, results suggest that T cell depletion may reduce the risk of early non-relapse mortality (29, 30).

Relapse is the major cause of death following transplantation for acute leukemia. Factors found to be significantly associated with risk for relapse include phase of disease at time of transplant and HLA-mismatch. Sierra, et al demonstrated a 2- to 5- fold reduction in risk for relapse for patients transplanted in remission compared to those in relapse (p=0.0001)(8). Of patients transplanted in relapse, patients with >30% leukemic blasts in the marrow have the highest risk for relapse (cumulative incidence > 70% vs. <50%, p=0.01). Recipients of HLA-A, -B, or DRB1 mismatched marrow had a decreased risk of relapse (RR: 0.5; CI: 0.3-0.9; p=0.01), consistent with a GVL effect, but this beneficial effect was negated by an increase in transplant-related mortality and EFS was not improved. EFS is approximately 50% for patients in remission at the time of transplant, compared to <15% for those with more advanced disease, and this outcome appears to be similar for patients with ALL or AML.(6, 8) Factors that favor leukemia free survival include transplantation during complete remission,(6-8) higher marrow cell dose, (8) CMV negative recipient, (8) younger age, (7) and HLA-A, -B, DRB1 match (7).

THE ROLE OF UNRELATED DONOR MARROW TRANSPLANTATION IN THE TREATMENT OF HEMATOLOGIC MALIGNANCIES OF CHILDHOOD

Acute Lymphoblastic Leukemia

Children with acute lymphoblastic leukemia (ALL) generally have a good prognosis, such that 75% of patients are expected to be cured with conventional chemotherapy (31). Certain groups of patients can be defined as high-risk, including those with the clonal cytogenetic abnormalities t(9;22) and t(4;ll) and those who have poor response to induction therapy (32); less than 30% of these patients can be cured with conventional chemotherapy. Marrow transplantation has been studied as a means to provide higher intensity therapy for high-risk ALL patients once remission is achieved. A conditioning regimen containing TBI followed by transplantation from matched sibling donors in first complete remission (CR1) appears to provide a survival advantage, with reports of 45-84% EFS at 3 years after transplantation (33-35). Transplantation may improve survival for infants considered to have very poor outcome with standard chemotherapy; in our experience 64% of high-risk infants transplanted during first remission survive without recurrent disease (Sanders, unpublished).

Unrelated marrow transplants have been performed for high-risk ALL patients who do not have suitably matched related donors. Studies in patients with Philadelphia-chromosome positive ALL have shown a 2-year EFS of 37-45% for those transplanted in first remission, approaching that found in those with matched sibling donors (36-37). Twelve children (<18 years) with ALL in CR1 have received unrelated marrow transplants at FHCRC, most of whom had high-risk features. These patients were conditioned with cyclophosphamide and TBI, and received marrow from matched (n=8) or 1-Ag mismatched (n=4) donors. Seven of these survive from >1 to >8 years after transplantation (Figure 4). Results from this study as well as others (38) suggest that unrelated marrow transplantation offers a significant survival advantage over conventional chemotherapy when an HLA-identical related donor is not available, but prospective studies should be performed to confirm these promising results.

Figure 4.

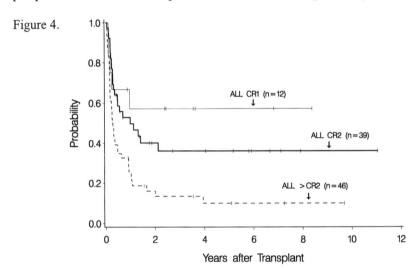

Prognosis for children who develop first marrow relapse depends on the duration of first remission. Patients with late relapse (> 2 years from diagnosis) may have relatively good outcome with conventional chemotherapy alone, although some studies continue to show potential for late second relapse (39). In contrast, children who relapse in the marrow within two years of diagnosis have poor outcome primarily due to treatment failure (40-41). Multiple studies have shown 40-50% EFS after marrow transplantation in second remission (42-43). These studies have been criticized for selection bias, since patients with aggressive disease die earlier and are not included in studies of marrow transplantation (44-45). To address this question, Barret et al., (39) performed a matched-pair analysis of CR2 patients treated with chemotherapy or transplanted from HLA-identical siblings, using data from the Pediatric Oncology Group and the International Bone Marrow Transplant Registry, respectively. Pairs were matched for variables found to be significantly associated with outcome, including duration of first and second remissions, WBC at time of diagnosis, and T cell phenotype. Patients who received marrow transplantation had significantly better EFS at 5 years compared to those treated with chemotherapy alone (40% vs. 17%; p<0.001). Marrow transplantation was associated with a reduced risk of relapse (45% vs 80%; p<0.001) that was not negated by increased treatment-related deaths (27% vs 14%). Transplantation resulted in better outcome for children with CR1 >36 months, as well as those with short duration CR1. Wheeler, et al., conducted a similar study of 489 patients who relapsed in the UKALL X trial and found that outcome after allogeneic marrow transplantation was superior only for those patients with early first relapse (46). Chemotherapy and marrow transplantation resulted in similar outcomes for patients with late medullary relapse or early extramedullary relapse.

While these and other studies support use of HLA-identical sibling marrow transplantation for treatment of ALL in CR2, particularly for those with early marrow relapse, the role of unrelated marrow transplantation has not been directly addressed. We have observed 56% disease-free survival at 3 years after unrelated marrow transplantation for children transplanted during CR2 (Figure 4), comparable to earlier reports of matched sibling marrow transplants (42). Weisdorf studied outcome of 106 unrelated recipients compared to 98 autologous patients transplanted in CR2, using data from NMDP, University of Minnesota, and Dana-Farber Cancer Institute. Univariate analysis showed that patients receiving unrelated marrow transplants had a higher probability of EFS at 2 years after transplantation (42% vs 20%; p=0.02), but multivariate analysis did not confirm that donor type significantly affected outcome (49). Recently, 50 patients treated on similar reinduction protocols and transplanted with T cell depleted unrelated marrow were reported to have an actuarial EFS of 53% at 2 years after transplantation (30). While these studies suggest that unrelated marrow provides similar results to matched related marrow transplantation, the analyses suffer from the immeasurable effects of selection bias.

The role of marrow transplantation in treatment of patients with isolated extramedullary relapse has not been determined, since many patients can achieve prolonged survival with chemotherapy alone. In these cases, unrelated marrow transplantation should be undertaken only on an established research protocol. On the other hand, patients who have refractory relapse and those who relapse after second remission have extremely poor outcome despite further treatment with conventional chemotherapy (32). Although allogeneic marrow transplantation might provide these patients with a survival advantage, the true

34

impact on EFS is difficult to assess because of selection bias. EFS in the range of 10-30% at 2-3 years after transplantation has been reported in multiple small series that include advanced stage ALL patients, and source of marrow (matched related vs unrelated) did not appear to affect outcome (26, 28, 47-49). Forty-six children have been transplanted with unrelated marrow at FHCRC for treatment of advanced stage ALL. At 3 years after transplantation, actuarial probability of EFS is approximately 10% (Figure 4). Importantly, for patients with advanced leukemia, disease burden is associated with outcome. Survival is significantly worse for patients with >30% marrow blasts, and particularly poor for those with circulating blasts (8).

Acute Myelogenous Leukemia

Despite intensive chemotherapy, less than half of all children with acute myelogenous leukemia (AML) will survive long term (50-51). Prospective cooperative group studies in newly diagnosed AML patients have addressed the question of whether post-remission myeloablative therapy followed by marrow transplantation might improve survival. Patients were conditioned for transplantation with BuCy or CyTBI and received marrow from HLA-identical relatives. These studies have shown 50-60% EFS after allogeneic marrow transplantation compared to 30-40% after autologous transplants or chemotherapy alone (51-53). Based on these studies allogeneic transplantation is recommended in first remission for AML patients with an HLA-identical related donor. The role of unrelated marrow transplantation in first remission remains unclear. Outcome has improved for patients treated with chemotherapy alone, and AML patients in first remission currently have a 40-50% risk of relapse (52-54). Additionally, marrow transplantation in early first relapse or second remission results in 30-40% EFS at 2 years after transplantation (55). Thus far, it is not apparent that the majority of AML patients would benefit from unrelated marrow transplantation in CR1 (51, unpublished data). Unrelated marrow transplantation in first remission might be considered for patients with high-risk features, such as extramedullary disease or poor prognosis cytogenetics, but transplantation should be undertaken only on an established research protocol. Specifically, infants with high-risk disease might benefit from unrelated marrow transplantation in CR1, since transplant-related mortality is ≤10%, regardless of donor source (57).

Marrow transplantation has an important role for treatment of relapsed AML patients because outcome is poor with chemotherapy alone. Two-year EFS is 30-40% for patients transplanted in early first untreated relapse or second remission (55, 58). Analyses that attempt to compare outcome based on treatment have shown a survival advantage for patients who receive marrow transplants compared to chemotherapy alone, particularly for younger patients and for those with longer first remission (59). Results of unrelated marrow transplantation have been similar to matched related marrow transplantation for treatment of advanced stage AML. While unrelated marrow transplants are associated with an increased risk of transplant-related mortality, the risk for relapse is lower, and 2-year EFS is 30-40% (60-61). Figure 5 shows outcome after unrelated marrow transplantation for treatment of children with advanced stage AML. Transplantation during second remission is associated with favorable survival compared to transplantation during more advanced phases of disease (6). Unrelated marrow transplantation may provide long term survival for patients with AML in relapse, particularly those in early untreated first relapse, but patients transplanted with >30% marrow blasts or circulating peripheral blasts have extremely poor outcome (8).

Figure 5.

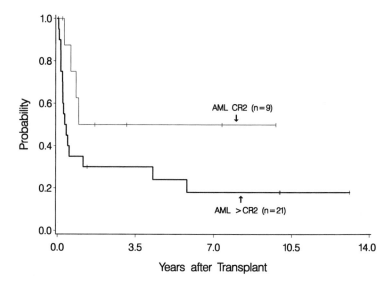

Myelodysplastic and myeloproliferative syndromes

Childhood myelodysplastic syndrome (MDS) is a stem cell disorder that can involve multiple hematopoietic lineages. Without treatment, the disease usually progresses rapidly, and virtually all patients succumb to complications of pancytopenia or leukemic transformation. Like other stem cell disorders, MDS responds poorly to conventional chemotherapy, particularly when therapy is initiated before leukemic transformation (62). For those patients who achieve complete remission, prospective studies have shown improved long-term survival after allogeneic marrow transplantation compared to chemotherapy alone, similar to AML patients. Marrow transplantation alone, without pre-transplant therapy, also has been shown to improve long-term survival for children with MDS, and the role of pre-transplant induction therapy must be re-evaluated particularly for patients in early phases of the disease (63-64).

In studies that include adults, MDS patients treated with marrow transplantation alone have a 4-year EFS of 40-45 % (65-66). Factors associated with favorable outcome include younger age and transplantation during early disease phase. The use of unrelated donors does not appear to compromise survival. Anderson, et al studied outcome for 52 MDS patients (median age 33 years) and reported 38% EFS at 2 years after transplantation, with a trend for improved EFS for patients with RA/RAEB compared to RAEBT/AML patients (47% vs. 26%, p=0.14) (67). HLA-compatibility was not found to affect survival significantly. Patients less than 20 years of age had 53% EFS. Other investigators have also reported that younger age and early phase disease are associated with improved outcome (27). Evidence for GVL effect has been suggested in several studies (27, 67) In an EBMT study of 118 patients, the probability of relapse was 26% for patients with grade II-IV acute GVHD compared to 42% for those with <grade II GVHD (27).

In our experience, marrow transplantation has shown promising results for children with MDS. Outcome for 47 consecutive patients has been recently analyzed, including 30 patients transplanted with related donor marrow and 17 transplanted with unrelated marrow (68). Graft failure occurred in 6 patients, including 3 unrelated donor grafts. EFS was 59% for RA patients, 56% for RAEB (OR: 1.5, CI: 0.6-3.8, p=0.4), and 14% for RAEB-T or CMML (OR: 2.8, CI: 1.0-8.0, p=0.06) at 2 years after transplantation. Patients with unrelated donors had survival similar to those with closely matched related donors, although the risk of severe GVHD was significantly higher (12% vs. 24%; OR: 6.4, CI: 2.1-19.3, p=0.001). Figure 6 shows outcome for 14 patients with RA or RAEB transplanted from unrelated donors at FHCRC. These results are supported by other studies that have shown similar survival for children transplanted with related or unrelated donor marrow (69, 70). Outcome for children with chronic myelomonocytic leukemia has been studied separately by Locatelli, et al. (64). In this study of 43 children, actuarial probability of EFS was 31% at 5 years after transplantation, comparable to results for patients with advanced MDS. Actuarial probability of EFS was 22% for patients with unrelated marrow donors compared to 38% for those with HLA-matched sibling donors (p<0.05). Patients transplanted early after diagnosis were found to have significantly better outcome in the univariate analysis. These studies support the use of unrelated marrow transplantation for treatment of MDS in early phase disease, but it must be kept in mind that no study has compared treatment outcomes prospectively (unrelated marrow transplantation vs. chemotherapy alone).

Figure 6.

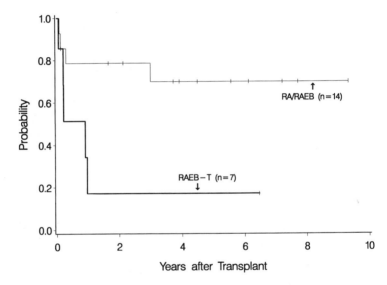

Juvenile CML (J-CML) is a lethal myeloproliferative/myelodysplastic stem cell disorder that occurs almost exclusively in childhood. Characteristics include hepatosplenomegaly, lymphadenopathy, eczematous rash, leukocytosis, thrombocytopenia, and hypercellular, dysplastic marrow. In vitro, the disease is characterized by spontaneous proliferation of leukemic progenitor granulocyte-macrophage colony-forming units. Some cases respond to therapy with isotrentinoin, (71) but marrow transplantation has been the only treatment reported to be curative (72). In several small series of patients, 40-50% EFS was observed at 2 years after marrow transplantation (72-76). In these studies, outcome with unrelated donors appeared comparable to outcome with closely matched related donors.

Chronic Myelogenous Leukemia

Allogeneic marrow transplantation from a matched sibling donor has been established as the best treatment for patients with chronic myelogenous leukemia (CML). Younger patients can expect a 4-year EFS of 75% if transplant is carried out within 1 year of diagnosis (77). In contrast, only 25% of patients survive 5 years with conventional therapy (78). Advances in treatment of CML with interferon-alpha (IFN-α), given alone or in combination with chemotherapy, has prolonged the time to disease progression and improved survival in a significant portion of patients (79-80). However, treatment with IFN-α is not curative for most patients, and survival is inferior when compared to marrow transplantation (7 year EFS: 32% vs 58%) (81). The use of unrelated marrow increases the opportunity for children to receive curative therapy, and in large studies that include adult patients, outcome with unrelated donors approaches the outcome with HLA-matched related donors (19, 82). Pretransplant regimens containing TBI and post-transplant immunosuppressive regimens containing cyclosporine and methotrexate produce superior outcome for unrelated marrow recipients (83). Analysis of 196 patients with chronic phase CML at FHCRC showed 57% 5-year survival. Transplant-related mortality accounted for most deaths and the cumulative incidence of relapse was 10% at 5 years. Patients less than 50 years of age who received an HLA-A, B, and DRB1 matched unrelated marrow transplant within 1 year after diagnosis had a 74% probability of surviving 5 years, comparable to results for patients transplanted with HLA-matched related marrow (19, 77). Outcome for children is similar to that for older patients (Figure 7). We have done unrelated marrow transplants for 24 children in chronic phase, using HLA-ABDRB1 matched (n=19) or 1-Ag mismatched (n=5) donors. Sixteen patients (67%), including 3 with mismatched donors, survive from >0.6 to 12 years after transplantation. Two studies that evaluated outcome after unrelated marrow transplantation for children in chronic phase showed 45-55% actuarial probability of EFS at 3 years after transplantation (84-85). Donors were HLA-A,-B, DRB1 identical or mismatched for 1 antigen; grades III-IV acute GVHD and extensive chronic GVHD occurred in 18-45% and 10-45% of patients, respectively. The majority of survivors had Karnofsky scores of >80%. Encouragingly, several studies have shown that patients transplanted in recent years have improved survival, (22, 83) possibly reflecting better methods of supportive care, such as prophylaxis for fungal and viral disease. Currently, marrow transplantation should be considered the optimal treatment for younger patients who have an HLA-A,B,DRB1 identical related or unrelated donor (86).

Figure 7.

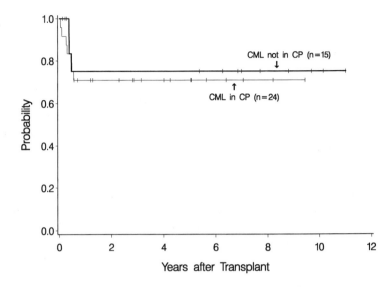

Factors that affect outcome need to be considered in determining when to initiate unrelated marrow transplantation. Variables associated with improved survival for chronic phase patients include younger age (87), higher marrow cell dose (84), HLA compatibility (19, 84, 87), shorter time from diagnosis to transplant (19, 87), and limited therapy with IFN-α(22, 88). Outcome is improved if transplantation is done within 1 year of diagnosis (86-87). In addition, the incidence of grades III-IV acute GHVD (55% vs 34%, p=0.01) and nonrelapse mortality (56% vs 38%, p=0.05) are higher for patients treated with INF-α for > 6 months as compared to those treated for < 6 months before transplantation (22). These studies indicate that patients with suitable unrelated donors should not be treated with INF-α for >6 months and should be transplanted within one year of diagnosis, if possible. This strategy must be modified, however, to take into account the benefit of an optimally matched unrelated donor, a procedure that remains time-consuming.

The value of optimizing the HLA match between the donor and recipient by use of advanced DNA-typing technology appears to be particularly important for chronic phase CML patients because survival is determined primarily by complications of graft-vs.-host disease (14, 19). Our studies have shown that

40

compatibility for HLA alleles improves survival for chronic phase CML patients. Examination of the effect of allele matching has demonstrated that a single class II mismatch (DRB1 or DQB1) is associated with an increased risk of grades III-IV GVHD (RR:1.8, CI:1.0-3.4, p=0.06). When a class II mismatch is associated with a class I allele mismatch, the risks of graft rejection (RR:9.8, CI:1.7-56.8, p=0.01), severe GVHD (OR:2.0, CI:1.2-3.4, p=0.01), and mortality (OR:3.0, CI:1.8-5.0, p<0.001) are significantly higher. Similarly, multiple class I allele disparities are associated with an increased incidence of graft failure (OR:10.5, CI:2.2-49.9, p=0.0003) and mortality (OR:3.5, CI:2.1-5.9, p<0.001) (14).

Overall survival for patients transplanted in accelerated phase, blast crisis, or second chronic phase has been estimated at 27-60%, 0-20 %, and 22-40%, respectively, with either related or unrelated donors (19, 87). Studies of children with advanced stage CML have shown 33%-45% actuarial probability of EFS at 3 years after unrelated marrow transplantation (84-85). In Seattle, 15 children with advanced CML have received unrelated marrow grafts, from HLA-A,B,DRB1 matched (n=11) or 1-antigen mismatched (n=4) donors. At time of transplant, 9 children were in accelerated phase, 4 in blast crisis and 2 in second chronic phase. Twelve patients survive from >0.1 to 11 years (median survival 6.9 years +/- 3.9) (Figure 7).

Relapse After Unrelated Marrow Transplantation

Risk for leukemic relapse is lower following unrelated marrow transplantation than that from closely matched related donors, presumably resulting from a more potent graft-vs leukemia (GVL) effect. One option for patients who relapse after unrelated marrow transplantation involves induction of a GVL effect, either by modification of the immunosuppressive regimen used to control GVHD or by infusion of donor lymphocytes (DLI). Potential for response to DLI depends on the type of leukemia. Patients with CML have response rates of 70-85%, while patients with ALL have much lower response rates (89, Flowers, unpublished). Patients that do not respond to or do not qualify for DLI may be eligible for a second marrow transplant. Younger patients and those transplanted more than one year after the first transplant have the best outcome after a second transplant (90). In our experience, 16 patients who relapsed after an unrelated marrow transplant have received a second transplant from a different (n=4) or the original (n=13) donor. Ten patients continue to survive, 5 of whom have lived longer after the second transplant than the interval between first transplant and relapse.

CONCLUSION

Unrelated marrow transplantation provides an important therapy in the management of childhood hematologic malignancies. Suitably matched unrelated donors are acceptable alternatives in the majority of instances in which marrow transplantation is indicated and HLA matched or closely matched related donors are not available. Outcome after unrelated marrow transplantation has improved over time with the development of better methods for supportive care and improved appreciation for the importance of HLA allele compatibility and marrow cell dose. The rapid growth of donor registries and efforts to recruit minority donors should increase the availability of unrelated marrow transplantation for treatment of children with leukemia.

REFERENCES

1. Hansen JA, Clift RA, Thomas ED, Buckner CD, Storb R, Giblett ER: Transplantation of marrow from an unrelated donor to a patient with acute leukemia. N Engl J Med 1980; 303:565-567.
2. McCullough J: Bone marrow transplantation from unrelated voluntary donors: summary of a conference on scientific, ethical, legal, financial and practical issues. Transfusion 1982; 22: 78.
3. Cleaver S: The Anthony Nolan Research Centre and other matching registries. In: Treleaven and Barret (eds.) Bone Marrow Transplantation in Practice. Edinburgh, Churchill Livingston 1992; 361-366.
4. McCullough J, Hansen J, Perkins H, Stroncek D, Bartsch G: The National Marrow Donor Program: How it works, accomplishments to date. Oncology 1989; 3: 63-74.
5. Oudshoorn M, Leeuwen A, Zanden HGMv, Rood JJv: Bone marrow donors worldwide: a successful exercise in international cooperation. Bone Marrow Transplant 1994; 14:3-8.
6. Balduzzi A, Gooley T, Anasetti C, Sanders JE, Martin PJ, Petersdorf, EW, Appelbaum FR, Buckner CD, Matthews D, Storb R. Unrelated donor marrow transplantation in children. Blood 1995; 86:3247-3256.
7. Kernan NA, Bartsch G, Ash RC, Beatty PG, Champlin R, Filipovich A, Gajewski J, Hansen JA, Henslee-Downey J, McCullough J. Analysis of 462 transplantations from unrelated donors facilitated by the National Marrow Donor Program. N Engl J Med 1993; 328:593-602.
8. Sierra J, Storer B, Hansen JA, Bjerke JW , Martin PJ, Petersdorf EW, Appelbaum FR, Bryant E, Chauncey TR, Sale G, Sanders JE, Storb R, Sullivan KM, Anasetti C. Transplantation of marrow cells from unrelated

donors for treatment of high-risk acute leukemia: the effect of leukemic burden, donor HLA-matching, and marrow cell dose. Blood 1997; 89:4226-4235.

9. Beatty PG, Anasetti C, Hansen JA, Longton GM, Sanders JE, Martin PJ, Mickelson EM, Choo SY, Petersdorf EW, Pepe MS, Apelbaum FR, Bearman SI, Buckner CD, Clift RA, Petersen FB, Singer J, Stewart PS, Storb RF, Sullivan KM, Tesler MC, Witherspoon RP, Thomas ED: Marrow transplantation from unrelated donors for treatment of hematologic malignancies: effect of mismatching for one HLA locus. Blood 1993; 81:249-253.

10. Slattery JT, Sanders JE, Buckner CD, Schaffer RL, Lambert KW, Langer, FP, Anasetti C, Bensinger WI, Fisher LD, Appelbaum FR. Graft-rejection and toxicity following bone marrow transplantation in relation to busulfan pharmacokinetics. Bone Marrow Transplant 1995; 16:31-42.

11. Terenzi A, Aversa F, Albi N, Galandrini R, Dembech C, Velardi A, et al. Residual clonable host cell detection for predicting engraftment of T cell depleted BMTs. Bone Marrow Transplant. 1993; 11:357-361.6.

12. Santamaria P, Reinsmoen NL, Lindstom, AL, Boyce-Jacino, MT, Barbosa, JJ, Faras AJ, et al. Frequent Hla Class I and DP Sequence Mismatches in Serologically (HLA-A, HLA-B, HLA-DR) and Molecularly (HLA-DRB1, HLA-DQA1, HLA-DQB1) HLA-Identical Unrelated Bone Marrow Transplant Pairs. Blood 1994; 83:280-287.

13. Petersdorf EW, Longton GM, Anasetti C, Mickelson EM, McKinney SK, Smith AG, et al. Association of HLA-C disparity with graft failure after marrow transplantation from unrelated donors. Blood 1997; 89:1818-1823.

14. Petersdorf, EW, Gooley TA, Anasetti C, Martin PJ, Mickelson E, Smith AG, Woolfrey AE, Hansen JA. Optimizing outcome after unrelated marrow transplantation by comprehensive matching of HLA class I and II alleles in the donor and recipient. Blood 1998; 92 (10): 3515-3520.

15. Anasetti C, Hansen JA. Bone marrow transplantation from HLA-partially matched related donors and unrelated volunteer donors. In: Forman SJ, Blume KG, Thomas ED, editors. Bone Marrow Transplantation. Boston, MA: Blackwell Scientific Publications, 1994:665-680.

16. Anasetti C, Tan P, Hansen JA, Martin PJ. Induction of specific nonresponsiveness in unprimed human T cell by anti-CD3 antibody and alloantigen. J.Exp.Med. 1990; 172:1691-1700.

17. Bjerke JW, Lorenz J, Martin PJ, Storb R, Hansen JA, Anasetti C: Treatment of graft failure with anti-CD3 antibody BD3, glucocorticoids and infusion of donor hematopoietic cells. Blood 1995; 86:107a.

18. Davies SM, Shu XO, Blazar BR, Filipovich AH, Kersey JH, Krivit W, McCullough J, Miller WJ, Ramsay NK, Segall M. Unrelated donor bone marrow transplantation: influence of HLA A and B incompatibility on outcome. Blood 1995; 86:1636-1642.

19. Hansen JA, Gooley TA, Martin PJ, Appelbaum F, Chauncey TR, Clift RA, Petersdorf EW, Radich J, Sanders JE, Storb RF, Sullivan KM, Anasetti. Bone marrow transplants from unrelated donors for patients with chronic myeloid leukemia. N Engl J Med 1998; 338:962-968.

20. Beatty PG, Hansen JA, Longton GM, Thomas ED, Sanders JE, Martin PJ, Bearman SI, Anasetti C, Petersdorf EW, Mickelson EM, Pepe MS, Appelbaum FR, Buckner CD, Clift RA, Petersen FB, Stewart PS, Storb RF, Sullivan KM, Tesler MC, Witherspoon RP: Marrow transplantation from HLA-matched unrelated donors for treatment of hematologic malignancies. Transplantation 1991; 51:443-447.

21. Morton AJ, Anasetti C, Gooley T, Flowers M, Deeg HJ, Hansen JA, Martin PJ, Sullivan KM: Chronic graft versus host disease following unrelated donor transplantation (submitted).

22. Morton AJ, Gooley T, Hansen JA, Appelbaum FR, Bjerke JW, Clift R, Martin PJ, Petersdorf EW, Sanders JE, Storb R, Sullivan KM, Woolfrey A, Anasetti C. Association between pre-transplant interferon-alpha and outcome after unrelated donor marrow transplantation for chronic myelogenous leukemia in chronic phase. Blood 1998; 92:394-401.

23. Petersdorf EW, Longton GM, Anasetti C, Martin PJ, Mickelson EM, Smith AG, Hansen JA: The significance of HLA-DRB1 matching on clinical outcome after HLA-A, B, DR identical unrelated donor marrow transplantation Blood 1995; 86:1606-1613.

24. Petersdorf EW, Longton GM, Anasetti C, Mickelson EM, Smith AG, Martin PJ, Hansen JA. Definition of HLA-DQ as a transplantation antigen. Proc Natl Acad Sci USA 1996; 93:15358-15363.

25. Sasazuki T, Juji T, Morishima Y, Kinukawa N, Kashiwabara H, Inoko H, Yoshida T, Kimura A, Akaza T, Kamikawaji N, Kodera Y, Takaku F, for the JMDP: Effect of matching of class I HLA alleles on clinical outcome after transplantation of hematopoietic stem cells from an unrelated donor. N Engl J Med 1998; 339:1177-1185.

26. Davies SM, Wagner JE, Shu XO, Blazar BR, Katsanis E, Orchard PJ, Kersey JH, Dusenbery KE, Weisdorf DJ, McGlave PB, Ramsay NK. Unrelated donor bone marrow transplantation for children with acute leukemia. J Clin Oncol 1997; 15:557-565.

27. Arnold R, deWitte T, vanBiezen A, Hermans J, Jacobsen N, Runde V, Gratwohl A, Apperley JF. Unrelated bone marrow transplantation in patients with myelodysplastic syndromes and secondary acute myeloid leukemia: an EBMT survey. European Blood and Marrow Transplantation Group. Bone Marrow Transplant 1998; 21:1213-1216.

28. Hongeng S, Krance RA, Bowman LC, Srivastava DK, Cunningham JM, Horwitz EM, Brenner MK, Heslop HE. Outcomes of transplantation with matched-sibling and unrelated-donor bone marrow in children with leukaemia. Lancet 1997; 350:767-771.

29. Cornish JM, Pamphilon DH, Potter MN, Steward CG, Goodman S, Green A, Goulden P, Goulden N, Knechtli C, Hale G, Waldmann H, Oakhill A. Unrelated donor bone marrow transplant in childhood ALL. The role of T-cell depletion. Bone Marrow Transplant 1996; 18 Suppl 2:31-35.

30. Oakhill A, Pamphilon DH, Potter MN, Steward CG, Goodman S, Green A, Goulden P, Goulden NJ, Hale G, Waldmann H, Cornish JM. Unrelated donor bone marrow transplantation for children with relapsed acute lymphoblastic leukaemia in second complete remission. Brit J Haematol 1996; 94:574-578.

31. Rivera GK, Pinkel D, Simone JV, Hancock ML, Crist WM: Treatment of acute lymphoblastic leukemia. 30 years' experience at St. Jude Children's Research Hospital. N Eng J Med 1993; 329:1289-1295.

32. Ortega JJ, Olive T. Haematopoietic progenitor cell transplant in acute leukaemias in children: indications, results and controversies. Bone Marrow Transplant 1998; 21(Suppl 2):S11-S16.

33. Bordigoni P, Vernant JP, Souillet G, Gluckman E, Marininchi D, Milpied N, Fischer A, Benz LE, Jouet JP, Reiffers J. Allogeneic bone marrow transplantation for children with acute lymphoblastic leukemia in first remission: a cooperative study of the Groupe d'Etude de la Greffe de Moelle Osseuse. Journal of Clinical Oncology 1989; 7:747-753.

34. Stockschlader M, Hegewisch-Becker S, Kruger W, Dieck A tom, Mross K, Hoffknecht M, Berger C, Kohlschutter B, Martin H, Peters S. Bone marrow transplantation for Philadelphia-chromosome-positive acute lymphoblastic leukemia. Bone Marrow Transplant 1995; 16:663-667.

35. Snyder DS, Chao NJ, Amylon MD, Taguchi J, Long GD, Negrin RS, Nademanee AP, O'Donnell MR, Schmidt GM, Stein AS: Fractionated total body irradiation and high-dose etoposide as a preparatory regimen for bone marrow transplantation for 99 patients with acute leukemia in first complete remission. Blood 1993; 82:2920-2928.

36. Sierra J, Radich J, Hansen JA, Martin PJ , Petersdorf EW, Bjerke J, Bryant E, Nash RA, Sanders JE, Storb R, Sullivan KM, Appelbaum FR, Anasetti C. Marrow transplants from unrelated donors for treatment of Philadelphia chromosome-positive acute lymphoblastic leukemia. Blood 1997; 90:1410-1414.

37. Marks DI, Bird JM, Cornish JM, Goulden NJ, Jones CG, Knechtli CJ, Pamphilon DH, Steward CG, Oakhill A. Unrelated donor bone marrow transplantation for children and adolescents with Philadelphia-positive acute lymphoblastic leukemia. J Clin Oncol 1998; 16:931-936.

38. Weisdorf DJ, Billett AL, Hannan P, Ritz J, Sallan SE, Steinbuch M, Ramsay NK. Autologous versus unrelated donor allogeneic marrow transplantation for acute lymphoblastic leukemia. Blood 1997; 90:2962-2968.

39. Barrett AJ, Horowitz MM, Pollock BH, Zhang MJ, Bortin MM, Buchanan, GR, Camitta BM, Ochs J, Graham-Pole J, Rowlings PA. Bone marrow transplants from HLA-identical siblings as compared with chemotherapy for children with acute lymphoblastic leukemia in a second remission. N Engl J Med 1994; 331:1253-1258.

40. Chessels JM, Leiper AD, Richards SM: A second course of treatment for childhood acute lymphoblastic leukemia: long-term follow-up is needed to assess results. Brit J Haematol 1994; 86:48-54.

41. Henze G, Fengler R, Hartmann R, Niethammer D, Schellong G, Riehm H: BFM group treatment results in relapsed childhood acute lymphoblastic leukemia. Hamatologie Bluttransfusion 1990; 33:619-626.

42. Sanders JE, Flournoy N, Thomas ED, Buckner CD, Lum LG, Clift RA, Appelbaum FR, Sullivan KM, Stewart P, Deeg HJ, Doney K, Storb R: Marrow transplant experience in children with acute lymphoblastic leukemia: an analysis of factors associated with survival, relapse and graft-versus-host disease. Med Pediatr Oncol 1985 13:165-172.

43. Brochstein JA, Kernan NA, Groshen S, Cirrincione C, Shank B, Emanuel D, Laver J, O'Reilly RJ: Allogeneic bone marrow transplantation after hyperfractionated total body irradiation and cyclophosphamide in children with acute leukemia. N Engl J Med 1987; 317:1618.

44. Pinkel D: Bone marrow transplantation in children. J Pediatr 1993; 122: 331-341.

45. Chessels JM, Rogers DW, Leiper AD, Blacklock H, Plowman PN, Richards S, Levinsky R, Festenstein H: Bone-marrow transplantation has a limited role in prolonging second marrow remission in childhood lymphoblastic leukaemia. Lancet 1986;1(8492):1239-1241.

46. Wheeler K, Richards S, Bailey C, Chessells J. Comparison of bone marrow transplant and chemotherapy for relapsed childhood acute lymphoblastic leukaemia: the MRC UKALL X experience. Medical Research Council Working Party on Childhood Leukaemia. Brit J Haematol 1998; 101:94-103.

47. Greinix HT, Reiter E, Keil F, Fischer G, Lechner K, Dieckmann K, Leitner G, Schulenburg A, Hoecker P, Haas OA, Knoebl P, Mannhalter C, Fonatsch C, Hinterberger W, Kalhs P. Leukemia-free survival and mortality in patients with refractory or relapsed acute leukemia given marrow transplants from sibling and unrelated donors. Bone Marrow Transplant 1998; 21:673-678.

48. Casper J, Camitta B, Truitt R, Baxter-Lowe LA, Bunin N, Lawton C, Murray K, Hunter J, Pietryga D, Garbrecht F. Unrelated bone marrow donor transplants for children with leukemia or myelodysplasia. Blood 1995; 85:2354-2363.

49. Weisdorf DJ: Bone marrow transplantation for acute lymphocytic leukemia (ALL). Leukemia 1997;11(4): S20-S22.

50. Wells RJ, Woods WG, Buckley JD, Odom LF, Benjamin D, Bernstein I, Betcher D, Feig S, Kim T, Ruymann F: Treatment of newly diagnosed children and adolescents with acute myeloid leukemia: a Childrens Cancer Group study. J.Clin.Oncol 1994; 12:2367-2377.

51. Woods WG, Kobrinsky N, Buckley J, Neudorf S, Sanders J, Miller L, Barnard D, Benjamin D, DeSwarte J, Kalousek D, Shina D, Hammond GD, Lange BJ: Intensively timed induction therapy followed by autologous or allogeneic bone marrow transplantation for children with acute myeloid leukemia or myelodysplastic syndrome: a Childrens Cancer Group pilot study. J.Clin.Oncol 1993; 11:1448.

52. Woods WG, Kobrinsky N, Buckley J, Lee JW, Sanders J, Neudorf S, Gold S, Barnard DR, DeSwarte J, Dusenbery K, Kalousek D, Arthur DC, Lange BJ: Timed-sequential induction therapy improves postremission outcome in acute myeloid leukemia: A report from the Children's Cancer Group. Blood 1996; 87:4979-4989.

53. Amadori S, Testi AM, Arico M, Comelli A, Giuliano M, Madon E, Masera G, Rondelli R, Zanesco L, Mandelli F: Prospective comparative study of bone marrow transplantation and postremission chemotherapy for childhood acute myelogenous leukemia. J Clin Oncol. 1993;11:1046-1054.

54. Stevens RF, Hann IM, Wheatley K, Gray RG. Marked improvements in outcome with chemotherapy alone in paediatric acute myeloid leukemia: results of the United Kingdom Medical Research Council's 10th AML trial. MRC Childhood Leukaemia Working Party. British Journal of Haematology 1998; 101:130-140.

55. Clift RA, Buckner CD, Appelbaum FR, Schoch G, Petersen FB, Bensinger WI, Sanders J, Sullivan KM, Storb R, Singer J, Hansen JA, Thomas ED: Allogeneic marrow transplantation during untreated first relapse of acute myeloid leukemia. J Clin Oncol 1992; 10:1723.

56. Chown SR, Marks DI, Cornish JM, Pamphilon DH, Potter MN, Steward CG, Oakhill A. Unrelated donor bone marrow transplantation in children and young adults with acute myeloid leukaemia in remission. British Journal of Haematology 1997; 99:36-40.

57. Woolfrey AE, Gooley TA, Sievers EL, Mulner LA, Andrews RG, Walters M, Hoffmeister P, Hansen JA, Anasetti C, Bryant E, Appelbaum FR, Sanders JE: Bone marrow transplantation for children less than two years of age with acute myelogenous leukemia or myelodysplastic syndrome. Blood, 1998;92:3546-3556.

58. Appelbaum FR, Clift RA, Buckner CD, Stewart P, Storb R, Sullivan KM, Thomas ED: Allogeneic marrow transplantation for acute nonlymphoblastic leukemia after first relapse. Blood 1983; 61:949-953.

59. Gale RP, Horowitz MM, Rees JK, Gray RG, Oken MM, Estey EH, Kim KM, Zhang MJ, Ash RC, Atkinson K, Champlin RE, Dicke KA, Gajewski JL, Goldman JM, Helbig W, Henslee-Downey PS, Hinterberger W,

Jacobsen N, Keating A, Klein JP, Marmont AM, Prentice HG, Reiffers J, Rimm AA, Bortin MM. Chemotherapy versus transplants for acute myelogenous leukemia in second remission. Leukemia 1996; 10:13-19.

60. Beatty PG, Anasetti C, Hansen JA, Longton GM, Sanders JE, Martin PJ, Mickelson EM, Choo SY, Petersdorf EW, Pepe MS: Marrow transplantation from unrelated donors for treatment of hematologic malignancies: effect of mismatching for one HLA locus. Blood 1993; 81:249-253.

61. Ash RC, Casper JT, Chitambar CR, Hansen R, Bunin N, Truitt RL, Lawton C, Murray K, Hunter J, Baxter-Lowe LA: Successful allogeneic transplantation of T-cell-depleted bone marrow from closely HLA-matched unrelated donors. N Engl J Med 1990; 322:485-494.

62. Hasle H, Kerndrup G, Yssing M, Clausen N, Ostergaard E, Jacobsen N, Brock Jacobsen B: Intensive chemotherapy in childhood myelodysplastic syndrome. A comparison with results in acute myeloid leukemia. Leukemia 1996;10:1269-1273.

63. Guinan EC, Tarbell NJ, Tantravahi R, Weinstein HJ: Bone marrow transplantation for children with myelodysplastic syndromes. Blood 1989; 73:619-622.

64. Locatelli F, Niemeyer C, Angelucci E, Bender-Gotze C, Burdach S, Ebell W, Friedrich W, Hasle H, Hermann J, Jacobsen N, Klingebiel T, Kremens B, Mann G, Pession A, Peters C, Schmid HJ, Stary J, Suttorp, Uderzo C, van't Veer-Korthof ET, Vossen J, Zecca M, Zimmermann M. Allogeneic bone marrow transplantation for chronic myelomonocytic leukemia in childhood: a report from the European Working Group on Myelodysplastic Syndrome in Childhood. Journal of Clinical Oncology 1997; 15:566-573.

65. Anderson JE, Appelbaum FR, Fisher LD, Schoch G, Shulman H, Anasetti C, Bensinger WI, Bryant E, Buckner CD, Doney K: Allogeneic bone marrow transplantation for 93 patients with myelodysplastic syndrome. Blood 1993; 82:677-681.

66. Appelbaum FR, Storb R, Ramberg RE, Shulman HM, Buckner CD, Clift RA, Deeg HJ, Fefer A, Sanders J, Stewart P: Allogeneic marrow transplantation in the treatment of preleukemia. Ann Intern Med 1984; 100:689-693.

67. Anderson JE, Anasetti C, Appelbaum FR, Schoch G, Gooley TA, Hansen, JA, Buckner CD, Sanders JE, Sullivan KM, Storb R. Unrelated donor marrow transplantation for myelodysplasia (MDS) and MDS-related acute myeloid leukaemia. British Journal of Haematology 1996; 93:59-67.

68. Frangoul HA, Gooley TA, Sanders JE: Allogeneic bone marrow transplantation (BMT) in children with de novo myelodysplastic syndrome (MDS). (Abstract) Blood (in press) .

69. Davies SM, Wagner JE, Defor T, Blazar BR, Katsanis E, Kersey JH, Orchard PJ, McGlave PB, Weisdorf DJ, Ramsay NK. Unrelated donor bone

marrow transplantation for children and adolescents with aplastic anaemia or myelodysplasia. British Journal of Haematology 1997; 96:749-756.

70. Locatelli F, Giorgiani G, Comoli P. Allogeneic transplantation of haematopoietic progenitors for myelodysplastic syndromes and myeloproliferative disorders. Bone Marrow Transplant 1998; 21 Suppl 2:S17-S20.

71. Castleberry RP, Emanuel PD, Zuckerman KS, Cohn S, Strauss L, Byrd RL, Homans A, Chaffee S, Nitschke R, Gualtieri RJ. A pilot study of isotretinoin in the treatment of juvenile chronic myelogenous leukemia [see comments]. New England Journal of Medicine 1994; 331:1680-1684.

72. Sanders JE, Buckner CD, Thomas ED, Fleischer R, Sullivan KM, Appelbaum FA , Storb R. Allogeneic marrow transplantation for children with juvenile chronic myelogenous leukemia. Blood 1988; 71:1144-1146.

73. Chown SR, Potter MN, Cornish J, Goulden P , Goulden N, Pamphilon D, Steward CG, Oakhill AO. Matched and mismatched unrelated donor bone marrow transplantation for juvenile chronic myeloid leukaemia. Brit J Haematol 1996; 93:674-676.

74. Locatelli F, Pession A, Comoli P, Bonetti F, Giorgiani G, Zecca M, Taibi RM, Mongini ME, Ambroselli F, de SP, Severi F, Paolucci. Role of allogeneic bone marrow transplantation from an HLA-identical sibling or a matched unrelated donor in the treatment of children with juvenile chronic myeloid leukaemia. British Journal of Haematology 1996; 92:49-54.

75. Bunin NJ, Casper JT, Lawton C, Murray K, Camitta BM, Greenwood M, Geil J, Ash RC. Allogeneic marrow transplantation using T cell depletion for patients with juvenile chronic myelogenous leukemia without HLA-identical siblings. Bone Marrow Transplantation 1992; 9:119-122.

76. Donadieu J, Stephan JL, Blanche S, Cavazzana-Calvo M, Baruchel A, Herbelin C, Benkerrou M, Thomas C, Girault D, Fischer A. Treatment of juvenile chronic myelomonocytic leukemia by allogeneic bone marrow transplantation [see comments]. Bone Marrow Transplantation 1994; 13:777-782.

77. Clift RA, Buckner CD, Thomas ED, Bensinger WI, Bowden R, Bryant E, Deeg HJ, Doney KC, Fisher LD, Hansen JA: Marrow transplantation for chronic myeloid leukemia: a randomized study comparing cyclophosphamide and total body irradiation with busulfan and cyclophosphamide. Blood 1994; 84:2036-2043.

78. Italian Cooperative Study Group on Chronic Myeloid Leukaemia. Evaluating survival after allogeneic bone marrow transplant for chronic myeloid leukaemia in chronic phase: a comparison of transplant versus no-transplant in a cohort of 258 patients first seen in Italy between 1984 and 1986. Brit J Haematol 1993; 85:292-299.

79. Italian Cooperative Study Group on Chronic Myeloid Leukemia. Interferon alfa-2a as compared with conventional chemotherapy for the treatment of chronic myeloid leukemia. The. N Engl J Med 1994; 330:820-825.

80. Tura S, Rosti G, Devivo A, Bonifazi F, Fiacchini M, Baccarani M, Russo D, Fanin R, Zuffa E, Montefusco E: Long-term follow-up of the Italian trial of interferon-alpha versus conventional chemotherapy in chronic myeloid leukemia. Blood 1998; 92:1541-1548.

81. Gale RP, Hehlmann R, Zhang MJ, Hasford J , Goldman JM, Heimpel H, Hochhaus A, Klein JP, Kolb HJ, McGlave PB, Passweg JR, Rowlings PA, Sobocinski KA, Horowitz MM. Survival with bone marrow transplantation versus hydroxyurea or interferon for chronic myelogenous leukemia. The German CML Study Group. Blood 1998; 91:1810-1819.

82. Marks DI, Cullis JO, Ward KN, Lacey S, Syzdlo R, Hughes TP, Schwarer, AP, Lutz E , Barrett AJ, Hows JM. Allogeneic bone marrow transplantation for chronic myeloid leukemia using sibling and volunteer unrelated donors. A comparison of complications in the first 2 years. Ann Int Med 1993; 119:207-214.

83. Dini G, Lamparelli T, Rondelli R, Lanino E, Barbanti M, Costa C, Manfredini L, Guidi S, Rosti G, Alessandrino EP, Locatelli F, Marenco, Soligo D, Di BP, Aversa F, La NG, Busca A, Majolino, De LA, Bacigalupo A. Unrelated donor marrow transplantation for chronic myelogenous leukaemia. Brit J Haematol 1998; 102:544-552.

84. Dini G, Rondelli R, Miano M, Vossen J, Gluckman E, Peters C, Bordigoni P, Locatelli F, Miniero R, Ljungman P, Saarinen U, Klingebiel T, Ortega J, Lanino E: Unrelated donor bone marrow transplantation for Philadelphia chromosome-positive chronic myelogenous leukemia in children: experience of eight European Countries. The EBMT Paediatric Diseases Working Party. Bone Marrow Transplant 1996; 18:80-85.

85. Gamis AS, Haake R, McGlave P, Ramsay NK. Unrelated-donor bone marrow transplantation for Philadelphia chromosome-positive chronic myelogenous leukemia in children. Journal of Clinical Oncology 1993; 11:834-838.

86. Lee SJ, Kuntz KM, Horowitz MM, McGlave PB, Goldman JM, Sobocinski KA , Hegland J, Kollman C, Parsons SK, Weinstein MC, Weeks JC, Antin JH. Unrelated donor bone marrow transplantation for chronic myelogenous leukemia: a decision analysis. Annals of Internal Medicine 1997; 127:1080-1088.

87. McGlave P, Bartsch G, Anasetti C, Ash R, Beatty P, Gajewski J, Kernan NA. Unrelated donor marrow transplantation therapy for chronic myelogenous leukemia: initial experience of the National Marrow Donor Program. Blood 1993; 81:543-550.

88. Beelen DW, Graeven U, Elmaagacli AH, Niederle N, Kloke O, Opalka B, Schaefer UW. Prolonged administration of interferon-alpha in patients with

chronic-phase Philadelphia chromosome-positive chronic myelogenous leukemia before allogeneic bone marrow transplantation may adversely affect transplant outcome. Blood 1995; 85:2981-2990.

89. Mackinnon S, Papadopoulos EB, Carabasi MH, Reich L, Collins NH, Boulad F, Castro-Malaspina H, Childs BH, Gillio AP, Kernan NA: Adoptive immunotherapy evaluating escalating doses of donor leukocytes for relapse of chronic myeloid leukemia after bone marrow transplantation: separation of graft-versus-leukemia responses from graft-versus-host disease. Blood 1995; 86:1261-1268.

90. Radich JP, Sanders JE, Buckern CD, Martin PJ, Peterson FB, Bensinger W, McDonald, GB, Mori M, Schoch G, Hansen JA: Second allogeneic marrow transplantation for patients with recurrent leukemia after initial transplant with total-body irradiation containing regimens. J Clin Oncol 1993; 11:304-313.

3

HAPLOIDENTICAL TRANSPLANTATION

P. Jean Henslee-Downey, M.D.

South Carolina Cancer Center University of South Carolina and Palmetto Richland Memorial Hospital Center for Cancer Treatment and Research Columbia, South Carolina, USA

INTRODUCTION

The majority of patients who could benefit from allogeneic stem cell transplantation (allo-SCT) will not have an HLA-matched sibling donor (MSD) to create access to potentially curative therapy. Pioneering efforts by clinical investigators have now made alternative sources of allogeneic stem cells a possibility (1-8). Currently, access to allo-SCT is available through three sources, which include: 1) half-matched family members, 2) adult volunteer unrelated donors, and 3) related or unrelated umbilical cord blood units (CBU). All alternative donors are mismatched with the single exception of a MSD CBU. While there are availability and logistical differences between these alternative donors, a clear preference in choosing an alternative donor for transplantation awaits prospective randomized trials.

In general, HLA genetic disparity is a feature of all alternative donors that is defined by major and minor histocompatibility antigens that evoke immunologic reactions between the donor and recipient. These differences create a barrier to successful transplantation that lead to greater risk of graft failure (1, 2, 9-14), graft-versus-host disease (GvHD) (1-3, 12-14) and/or prolonged disruption of the immune system (15-18). In general, these complications are associated with higher rates of transplant-related mortality, thus worsen the probability of long-term survival (18,14). This chapter will focus on the use of partially mismatched related donors (PMRD) with particular attention to overcoming immunologic responses that cause rejection and GvHD.

HISTOCOMPATIBILITY OF ALTERNATIVE DONORS

Polymorphic cell surface molecules known as human leukocyte antigens (HLA) arise from the major histocompatibility complex (MHC) contained on the short arm of chromosome 6 in man. These HLA specificities govern immunologic responses and determine histocompatibility between an allogeneic donor and recipient. The class I and II antigens, particularly alleles for HLA-A, B, and DR, are considered primary to immune reactions involved in cellular transplantation. The class I antigens are shown to activate CD8[+] cytotoxic T cells responsible for rejection of foreign tissue, while class II antigens activate CD4[+] T lymphocytes, which have either helper or cytotoxic functions (19, 20). Thus, HLA-restricted antigen presentation of immunogenic peptides occurs through the binding of HLA molecules to T-lymphocytes, which initiates cellular reactions that can result in rejection and/or GvHD (21,22). Although the Class I and II major-HLA antigens are considered prominent in evoking these immune responses, a wide range of so-called "minor" histocompatibility antigens that have been identified on other chromosomes are also felt to be operative in stem cell transplantation (23-25).

In man there are two HLA haplotypes, each inherited en bloc from two parents, and designated by numbers to denote specificities for the major HLA. Therefore, in accordance with Mendelian genetics, offspring from the same parents have a 25% chance to inherit the same two of four distinct haplotypes, thereby producing histocompatible siblings. There will be an approximate 75% chance to inherit one haplotype in common (genotype haploidentity) and a 25% chance to inherit no haplotype in common (complete mismatch). Unless genetic information becomes crossed during DNA transcription, all parents will be haploidentical with their children and visa versa. Furthermore, genetic haploidentity can be found in many extended family members. When parents or family members happen to share HLA specificities, additional phenotypic "matching" on the chromosome not inherited in common, or the appearance of homozygosity, will reduce the degree of major HLA mismatch.

Transplants performed between an unrelated donor and recipient involve individuals who share similar appearing major HLA-A, B, and Dr loci as determined by serologic testing. However, the antigens can actually be mismatched, as shown through molecular DNA typing (26,27). Matching between unrelated individuals is usually based only on the three major HLA loci and thus defined as a 6 of 6 or less "match". However, the term "match" can not be considered in the same context as when it is used to describe a matched sibling. When the term "match" is used to define histocompatibility between related individuals it represents identity of one or both 6th chromosomes (i.e., fully matched for the entire MHC complex).

Techniques are not yet developed to measure the vast array of non major-HLA and minor histocompatibility antigens, which are highly apt to be mismatched between unrelated persons. Due to the existence of genetic haploidentity and the possibility of inheriting, MHC non-HLA, and minor histocompatibility antigens in common, family members may be more "compatible" than "matched" unrelated donors who are shown to be phenotypically similar, or even molecularly matched for major-HLA loci. In the absence of genetic sharing, the use of extensive molecular typing for HLA antigens between unrelated donors diminishes post-transplant immunologic complications while decreasing donor availability (28).

The terminology used to describe haploidentical related donors defines both genotypic and phenotypic matching of the major-HLA antigens A, B, and Dr. Thus, a family member who has both genotypic and phenotypic identity is considered matched (6/6, i.e. 0-antigen mismatch). However, usually the unshared haplotype contains a mismatch at one or more of the three major-HLA antigens (5/6, i.e. 1-antigen mismatch; 4/6, i.e. 2-antigen mismatch; or 3/6, i.e. 3-antigen mismatch). Conventionally, the degree of mismatch of a PMRD transplant refers to the number of major-HLA mismatched antigens found in the patient (GvHD direction), rather than the number of mismatches in the donor (rejection direction). It is more instructive to use a bidirectional descriptor and, when this is done, the recipient mismatch is still often given first (i.e. 1/3 PMRD refers to a 1-antigen mismatched recipient and a 3-antigen mismatched donor). Since there are usually many family donors available to a given patient, this enhanced description of haploidentical donors can be helpful in the process of selecting the optimal donor for transplantation.

ACCESS TO ALTERNATIVE DONORS

Comparisons between related and unrelated donor availability are shown in Figure 1. In searching for unrelated donors, "finding a donor" does not always mean that a transplant is available, particularly for non-Caucasian patients. A range in donor availability is a function of whether the HLA haplotypes of the patient are commonly expressed in the donor pool. In contrast, full and immediate access to transplant is available through the use of a 3/6 (half-matched, half-mismatched) haploidentical family member. Almost every individual who can identify biologic family members will have such a donor and thus, immediate access to transplant should exceed 95%. Taking advantage of this universal donor pool is limited in many centers due to a policy to accept only a zero or 1-antigen mismatched haploidentical donor. When that criteria is used, a probabilistic model developed by Kaufman indicates that there may be a 25% chance of finding a 6 of 6 PMRD when extensive family typing is pursued

(29). Of interest, Vowels, and coworkers, reported that extensive family donor searches resulted in identification of a zero or 1-antigen PMRD for 46% of their patients (30). The ability to identify a 2-antigen PMRD probably exceeds 50% when family members beyond the immediate family are typed. As transplant techniques become successful in overcoming major HLA differences making 3-antigen PMRD acceptable, donor availability will no longer limit access to transplant. Furthermore, family members are extremely willing donors and usually available for harvesting when needed by the patient.

Figure 1.

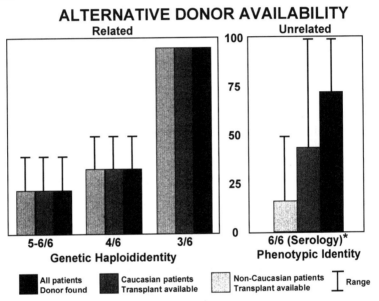

Based on serologic HLA typing, filled hatched bars indicate general probabilities and extension bars indicate potential probabilities for a given patient. * Availability of an unrelated donor is expected to decrease using DNA HLA typing and would potentially increase if mismatch is acceptable.

Access to unrelated alternative donors has been tremendously expanded through the development of volunteer donor registries and cord blood banks (31, 32). The availability of an unrelated donor can vary drastically for individual patients depending upon the size of the donor pool and the distribution frequency of HLA haplotype combinations, as expressed in the patient and the donor pool (33). Unfortunately, many patients who originate from a highly diverse population base, often representing ethnic or racial minorities, are unlikely to find a donor (34). The range for non-Caucasian patients can be broad, the highest success often found in Native Americans and some Orientals, while the worst chance is encountered by African Americans and Hispanics. With the continued growth in the number of donors available through international registries, there has been an increase in the proportion of patients who can identify a potentially acceptable donor. However, even when a donor is identified, delays in confirming the donor and/or arranging for stem cell harvest have generally limited access to less than 40% of patients who seek a donor. Using molecular techniques to improve major-HLA matching between unrelated individuals will, unfortunately, cause a substantial decline in donor availability. On the other hand, the development of unrelated cord blood transplantation, where greater major-HLA mismatch in an unrelated donor might be tolerated, may increase access to transplant.

CHOOSING ALTERNATIVE DONORS

Numerous donors are usually available from within a family and how to select the best donor changes as additional information becomes available. Although in the past, the degree of recipient major-HLA mismatch (GvHD direction) has been considered of utmost importance, more recent data suggests that the donor with less major-HLA mismatch (rejection direction) should be favored. Even more critical, is the absence of HLA antibody production shown to be directed against specific HLA differences found in the donor. This should also include a negative crossmatch screen using patient serum and donor T and B lymphocytes. Other considerations, in order of preference, include: 1) donor CMV seronegative status for a CMV-negative recipient, 2) youngest possible donor age, 3) same sex, 4) avoidance of multiparous female donor, and 5) donor health and psychosocial issues.

An ever-increasing number of patients who identify an unrelated volunteer donor will also have numerous donors from which to select. It is clear that high resolution DNA typing should be employed to select the donor with the highest-resolved identity for major-HLA loci, beginning with molecular matching at the Dr locus (35). The absence of cytotoxic donor T-cell activity has also been associated with a reduction in post transplant complications and mortality (36). Again, T and B cell crossmatch studies should be performed and positive donors avoided. When the information is available on remaining donors, consideration should be given to CMV status, age, sex, and health of the donor. When selecting a cord blood unit, information for consideration may include sterility, HLA and RBC typing, infectious disease testing, and cell dose. The later is the only parameter for which there is clinical data to support the selection process, with a current recommendation that the nucleated cell dose should be above > 37 million per kg recipient weight (11).

CLINICAL TRANSPLANTATION USING ALTERNATIVE DONORS

Engraftment

Allogeneic stem cell engraftment is a result of the competitive interaction between what remains of host and donor immune capabilities following host conditioning therapy and graft manipulation (37).   When using alternative donors, particularly 3-antigen mismatched PMRD; establishing stable engraftment is challenged by the heightened immune response brought on by the presence of mismatched major and/or minor histocompatibility antigens.   In general, higher graft failure rates, often influenced by transplant techniques, occur in alternative donor recipients (9,13,14, 38-42).   Both host and donor immunoablation, achieved through pre-transplant conditioning therapy and graft engineering, modifies the immune response and often influences either rejection or successful establishment of a functional hematopoietic chimera.

The most lethal early post-transplant complication using alternative donors is graft failure (39).   Evidence of host-mediated rejection is the most worrisome cause for graft failure as it may be difficult to achieve secondary engraftment consistent with long-term survival.   A higher rejection rate is seen in PMRD recipients who are conditioned with a non-TBI regimen (43).   Approaches to the management of rejection include the use of secondary conditioning therapy, administration of high-dose hematopoietic growth factors, and stem cell grafts from the primary or a secondary donor (44-47).   Unfortunately, death often occurs due to infection secondary to prolonged aplasia, multi-organ failure partially related to secondary cytotoxic therapy, and severe acute GvHD, particularly, if larger numbers of alloreactive lymphocytes are given in the secondary graft.   When persistent malignant disease is a feature of graft failure, death from the underlying disease usually occurs.   On the other hand, graft failure related to infection or toxins can be overcome using therapeutic measures, including discontinuation of myelosuppressive drugs, effective anti-viral   therapy,   intravenous   immunoglobulin   therapy,   high   dose immunosuppressive therapy, and the use of hematopoietic growth factors.

To improve engraftment, many investigators have increased host conditioning therapy, particularly when graft manipulation using T-cell depletion (TCD) is used to prevent graft-versus-host disease (GvHD) (48-56).   While a higher dose of total body irradiation (TBI) and/or combination high-dose chemotherapy and immunosuppression have resulted in improved engraftment in both animal and human studies, an increase in organ toxicity and infection rates has also been observed (4, 42, 57-58).   It is often difficult to assess the correlation between the conditioning therapy and post-transplant mortality in PMRD recipients since most patients are inherently at higher risk for toxicity and infection due to advanced or refractory disease. Despite the combined use of high-dose TBI, chemotherapy and immunosuppression, Henslee-Downey, and coworkers, observed a 7% risk of early (<60 days post-BMT) regimen-related mortality, which occurred exclusively in high-risk patients (41).

Total body irradiation as a primary component of the conditioning regimen has been used more often for PMRD transplants compared to a MSD (14). The total dose of TBI and the method of delivery have been associated with the success of achieving a full donor chimera, particularly following TCD (9, 41, 59-63). Additional total-nodal irradiation has also been shown to improve engraftment (64-66). Adding other myeloablative drugs to the conditioning regimen, e.g. thiotepa, dimethyl myleran, fludarabine and busulfan, or immunosuppressants, e.g. anti-T-cell antibodies or antithymocyte globulin, has also been helpful in improving engraftment of TCD marrow grafts (41, 48-58, 65-76). Although non-TBI busulfan-containing regimens have been associated with higher graft failure rates, consistent engraftment has now been demonstrated using the combination of busulfan, thiotepa, cyclophosphamide and methylprednisolone prior to a partially TCD PMRD transplant (77-79).

There is a well recognized inverse relationship between the potency of TCD and the success of engraftment, particularly, using an HLA-mismatched graft (80). A highly effective technique combining agglutination with soybean lectin and E-rosetting produces successful engraftment in immunodeficient patients who inherently offer less graft resistance; however, graft failure can increase up to 50% in patients with hematologic malignancies or metabolic disorders (37, 81-84). Higher rates of engraftment have been associated with less rigorous methods of TCD; however, this can be accompanied by increased rates of acute GvHD (40, 85).

Based on experience in murine models, Reisner, and co-workers, have explored the use of large doses of stem cells (coined as "mega-dose"), in conjunction with TCD, in an effort to improve engraftment across HLA-barriers (86, 87). In an early publication, prompt engraftment using 3-antigen PMRD appeared to follow the combination of lectin-agglutinated and E-rosetted marrow combined with G-CSF stimulated peripheral blood stem cells (PBSC) (53). However, the time to engraftment was not quicker than that previously reported by Henslee-Downey, and co-workers, who combined moderate TCD of the graft with post-transplant immunosuppression (52). Subsequent follow-up data indicated that late graft failures could occur following "mega-dose" PMRD stem cell transplants (42, 57). More recently these investigators have obtained better results by reducing the toxicity of the conditioning therapy and further enriching the primitive stem cell content of the graft by tandem infusions of e-rosette depleted, CD34+ selected G-CSF mobilized leukopheresis PBSC collections (58). With this approach only 2 patients developed rejection for a 95% sustained engraftment rate and acute GvHD was not observed. However, infection and lymphoproliferative disease was a cause of death in 30% of the patients suggesting that the immunoablative condition regimen combined with extensive T-cell depletion may significantly hamper immune recovery.

In a multi-center PMRD trial using CD34$^+$ selection, despite extraordinarily high stem cell doses, rejection and severe acute GvHD were observed (88, 89). Haploidentical bone marrow, instead of peripheral blood, was enriched for CD34$^+$ cells using immunomagnetic positive selection, and was shown to result in successful engraftment in a patient who rejected an unrelated graft (90). The use of unmodified but G-CSF mobilized peripheral blood from haploidentical donors produced slower engraftment and a higher rate of GvHD compared to matched donors. However, the mismatched recipients experienced a lower rate of relapse and thus, achieved a similar rate of leukemia free survival (91).

Full haplotype mismatch in a PMRD donor and/or a positive antibody crossmatch in any alternative donor remain the most difficult deterrents to successful engraftment. Despite 3-loci major-HLA disparity, investigators at the University of South Carolina have shown rapid engraftment in a large series of 210 haploidentical recipients, as shown in Figure 2 (55, 56). In this analysis, 99% of patients given antithymocyte globulin as a part of condition therapy achieved stable engraftment with a median time to a white count of 1000/mm^3 for 3 consecutive days occurring on day 16 following SCT. Engraftment was not effected by the degree of donor HLA mismatch nor the nucleated cell dose. These results suggest that it is possible to obtain engraftment rates that are comparable to a MSD, even when using a 3-antigen mismatched PMRD, although, clearly more intensive immunoablation is required. These same investigators have also succeeded in achieving engraftment in PMRD recipients who are crossmatch positive with the donor by utilizing pre-transplant Prosorba column absorption combined with pre and post-transplant plasmapheresis (92).

Figure 2. Engraftment following Haploidentical Transplant

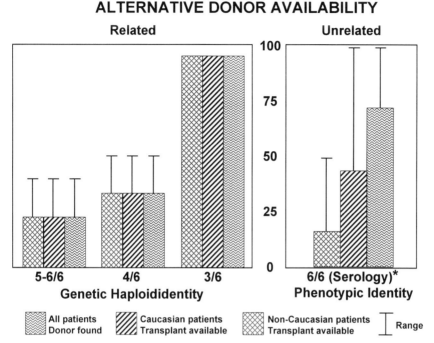

Estimate of engraftment in 110 patients who received additional pre-transplant conditioning using antithymocyte globulin and OKT3 TCD haploidentical donor grafts: a.) median time to engraftment measured at a WBC > 1000/mm^3 for 3 consecutive days , b.) probability of engraftment following a graft from a donor who was 0 – 1 antigen, 2 antigen or 3 antigen mismatched, c.) probability of engraftment in patients receiving a nucleated cell dose above or below the median per kg recipient weight, d.) probability of engraftment in patients receiving a CD34+ cell dose above or below the median per kg recipient weight.

Investigators and patients should be aware of the observation made by Bishop, and coworkers, who showed an increased risk of graft failure following PMRD SCT in patients with chronic myelogenous leukemia, particularly, in those with advanced disease (93). Reports from Lamb, and coworkers, also identified the diagnosis of CML as being associated with graft failure following PMRD SCT (94, 95). In their early studies, three antigen major-HLA mismatch in the donor was associated with graft rejection but graft characteristics, including nucleated cell, T lymphocyte, and CFU-GM doses were not. Immunophenotype analysis of peripheral blood from patient's experiencing graft rejection revealed a predominance of $CD3^+CD8^+$ cytotoxic cells, which paralleled the findings seen in graft failure using unrelated donors (96). Although there is, in general, an increased risk of graft failure associated with unrelated donors, less resistance to engraftment is evidenced by a greater ability to use non-TBI conditioning therapy.

ACUTE GRAFT VERSUS HOST DISEASE

The use of alternative donors is often discouraged, or even avoided, due to an expected high risk of developing acute GvHD. Moderate or severe GvHD has been reported in over 70% and 50% of patients, respectively, and thus it is considered another major impediment to successful transplantation (1-4, 12, 13,14, 40, 97-102). Many investigators explored TCD in an effort to control GvHD and, in fact, this was largely successful and, when highly efficient TCD was used, the incidence of acute GvHD could be reduced to ~ 10%; however, as previously discussed, this can be at the expense of successful engraftment (103, 104). In pooled analysis of alternative donor transplantation, TCD is the only factor that appears to decrease the probability of moderate to severe acute GvHD (3, 13, 99). However, there has been a reluctance to use TCD because of the results in MSD transplant that showed an inferior disease-free survival, primarily due to higher relapse rates that was thought to be due to an interference with a graft-versus-leukemia (GVL) effect (105). This remains controversial in T-depleted PMRD SCT where relapse appears to more closely correlate with disease risk rather than graft preparation (6-8, 11, 40, 41, 55-57, 106-110).

The risk of developing acute GvHD has been clearly shown to be associated with the dose of alloreactive T-lymphocytes (111-113). Nonetheless, to balance engraftment and GvHD, there has been a tendency to use less rigorous methods of TCD and add post-transplant immunosuppression (51, 52, 40, 41, 48, 50, 55, 56, 71, 72, 74, 75, 78, 79, 80, 85, 93,107, 110, 114-19). Henslee-Downey, and co-workers, used T-cell lytic, monoclonal antibody products, ex vivo and in vivo, given in sequence, to achieve engraftment in over 90% of haploidentical recipients while significantly reducing the risk of grade II-IV acute GvHD to < 40% and grade III-IV to <20% (40). In a separate analysis of patients with acute lymphoblastic leukemia, these investigators showed that recipients of PMRD SCT, when compared to non-TCD MSD, experienced comparable rates of engraftment (91% vs 94%, respectively) and grade 0-II and III-IV acute GvHD (71% vs 73% and 29% vs 27%, respectively) (119). There were no differences seen in relapse, survival, or disease-free survival rates in comparison between

MSD and PMRD recipients, nor did HLA mismatch effect outcome in the later group.

Henslee-Downey, and co-workers, examined a series of patients who were given PMRD marrow grafts prepared in a similar fashion using the anti-heterodimer monoclonal antibody, T10B9, for ex vivo TCD. However, post transplant immunosuppression was changed to use FDA-approved lymphocyte-specific anti-sera (Atgam®), which was combined with low-dose steroid and cyclosporin therapy (41,120). This approach was highly successful in reducing the risk of acute GvHD to 16% with only 8% of patients developing grade III-IV disease. In multivariate analysis, the only prognostic factor associated with an increase in acute GvHD was a higher T-cell dose, while the degree of major-HLA mismatch had no effect. Other investigators have used T10B9 for ex vivo TCD of unrelated donor grafts and reduced the risk of grade II-IV acute GvHD to between 33 and 46 percent (107,114,115). In subsequent trials where approximately 80% of patients were 2 or 3-antigen mismatched, a FDA-approved anti-CD3 monoclonal antibody, Orthoclone (OKT®3), has been used instead of T10B9 for TCD, and the incidence of acute GvHD remained low (55, 56, 110). Taken together with the observation of no GvHD reported by Aversa and co-workers (58), the current results indicate that techniques are available to effectively control acute GvHD following haploidentical PMRD SCT. However, further studies are needed to determine the safest approach for controlling GvHD while preserving effective GVL reactivity and promoting prompt immune reconstitution.

Molecular HLA typing decreases acute GvHD following unrelated HSCT (28, 121) but this correlation is observed in PMRD SCT by prophylactic techniques (40, 41, 51-57, 122). Younger recipient age does not appear to protect children from acute GvHD following alternative donor SCT (101, 102). In adult patients, older age of either recipient or donor and advanced disease stage appears to increase the risk of GvHD (102). Also similar to MSD SCT, severe regimen-related toxicity and infection are thought to play a role in GvHD development.

When acute GvHD occurs following alternative donor transplant it is more difficult to manage and more often becomes refractory to therapy and is often associated with fatal complications (13, 14, 123). Effective management appears to require prompt institution of lympholytic, as well as broad-spectrum immunosuppressive therapy, which can be difficult to discontinue (124). In an attempt to ablate and avoid clonal proliferation of alloreactive T-cells, high-dose methylprednisolone therapy is given at a dose of 500 mg/m^2 recipient weight every 12 hours for two doses and repeated in 48 to 72 hours if symptoms persist. Such prompt intervention can abrogate the evolution of acute GvHD and may be integral to the long-term successful control of GvHD.

TRANSPLANT RELATED COMPLICATIONS AND SURVIVAL

In recipients of alternative donor SCT, major challenges beyond engraftment and acute graft versus host disease, can reduce survival, including: 1.) overwhelming infection, particularly opportunistic infection, 2.) major organ dysfunction or failure, 3.) chronic GvHD, 4.) delayed immune reconstitution, 5.) relapse in high-risk patients, and 6.) secondary malignancy, particularly lymphoproliferative disorder (4, 8, 13, 15, 16, 57, 125-132). These problems, in large part, are related to 1.) the condition of the patient and status of the underlying disease at time of transplant; 2.) the immunologic barriers created by HLA disparity; 3.) the intensity of conditioning and immunosuppressive therapy given to the patient; and 4.) the slow and, sometimes incomplete, process of immune reconstitution. In addition to meticulous medical management and broad-spectrum preventative therapy, methods are now being explored to develop post-transplant cellular therapy to enhance immune recovery and promote GvL effects (133-139).

In single center analysis, it is clear that, for all donor types and for all endpoints including survival, results are best in patients who are transplanted earlier in their disease course, while in good medical condition (8,11, 41, 56-8, 75, 99-102,108-110, 114-, 115, 117, 119, 121, 122, 140). Survival is particularly difficult to examine following haploidentical transplant since patients are almost exclusively referred due to high-risk disease characteristics even when in remission. That considered, estimates of 2-year survival have ranged from 25 to 53% in patients transplanted in remission and 15 to 23% in patients transplanted in relapse (3, 13, 14, 40, 41, 58, 75, 88, 119). From trials initiated over a decade ago, patients surviving today with Karnosky scores of 90 to 100% are the ultimate demonstration of the feasibility of haploidentical transplantation (40-42, 52).

SUMMARY AND CONCLUSIONS

When allogeneic transplant is indicated and a MSD is not available, most centers first seek an unrelated donor. However, one must avoid undue delays when a donor is not available and family members should be typed to identify the preferred donor amongst the family. Since a family donor can provide access to transplant for almost every patient, a greater effort should be encouraged to improve and expand haploidentical transplantation. The advantages, outlined in Table 1, suggest compelling reason to perfect the use of haploidentical related donors.

Table 1. Advantages Using Haploidentical Related Donors

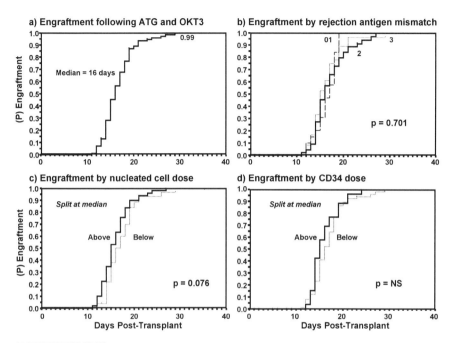

a) Engraftment following ATG and OKT3
b) Engraftment by rejection antigen mismatch
c) Engraftment by nucleated cell dose
d) Engraftment by CD34 dose

REFERENCES

1. O'Reilly RJ, Dupont B, Pahwa S, et al. Reconstitution in severe combined immunodeficiency by transplantation of marrow from an unrelated donor. N Engl J Med 1977;297:1311-1318.
2.   Hansen JA, Clift RA, Thomas ED, et al. Transplantation of marrow from an unrelated donor to a patient with acute leukemia. N Engl J Med 1980; 303:565-567.
3. Beatty PG, Clift RA, Mickelson EM, et al. Marrow transplantation from related donors other than HLA-identical siblings.   N Engl J Med 1985;313:765-771.
4. Kernan NA, Bartsch G, Ash RC, et al. Analysis of 462 transplantations from unrelated donors facilitated by the National Donor Program. N Engl J Med 1993;328:593-602.

5. Henslee PJ, Byers VS, Jennings E, et al. A new approach to the prevention of graft-versus-host disease using XomaZyme-H65 following histo-incompatible partially T-depleted marrow grafts. Transplantation Proceedings 1989;21:3004-3007.
6. Wagner JE, Rosenthal J, Sweetman R, et al. Successful transplantation of HLA-matched and HLA-mismatched umbilical cord blood from unrelated donors: analysis of engraftment and acute graft-versus-host disease. Blood 1996;88(3):795-802.
7. Kurtzberg J, Laughlin M, Graham M, et al. Placental Blood as a source of hematopoietic stem cells for transplantation into unrelated recipients. N Engl J Med 1996; 335:157-66.
8. Gluckman E, Vanderson R, Boyer-Chammard A, et al. Outcome of cord-blood transplantation from related and unrelated donors. N Engl J Med 1997;337:373-381.
9. Anasetti C, Amos D, Beatty PG, et al.. Effect of HLA compatibility on engraftment of bone marrow transplants in patients with leukemia or lymphoma. N Engl J Med 1989;320:197-204.
10. Davies SM, Ramsay NKC, Haake RJ, et al.. Comparison of engraftment in recipients of matched sibling or unrelated donor marrow allografts. Bone Marrow Transplant 1994;13:51-57.
11. Gluckman E, Rocha V, Boyer-Chammard A, et al. Outcome of cord-blood transplantation from related and unrelated donors. N Engl J Med 1997;337:373-381.
12. Hows J, Bradley BA, Gore S, et al. on behalf of the International Marrow Unrelated Search and Transplant (IMUST) Study. Prospective evaluation of unrelated donor bone marrow transplantation. Bone Marrow Transplant 1993;12:371-380.
13. Ash RC, Horowitz MM, Gale RP, et al.. Bone marrow transplantation from related donors other than HLA-identical siblings: effect of T-cell depletion. Bone Marrow Transplant 1991;7:443-452.
14. Szydlo R, Goldman JM, Klein JP, et al.. Results of allogeneic bone marrow transplants for leukemia using donors other than HLA-identical siblings. J Clin Oncol 1997; 15:1767-1777.
15. Sullivan KM, Mori M, Sanders J, et al.. Late complications of allogeneic and autologous marrow transplantation. Bone Marrow Transplant 1992;10(Suppl 1):127-134.
16. Ochs L, Shu XO, Miller J, et al.. Late infections after allogeneic bone marrow transplantation: comparison of incidence in related and unrelated donor transplant recipients. Blood 1995;10:3979-3986.

17. Kook H, Goldman F, Padley D, et al.. Reconstruction of the immune system after unrelated or partially matched T-cell-depleted bone marrow transplantation in children: immunophenotypic analysis and factors affecting the speed of recovery. Blood 1996;88:1089-1097.

18. Lamb LS, Henslee-Downey PJ, Hazlett L, et al. Phenotypic and functional reconstitution of peripheral blood lymphocytes following T-cell depleted bone marrow transplantation from partially mismatched related donors. Bone Marrow Transplant 1998; 21(5):461-471.

19. Zinkernagel RM, Doherty PC. MHC-restricted cytotoxic T cells: studies on the biological role of polymorphic major transplantation antigens determining T cell restriction specificity, function, and responsiveness. Adv Immunol 1979;27:151-177.

20. Benacerraf B, McDevitt HO. Histocompatibility-linked immune response genes. Science 1972;175:273-79.

21. Bach FH, Sachs DH. Transplantation immunology. N Engl J Med 1987;317:489-492.

22. van Rood JJ. The impact of the HLA system in clinical hematology. Blut 1989;59:214-220.

23. Martin PJ. Increased disparity for minor histocompatibility antigens as a potential cause of increased GVHD risk in marrow transplantation from unrelated donors compared with related donors. Bone Marrow Transplant 1991;8:217-223.

24. Theobald M. Allorecognition and graft-versus-host disease. Bone Marrow Transplant 1995;15:489-498.

25. Goulmy E, Schipper R, Pool J, et al.. Mismatches of minor histocompatibility antigens between HLA-identical donors and recipients and the development of graft-versus-host disease after bone marrow transplantation. N Engl J Med 1996;334(5):281-285.

26. Keever CA, Leong N, Cunningham I, et al.. HLA-B44-directed cytotoxic T cells associated with acute graft-versus-host disease following unrelated bone marrow transplantation. Bone Marrow Transplant 1994;14:137-145.

27. Baxter-Lowe LA. Molecular techniques for typing unrelated donors: potential impact of molecular typing disparity on donor selection. Bone Marrow Transplant 1995;14(Suppl 4):542-550.

28. Sasazuki T, Juji T, Morishima Y, et al. Effect of matching of Class I HLA alleles on clinical outcome after transplantation of hematopoietic stem cells from an unrelated donor. N Engl J Med 1998;339:1177-1185.

29. Kaufman R. A generalized HLA prediction model for related donor matches. Bone Marrow Transpl 1996;17:1013-1020.

30. Vowels M, Honeyman M, Ziegler J, White L, Doran T, Lane J, Lam-Po-Tang R. Searches for matched and closely matched marrow donors undertaken in a paediatric unit. Transplant Proc 1990;22:2171.

31. Stroncek D, Bartsch G, Perkins HA, et al.. The National Marrow Donor Program. Transfusion 1993;33:567-77.
32. Rubinstein P, Rosenfield RE, Adamson JW, Stevens CE. Stored placental blood for unrelated bone marrow reconstitution. Blood 1993;81:1679-1690.
33. Sonnenberg FA, Eckman MH, Pauker SG. Bone marrow donor registries: the relation between registry size and probability of finding complete and partial matches. Blood 1989;74:2569-2578.
34. Beatty PG, Mori M, Milford E. Impact of racial genetic polymorphism on the probability of finding an HLA-matched donor. Transplantation 1995;60(8):778-783.
35. Petersdorf EW, Longton GM, Anasetti C, et al.. The significance of HLA-DRB1 matching on clinical outcome after HLA-A, B, DR identical unrelated donor marrow transplantation. Blood 1995;88:1606-1613.
36. Speiser DE, Loliger CC, Siren MK, Jeannet M. Pretransplant cytotoxic donor T-cell activity specific to patient HLA class I antigens correlating with mortality after unrelated BMT. Br J Haematol 1996;93:935-939.
37. Martin PJ. The role of donor lymphoid cells in allogeneic marrow engraftment. Bone Marrow Transplant 1990;6:283-289.
38. Kernan NA, Flomenberg N, Dupont B, O'Reilly RJ. Graft rejection in recipients of T-cell-depleted HLA-nonidentical marrow transplants for leukemia: identification of host-derived antidonor allocytotoxic T lymphocytes. Transplantation 1987;43(6):842-847.
39. O'Reilly RJ, Collins NH, Kernan NA, et al.. Transplantation of marrow depleted T cells by soybean lectin agglutination and E-rosette depletion: major histocompatibility complex-related graft resistance in leukemic transplant patients. Transplant Proc 1985;17:455-459.
40. Henslee-Downey PJ, Parrish RS, Macdonald JS, et al.. Combined in vitro and in vivo T-lymphocyte depletion for the control of graft-versus-host disease following haplo-identical marrow transplant. Transplantation 1996;61(5):738-745.
41. Henslee-Downey PJ, Abhyankar SH, Parrish RS, et al.. Use of partially mismatched related donors extend access to allogeneic marrow transplant. Blood 1997; 89(10):3864-3672.
42. O'Reilly R, Hanson JA, Kurtzberg J, et al. Allogeneic marrow transplants: approaches for the patient lacking a donor. Hematology 1996, Eds: Schechter GP and McArthur JR, The American Society of Hematology, Seattle: 1996, 132-146.
43. Polchi P, Lucarelli G, Galimberti M, et al.. Haploidentical bone marrow transplantation from mother to child with advanced leukemia. Bone Marrow Transplant 1995; 16:529-535.
44. Nemunaitis J. Overview of the role of hematopoietic growth factors in bone marrow transplant recovery and bone marrow transplant failure. Support Care Cancer 1994; 2(6):374-376.

45. Molina L, Chabannon C, Viret F, et al.. Granulocyte colony-stimulating factor-mobilized allogeneic peripheral blood stem cells for rescue graft failure after allogeneic bone marrow transplantation in two patients with acute myeloblastic leukemia in first complete remission. Blood 1995; 85:1678-1679.

46. Godder KT, Abhyankar SH, Lamb LS, et al.. Donor leukocyte infusion for treatment of graft rejection post partially mismatched related donor bone marrow transplant. Bone Marrow Transplant 1998; 22:111-113.

47. Zecca M, Perotti C, Marradi P, et al.. Recombinant human G-CSF-mobilized peripheral blood stem cells for second allogeneic transplant after bone marrow graft rejection in children. Br J Haematol 1996; 92:432-434.

48. Trigg M, Gingrich R, Goeken N, et al.. Low rejection rate when using unrelated or haploidentical donors for children with leukemia undergoing marrow transplantation. Bone Marrow Transplant 1989;4(4):431-437.

49. Champlin RE, Ho WG, Mitsuyasu R, et al.. Graft failure and leukemia relaspe following T lymphocyte-depleted bone marrow transplants: effect of intensification of immunosuppressive conditioning. Transplant Proc 1987;19(1):2616-2619.

50. Sondel PM, Bozdech MJ, Trigg ME, et al.. Additional immunosuppression allows engraftment following HLA-mismatched T cell-depleted bone marrow transplantation for leukemia. Transplant Proc 1985;17:460-461.

51. Henslee PJ, Byers VS, Jennings CD, et al.. A new approach to the prevention of graft-versus-host disease using Xomazyme-H65 following histo-incompatible partially T-depleted marrow grafts. Transplant Proc 1989;21:3004-3007.

52. Henslee-Downey PJ, Romond E, Harder E, et al.. Successful engraftment and control of graft-versus-host disease following 3-antigen mismatched haploidentical marrow transplant. Blood 1991;78(Suppl 10):231a.

53. Aversa F, Tabilio A, Terenzi A, et al.. Successful engraftment of T-cell-depleted haploidentical "three loci" incompatible transplants in leukemia patients by addition of recombinant human granulocyte colony-stimulating factor-mobilized peripheral blood progenitor cells to bone marrow inoculum. Blood 1994;84(11):3948-3955.

54. Oakhill A, Pamphilon DH, Potter MN, et al.. Unrelated donor bone marrow transplantation for children with relapsed acute lymphoblastic leukeaemia in second remission. Br J Haematol 1996; 94:574-578.

55. Lee C, Brouillette M, Hazlett L, et al.. Comparison of engraftment and acute GvHD following transplantation or partially mismatched grafts T cell depleted with OKT3 or T10B9 monoclonal antibody. J Hematother 1997; 6(4):395.

56. Henslee-Downey PJ, Lee CG, Hazlett LJ, et al. Rare failure to engraft following haploidentical T-cell depleted marrow transplantation using enhanced host immunoablation and OKT3 graft purging. Experimental Hematol 1997; 25(8):183a.

57. Aversa F, Martelli MM, Reisner Y. Use of stem cells from mismatched related donors. Curr Opin Hematol 1997;4(6):419-422.

58. Aversa F, Tabilio A, Velardi A, et al. Treatment of high-risk acute leukemia with T-cell-depleted stem cells from related donors with one fully mismatched HLA haplotype. N Engl J Med 1998;339:1186-1193.

59. Martin PJ, Hansen JA, Torok-Storb B, et al.. Graft failure in patients receiving T cell-depleted HLA-identical allogeneic marrow transplants. Bone Marrow Transplant 1988;3:445-456.

60. Smith CV, Suzuki T, Guzzetta PC, et al.. Bone marrow transplantation in miniature swine: IV. Development of myeloablative regimens that allow engraftment across major histocompatibility barriers. Transplantation 1993;56(3):541-549.

61. Patterson J, Prentice HG, Brenner MK, et al.. Graft rejection following HLA matched T-lymphocyte depleted bone marrow transplantation. Br. J Haematol 1986;63:221-230.

62. Guyotat D, Dutou L, Erhsam A, et al.. Graft rejection after T cell-depleted marrow transplantation. Role of fractionated irradiation. Br J Haematol 1987;65:499-507.

63. van Os R, Konings AW. Compromising effect of low dose-rate total body irradiation of allogeneic bone marrow engraftment. Int J Radiat Biol 1993;64(6):761-770.

64. Slavin S, Naparstek E, Aker M, et al.. The use of total lymphoid irradiation for prevention of rejection of T-lymphocyte depleted bone marrow allografts in non-malignant hematologic disorders. Transplant Proc 1989;21:3053-3054.

65. James ND, Apperley JF, Kam KC, et al.. Total lymphoid irradiation preceding bone marrow transplantation for chronic myeloid leukaemia. Clin Radiology 1989;40:195-198.

66. Soiffer RJ, Mauch P, Tarbell NJ, et al.. Total lymphoid irradiation to prevent graft rejection in recipients of HLA non-identical T-cell-depleted allogeneic marrow. Bone Marrow Transplant 1991;7(1):23-33.

67. Terenzi A, Lubin I, Lapidot T, et al.. Enhancement of T cell-depleted bone marrow allografts in mice by thiotepa. Transplantation 1990;20:717-720.

68. Mackinnon S, Barnett L, Bourhis JH, et al.. Myeloid and lymphoid chimerism after T-cell-depleted bone marrow transplantation: evaluation of conditioning regimens using the polymerase chain reaction to amplify human minisatellite regions of genomic DNA. Blood 1992;80(12):3235-3241.

69. Lapidot T, Terenzi A, Singer TS, et al.. Enhancement by dimethyl myleran of donor type chimerism in murine recipients of bone marrow allografts. Blood 1989;73(7):2025-2032.

70. Cahn JY, Herve P, Flesch M, et al.. Marrow transplantation from HLA non-identical family donors for the treatment of leukaemia: a pilot study of 15 patients using additional immunosuppression and T-cell depletion. Br J Haematol 1988;69:345-349.

71. Fischer A, Blanche S, Veber F, et al.. Prevention of graft failure by an anti-HLFA-1 monoclonal antibody in HLA-mismatched bone marrow transplantation. Lancet 1986; 2(8515):1058-1061.

72. Hale G, Waldmann H. Control of graft-versus-host disease and graft rejection by T cell depletion of donor and recipient with Campath-1 antibodies: results of matched sibling transplants for malignant diseases. Bone Marrow Transplant 1994;13(5):597-611.

73. Kernan NA, Emanuel D, Castro-Malaspina H, et al.. Posttransplant immunosuppression with antithymocyte globulin and methylprednisolone prevents immunologically mediated graft failure following a T-cell depleted marrow transplant. Blood 1989;74(Suppl1):123a.

74. Malilay G P, Sevenich EA, Condie RM, Filipovich AH. Prevention of graft rejection in allogeneic bone marrow transplantation: I. Preclinical studies with antithymocyte globulins. Bone Marrow Transplant 1989;4:107-112.

75. Lee C, Henslee-Downey PJ, Brouillette M, et al.. Comparison of OKT3 and T10B9 for ex vivo T-cell depletion of partially mismatched related donor bone marrow transplants. Blood 1995;86(10Suppl1):625a.

76. Terenzi A, Aristei C, Chionne F, et al.. Preliminary results of fludarabine as an immunosuppressor in bone marrow transplantation conditioning. Bone Marrow Transplant 1996;17(1):abstr 89.

77. Schultz KR, Ratanatharathorn V, Abella E, et al.. Graft failure in children receiving HLA-mismatched marrow transplants with busulfan-containing regimens. Bone Marrow Transplant 1994;13:817-822.

78. Godder K, Pati AR, Abhyankar S, et al.. Partially mismatched related donor transplants as salvage therapy for patients with refractory leukemia who relapse post-BMT. Bone Marrow Transplant 1996;17:49-53.

79. McGuirk J, Godder K, Pati AR, et al.. Salvage of relapsed acute myelogenous leukemia post-transplant using a partially mismatched related donor for second bone marrow transplant. Blood 1996;88(10 Suppl 1): 269a.

80. Sondel PM, Hank JA, Trigg ME, et al.. Transplantation of HLA-haploidentical T cell-depleted marrow for leukemia: autologous marrow recovery with specific immune sensitization to donor antigens. Exp Hematol 1986;14:278-286.

81. Reisner Y, Kapoor N, Kirkpatrick D, et al.. Transplantation for severe combined immunodeficiency with HLA-A, B, D, DR incompatible parental marrow cells fractionated by soybean agglutinin and sheep red cells. Blood 1983;61:341-348.

82. Reisner Y, Kapoor N, Kirkpatrick D, et al.. Transplantation for acute leukaemia with HLA-A and B nonidentical parental marow cells fractionated with soybean agglutinin and sheep red blood cells. Lancet 1981; 2(8242): 327-331.

83. Matthay KK, Wara DW, Ammann AJ, et al.. Mismatched bone marrow transplantation using soybean agglutinin processed T-cell depleted marrow. In Progress in Bone Marrow Transplantation, Eds: Gale RP, Champlin RE; Alan R Liss, Inc., New York:1987, 343-351.

84. Peters C, Balthazor M, Shapiro E, et al.. Outcome of unrelated donor bone marrow transplantation in 40 children with Hurler syndrome. Blood 1996;87:4894-4902.

85. Prentice HG, Blacklock HA, Janossy G, et al.. Use of anti-T cell monoclonal antibody OKT3 to prevent acute graft-versus-host disease in allogeneic bone-marrow transplantation for acute leukemia. Lancet 1982; 1(8274):700-703.

86. Reisner Y, Martelli MF. Bone marrow transplantation across HLA barriers by increasing the number of transplanted cells. Immunology Today 1995;16(9):437-440.

87. Reisner Y, Rachamim N, Bachar-Lustig E, et al.. Human CD34 stem cells exhibit potent veto activity in vitro: relevance to 'mega dose' stem cell transplants in mismatched leukemia patients. Blood 1996;88(10Suppl1):298a.

88. Yaeger AM, Anasetti C, Chauncey T, et al.. Transplantation of positively selected CD34+ bone marrow and mobilized peripheral blood cells from haploidentical related donors for high-risk hematologic malignancies. Blood 1996;88(10Suppl2):281b.

89. Mogul MJ, Forte KJ, Holland HK, et al.. Steroid-refractory cutaneous graft-versus-host disease after transplantation of haploidentical parental CD34+ cells in children with Down's Syndrome and recurrent acute leukemia. J Ped Hem/Onc 1997; 19(1):142-144.

90 Fujimori Y, Kanamaru A, Hashimoto N, et al.. Second transplantation with CD34+ bone marrow cells selected from a two-loci HLA-mismatched sibling for a patient with chronic myeloid leukemia. Brit J Haematol 1996; 94:123-125.

91. Russell JA, Desai S, Herbut B, et al.. Partially mismatched blood cell transplants for high-risk hematologic malignancy. Bone Marrow Transplant 1997; 19:861-866.

92. Abhyankar SH, Geier SS, Parrish R, et al.. Effect of crossmatch reactions and HLA typed cell panel antibody response on engraftment using plasmapheresis and Prosorba column absorption during partially mismatched related donor BMT. Blood 1995;86(10 Suppl 1):564a.

93. Bishop MR, Henslee-Downey PJ, Anderson JR, et al.. Long-term survival in advanced chronic myelogenous leukemia following bone marrow transplantation from haploidentical related donors. Bone Marrow Transplant 1996;18:747-753.

94. Lamb LS, Szafer F, Henslee-Downey PJ, et al.. Characterization of acute bone marrow graft rejection in T cell-depleted, partially mismatched related donor bone marrow transplantation. Exp Hematol 1995;23:1595-1600.

95. Lamb L, Gee A, Parrish R, et al.. Acute rejection of marrow grafts in patients transplanted from a partially mismatched related donor: clinical and immunologic characteristics. Bone Marrow Transplant 1996;17:1021-1027.

96. Donohue J, Homge M, Kernan NA. Characterization of cells emerging at the time of graft failure after bone marrow transplantation from an unrelated marrow donor. Blood 1993;82(3):1023-1029.

97. Beatty PG, Hansen JA, Longton GM, et al.. Marrow transplantation from HLA-matched unrelated donors for treatment of hematologic maligancies. Transplantation 1991;51:443-447.

98. Gajewski JL, Ho WG, Feig SA, et al.. Bone marrow transplantation using unrelated donors for patients with advanced leukemia or bone marrow failure. Transplantation 1990;50: 244-249.

99. McGlave P, Bartsch G, Anasetti C, et al.. Unrelated donor marrow transplantation therapy for chronic myelogenous leukemia: initial experience of the National Marrow Donor Program. Blood 1993;81:543-550.

100. Balduzzi A, Gooley T, Anasetti C, et al.. Unrelated donor marrow transplantation in children. Blood 1995;86:3247-3256.

101. Davies SM, Wagner JE, Shu X-O, et al.. Unrelated donor bone marrow transplantation for children with acute leukemia. J Clin Oncol 1997;15:557-565.

102. McGlave P. Unrelated donor transplant therapy for chronic myelogenous leukemia. Hem/Onc Clin of N Amer 1998;12(1):93-105.

103. O'Reilly RJ, Kernan N, Cunningham I, et al.. Soybean lectin agglutination and E-rosette depletion for removal of T-cells from HLA-identical and non-identical grafts administered for the treatment of leukemia. In T-Cell Depletion in Allogeneic Bone Marrow Transplantation, Eds: Martelli MF, Grignani F, Reisner Y; Ares-Serono Symposia, Rome Italy:1988,123-129.

104. Martin PJ, Kernan NA. T-cell depletion for the prevention of graft-vs.-host disease. In Graft-vs.Host Disease: Immunology, Pathophysiology, and Treatment, Eds: Burkoff SJ, Deeg HJ, Ferrara J, Atkinson K; Marcel Dekker, New York, NY: 1990, 371-387.

105. Horowitz MM, Gale RP, Sondel PM, et al.. Graft-versus-leukemia reactions after bone marrow transplantation. Blood 1990;75: 555-562.

106. Marmont AM, Horowitz MM, Gale RP, et al.. T-cell depletion of HLA-identical transplants in leukemia. Blood 1991; 78(8):2120-2130.

107. Drobyski WR, Ash RC, Casper JT, et al.. Effect of T-cell depletion as graft-versus-host disease prophylaxis on engraftment, relapse, and disease-free survival in unrelated marrow transplantation for chronic myelogenous leukemia. Blood 1994;83(7):1980-1987.

108. Hessner MJ, Endean DJ, Casper JT, et al.. Use of unrelated marrow grafts compensates for reduced graft-versus-leukemia reactivity after T-cell-depleted allogeneic marrow transplantation for chronic myelogenous leukemia. Blood 1995;86(10):3987-3996.

109. Speiser DE, Hermans J, van Biezen A, et al.. Haploidentical family member transplants for patients with chronic myeloid leukaemia: a report of the Chronic Leukaemia Working Party of the European Group for Blood and Marrow Transplantation (EBMT). Bone Marrow Transplant 1997; 19:1197-1203.

110. Lee C, Henslee-Downey PJ, Christiansen N, et al.: Consistent prompt engraftment and low risk of acute graft-versus-host disease following haploidentical transplant. J Hematotherapy, 1998;7(3):274.

111. Lowenberg B, Wagemaker E, van Beckkum DW, et al.. Graft-versus-host disease following transplantation of "one log" versus "two log" T-lymphocyte depleted bone marrow from HLA-identical donors. Bone Marrow Transplant 1986;1:133-140.

112. Kernan NA, Collins NH, Juliano L, et al.. Clonable T lymphocytes in T cell-depleted bone marrow transplants correlate with development of graft-versus-host disease. Blood 1986;68:770-773.

113. Atkinson K, Farrelly H, Cooley M, et al.. Human marrow T cell dose correlates with severity of subsequent acute graft-versus-host disease. Bone Marrow Transplant 1987;2:51-57.

114. Ash RC, Casper JT, Chitambar CR, et al.. Successful allogeneic transplantation of T-cell depleted bone marrow from closely HLA-matched unrelated donors. N Engl J Med 1990;322:485-494.

115. Casper J, Camitta B, Truitt R, et al.. Unrelated bone marrow donor transplants for children with leukemia or myelodysplasia. Blood 1995;85(9):2354-2363.

116. Cullis JO, Szydlo RM, Cross NC, et al.. Matched unrelated donor bone marrow transplantation for chronic myeloid leukemia in chronic phase: comparison of ex vivo and in vivo T-cell depletion. Bone Marrow Transplant 1993;11(Suppl1):107-111.

117. Henslee-Downey PJ, Gee AP, Godder K, et al.. Minimal risk of graft versus host disease following haploidentical but partially mismatched related donor bone marrow transplantation. Exp Hematol 1994;22:716a.

118. Bunin NJ, Casper JT, Lawton C, et al.. Allogeneic marrow transplantation using T cell depletion for patients with juvenile chronic myelogeneous leukemia without HLA-identical siblings. Bone Marrow Transplant 1992;9:119-122.

119. Fleming DR, Henslee-Downey PJ, Romond EH, et al.. Allogeneic bone marrow transplantation with T cell-depleted partially matched related donors for advanced acute lymphoblastic leukemia in children and adults: a comparative matched cohort study. Bone Marrow Transplant 1996;17:917-922.

120. Lee C, Brouillete M, Lamb L, et al.. Use of a closed system for V ab-positive T-cell depletion of marrow for use in partially mismatched related donor transplantation. In Progress in Clinical and Biological Research, Eds, Gee A, Gross S, Worthington-White D; Wiley Liss, New York, NY:1994,523-532.

121. Nademanee A, Schmidt GM, Parker P, et al.. The outcome of matched unrelated donor bone marrow transplantation in patients with hematologic malignancies using molecular typing for donor selection and graft-versus-host disease prophylaxis regimen of cyclosporin, methotrexate, and prednisone. Blood 1995;86:1228-1234.

122. Soiffer RJ, Mauch P, Fairclough D, et al.. CD6+ T cell depleted allogeneic bone marrow transplantation from genotypically HLA non-identical related donors. Biol Bld and Mar Transplant 1997; 3:11-17.

123. Roy J, McGlave PB, Filipovich AH, et al.. Acute graft-versus-host disease following unrelated donor marrow transplantation: failure of conventional therapy. Bone Marrow Transplant 1992;10:77-82.

124. Hings IM, Severson R, Filipovich AH, et al.. Treatment of moderate and severe acute GvHD after allogeneic bone marrow transplantation. Transplantation 1994;58:437-442.

125. Busca A, Anasetti C, Anderson G, et al.. Unrelated donor or autologous marrow transplantation for treatment of acute leukemia. Blood 1994;83(10):3077-3084.

126. Marks DI, Cullis JO, Ward KN, et al.. Allogeneic bone marrow transplantation for chronic myeloid leukemia using sibling and volunteer unrelated donors: a comparison of complications in the first 2 years. Ann Intern Med 1993;119:207-214.

127. Enright H, Davies S, McGlave P. Bone marrow transplantation for chronic myelogenous leukemia: clinical outcomes. Clin Transpl 1994;283-293.

128. Gerritsen EJ, Stam ED, Hermans J, et al.. Risk factors for developing EBV-related B cell lymphoproliferative disorders (BLPD) after non-HLA-identical BMT in children. Bone Marrow Transplant 1996;18:377-382.

129. Bhatia S, Ramsay NK, Steinbuch M, et al.. Malignant neoplasms following bone marrow transplantation. Blood 1996;87(9):3633-3639.

130. Godder K, Pati AR, Abhyankar SH, et al.. De novo chronic graft-versus-host disease presenting as hemolytic anemia following partially mismatched related donor bone marrow transplant. Bone Marrow Transplant 1997; 19:813-817.

131. Schultz KR, Green GJ, Wensley D, et al.. Obstructive lung disease in children after allogeneic bone marrow transplantation. Blood 1994;84 (9):3212-3220.

132. Atkinson K, Farewell V, Storb R, et al.. Analysis of late infections after human bone marrow transplantation: role of genotypic nonidentity between marrow donor and recipient and of nonspecific suppressor cells in patients with chronic graft-versus-host disease. Blood 1982;60(3):714-720.

133. Riddell SR, Watanabe K, Goodrich J, et al. Restoration of viral immunity in immunodeficient humans by the adoptive transfer of T cell clones. Science 1992;257:238-241.

134. Walter E, Greenberg P, Gilbert M, et al.. Reconstitution of cellular immunity against cytomegalovirus in recipients of allogeneic bone marrow by transfer of T-cell clones from the donor. N Engl J Med 1995;16:1038-1044.

135. Rooney CM, Smith CA, Ng CYC, et al.. Use of gene-modified virus-specific T lymphocytes to control Epstein-Barr-virus-related lymphoproliferation. Lancet 1995;345:9-13.

135. Heslop HE, Ng CY, Li C, et al.. Long-term restoration of immunity against Epstein-Barr virus infection by adoptive transfer of gene-modified virus-specific T lymphocytes. Nat Med 1996;5:551-555.

136. Kline RM, Stiehm ER, and Cowan MJ. Bone marrow 'boosts' following T cell-depleted haploidentical bone marrow transplantation. Bone Marrow Transplant 1996; !7(4):543-548.

137. Sullivan KM, Kopecky Jocom J, Fisher L, et al.. Immunomodulatory and antimicrobial efficacy of intravenous immunoglobulin in bone marrow transplantation. N Engl J Med 1990;323:705-712.

138. Slavin S, Naparstek E, Nagler A, et al.. Allogeneic cell therapy for relapsed leukemia after bone marrow transplantation with donor peripheral blood lymphocytes. Exp Hematol 1995;23(14):1553-1562.

139. van Rhee F, Lin F, Cullis JO, et al.. Relapse of chronic myeloid leukemia after allogeneic bone marrow transplant: the case for giving donor leukocyte transfusions before the onset of hematologic relapse. Blood 1994;11:3377-3383.
140. Pati AR, Godder K, Parrish R, et al.. Pre-emptive therapy with donor leukocyte infusions to prevent relapse following partially mismatched related donor bone marrow transplantation. Blood 1996;88(10Suppl1):259a.
141. Hansen JA, Gooley TA, Martin PJ, et al.. Bone marrow transplants from unrelated donors for patients with chronic myeloid leukemia. N Engl J Med 1998; 338:962-968.

4

UMBILICAL CORD BLOOD HEMATOPOIETIC STEM CELL TRANSPLANTATION

Gluckman E, Rocha V, Chastang CL, on behalf of Eurocord-Cord blood
transplant group
Hôpital Saint Louis,1 Ave Claude Vellefaux, 75475 Paris Cedex 10. France

INTRODUCTION

The principal limitations of allogeneic bone marrow transplantation are the lack of suitable HLA-matched donors and the complications of graft versus host disease associated with HLA disparities. In the absence of a suitable HLA identical sibling donor, alternative donors such as mismatched related or matched unrelated donors are searched. In these transplants, major and minor histocompatibility differences are often unrecognized by current matching tests, explaining the relatively high frequency of graft failure, graft versus host disease and delayed immune reconstitution. New more sensitive techniques of typing by molecular biology has decreased the probability of finding a fully matched donor for class I and class II HLA antigens (1-5). Despite a bone marrow donor registry which contains more than 4 million bone marrow donors worldwide, some patients cannot be transplanted because of the lack of an HLA identical donor.

Cord blood has many theoretical advantages due to the relative immaturity of newborn cells compared to adult cells. Hematopoietic progenitors from cord blood are enriched in the most primitive stem cells (6, 7) which are able to produce in vivo long-term repopulating stem cells. Compared to adults cells, cord blood hematopoietic stem cells grow larger colonies in presence of growth factors, have different growth factor requirements, are able to expand upon long term culture in vitro, to engraft SCID-Human mice in the absence of additional human growth factors and have longer telomeres than adult cells (8-10). The properties of cord blood cells should compensate the relatively low number of cells contained in a single cord blood.

The second advantage of cord blood is the relative immaturity of the immune system at birth (11). Cord blood lymphocytes are enriched in double negative CD3+ cells, have a naive phenotype, produce less cytokines, express mRNA transcripts for INFγ, IL-4and IL-10 but very little IL-2, have a fully constituted polyclonal T cell repertoire (12) and could be protected from apoptosis due to low levels of CD95. NK function is reduced. Most of these functions are inducible through in vitro or in vivo activation, as a consequence, early NK and T cell cytotoxicity is impaired but secondary activation can occur. Therefore, we can speculate that despite reduced graft versus host disease (GVHD), graft versus leukemia (GVL) should be maintained (13-15). Acute graft versus host disease is an early event after allogeneic BMT; and it is in part triggered by cytokines release. It is reasonable to postulate that cord blood transplant induces less frequent and less severe acute GVHD than adult hematopoietic stem cell transplants which contain a higher number of activated T cells. These properties should lead to less stringent criteria for HLA donor recipient selection.

The main practical advantages of using cord blood as an alternative source of stem cells are the relative ease of procurement, the absence of risks to donors, the reduced risk of transmitting infection and the prompt availability of cryopreserved samples. These advantages were first recognized in cord blood transplant using related donors, secondarily, large unrelated cord blood banks established criteria for standardization of cord blood collection, banking, processing and cryopreservation (16,17). More than 15,000 units of frozen cord blood are currently available and this number is increasing rapidly worldwide. Netcord is a non profit organization for establishing criteria of qualification and accreditation of cord blood banks.

Since the first cord blood transplant performed in 1988, cord blood is increasingly used as a new source of hematopoietic stem cells and more than 700 transplants have been reported worldwide. In order to analyze factors associated with outcome of cord blood transplants, Eurocord-Cord Blood Transplant Group collected data on 300 cord blood transfusion (CBT) coming from more than 80 centers worldwide.

Analysis of the clinical results has shown that related cord blood gives better results than unrelated CBT. Factors associated with better survival in related and unrelated CBT were younger age, and diagnosis with better results in inborn errors and children with acute leukemia in 1st or 2nd remission. Higher number of nucleated cells in the transplant and recipient negative CMV serology were also favorable risk factors for survival.

RESULTS OF RELATED CORD BLOOD TRANSPLANT

The first CBT was performed in 1988 in a patient with Fanconi anemia (18). This patient had a healthy HLA identical sibling whose cord blood was collected at birth, cryopreserved and used after thawing for transplantation. This patient had a prompt engraftment after receiving low dose cyclophosphamide and lymphoid irradiation. He had no GVH and is now currently healthy with a complete hematologic and immunologic donor reconstitution for more than 10 years after the CBT.

Eurocord has analyzed the outcome of 102 patients transplanted with a related cord blood between October 1988 and January 1998 in 19 countries and 44 transplant centers (19,20). The median follow-up time was 30 months (0,1-111). The median age was 5 years (0.2-20), median weight 19 Kg (5-50). Sixty one patients had a malignant disease: 43 acute leukemia (AL), 25 were in 1st or 2nd complete remission(CR) and 18 were in $>2^{nd}$ CR or resistant relapse (7 chronic myeloid leukemia (CML), 7 myelodysplastic syndrome, 2 neuroblastoma and 2 NHL). Forty one patients had a non-malignant disease: 19 patients had a bone marrow failure syndrome (BMFS), 15 had hemoglobinopathies (3 sickle cell anemia(SCA), 12 thalassemia and 7 had inborn errors. The donor was an HLA identical sibling in 80 cases and an HLA mismatched donor in 22 cases. Five patients had 1 HLA difference, 6 patients 2 HLA differences , 10 patients 3 HLA differences and 1 patient 4 HLA differences. The median number of nucleated cells (NC) infused/kg was $4.0x10^7$ (0.7-18). Median days for neutrophil engraftment was 28 days (8-49) and 48 days (14-180) for platelet engraftment. Eighteen patients did not engraft and 10 died before day 60.

One-year overall survival was 64%. HLA identical transplants had a 1-year survival of 73% while, it was 50% for patients transplanted with a HLA mismatched CB (p=0.006). According to the initial diagnosis 1-year survival was 55% in patients with malignancies, 67% in patients with BMFS, 100% in patients with hemoglobinopathies and 71% in patients with Inborn Errors. Other factors affecting favorable survival were: age (<6y), weight (<20 kg), negative cytomegalovirus (CMV) serology in the recipient, sex match and number of cells infused ($\geq 3.7\ 10^7$/kg). There was a correlation between the number of cells infused and engraftment. The incidence of grade II-IV GVHD was 24%, 7 patients had acute GVHD grade III-IV and chronic GVHD was observed in 3/43. HLA differences were the major prognostic factor for acute GVHD. HLA identical CBT had an incidence of acute GVHD of 9% compared to 50% in mismatched CBT (p=0.001).

RESULTS OF UNRELATED CORD BLOOD TRANSPLANTATION

As of April 1998, 158 unrelated cord blood transplants were reported to Eurocord Registry by 39 transplant centers from 15 countries (19,21). There were 112 children and 46 adults. One hundred two children given an unrelated CBT from July 1994 to January 1998 were analyzed. The median age was 5 years (range 0.2-14), median weight 19 kg (range 5-46) and median follow-up time 12 months (range 0.3-42). 72 patients had a diagnosis of malignancy including 40 ALL, 20 AML (41 in CR1 or CR2 and 19 in more advanced stage of the disease), 5 patients had MDS, 5 juvenile CML and 2 NHL. 12 patients had a bone marrow failure syndrome and 18 patients had an inborn error. Cord blood was provided by a European cord blood bank in 59 cases and by the New-York cord blood bank in 43 cases. The median number of NC infused was $4x10^7$/kg. 14 patients received an HLA matched CBT 64 a 1 HLA, 23 had 2 HLA differences and 1 had 3 HLA differences CBT. The overall 1 year survival was 37%. Factors associated with improved survival were CMV negative status before CBT (p=0.02) and ABO match (p=0.01). Age, weight, number of cells infused, HLA and sex differences were not significantly associated with survival. Neutrophil engraftment was observed in 74% of the cases. The incidence of acute GVHD grade II-IV was 38%. There was no correlation between GVHD and the number of HLA mismatches. In patients with malignancies, the overall survival was 35%. In bone marrow failure syndromes, only 10% of patients survived and in inborn errors survival was 70% (Figure 1).

In 42 adults with malignancies, the overall survival was 17%. Most of the patients received less than $3x10^7$/kg nucleated cells, the donor was HLA identical in 6 cases, with 1 HLA difference in 17 cases, 2 HLA differences in 14 cases and 3 HLA differences in 5 cases. The number of cells infused and disease status before transplant were the main prognostic factors but the small number of patients and the heterogeneity of the diagnosis precludes any statement on the indications and methods of CBT in adults. Of note the use of steroids was a good prognostic factor while the use of Methotrexate was associated with poorer survival.

Figure 1. Kaplan Meier estimate of one year survival for children given an unrelated cord blood transplant according to diagnosis.

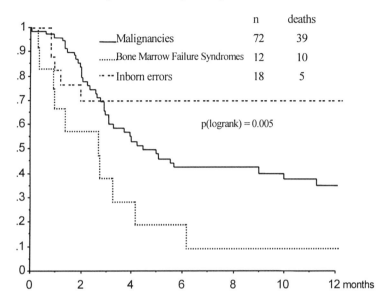

These results show that unrelated cord blood transplants give good results in children mainly if they are transplanted for acute leukemia in remission, inborn errors and immune deficiencies. Results must improve in patients with bone marrow failure syndrome and in adults patients. HLA disparity is not a limiting factor but the number of cells infused is important. Currently the use of less than 1×10^7 Aurleatal cells/kg is not recommended. Several questions remain including the criteria for choosing a donor, the indications in children and in adults, the comparison of cord blood transplants to other sources of hematopoietic stem cells and the role of growth factors and expansion for improving the speed of engraftment.

INDICATIONS AND RESULTS OF CORD BLOOD TRANSPLANTATION ACCORDING TO INITIAL DIAGNOSIS

Results varied according to diagnosis, therefore, we analyzed some subgroups of patients in order to better delineate the indications of cord blood transplant.

Cord blood transplantation in children with acute leukemia

We have analyzed factors associated with outcome in 102 children with acute leukemia reported to the Eurocord Registry in order to investigate the role of

CBT in this patients population (22). Seventy patients with acute lymphoblastic and 32 with acute myeloid leukemia were given either a related (n=42) or an unrelated (n=60) CBT. Children given CBT during 1st or 2nd complete remission were considered as belonging to the good risk group (n=66), whereas patients transplanted in more advanced stage of the disease were assigned to the poor risk group (n=36). In the related group (RCBT), 12 out of 42 patients received an HLA mismatched CBT whereas in the unrelated group (UCBT) 54 out of 60 received an HLA mismatched CBT. Kaplan-Meier estimates for neutrophil recovery at day 60 was $84\pm7\%$ in RCBT and $79\pm6\%$ in UCBT (p=0.16). In a multivariate analysis, the most important factor influencing neutrophil engraftment in UCBT was a nucleated cell dose greater than 3.7×10^7/Kg (p=0.05). The incidence of grade II-IV GVHD was $41\pm8\%$ in the RCBT group and $37\pm6\%$ in the UCBT group (Figure 2). Kaplan-Meier estimates of 2-year event-free-survival (EFS) after related or unrelated CBT were $39\pm8\%$ and $30\pm7\%$, respectively (p=0.19). In a multivariate analysis, the most important factor influencing EFS was disease status at time of transplantation. Good-risk patients had a 2-year EFS of $49\pm$ 7% as compared to $8\pm5\%$ in patients with more advanced disease (p=0.0003). This was a consequence of both an increased one-year transplant related mortality and a higher 2-year relapse rate in the poor risk group ($65\pm9\%$ and 77 ± 14 % respectively) as compared to good risk patients ($34\pm6\%$ and 31 ± 9 % respectively).

Fig 2 Kaplan Meier estimate of acute GVHD in children given a related and unrelated cord blood transplant for acute leukemia

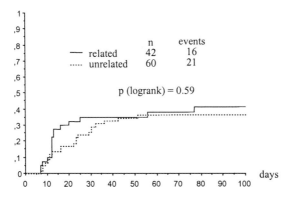

These data confirm that allogeneic CBT from either a related or an unrelated donor is feasible and cures a significant proportion of children with acute leukemia with standard risk factors.

Unrelated umbilical cord blood transplants in adults with hematologic malignancies.
Cord blood cells have been used as a source of hematopoietic stem cells in the unrelated transplant setting, mainly in pediatric patients, while in adults the number of cases is smaller because of concern on engraftment. We have analyzed 42 patients with malignancies transplanted from December 1994 to February 1998 reported to Eurocord Registry. Median age was 26 years (15-50), median weight was 56 kg (35-90) and median follow-up time was 14 months (2-40). Sixteen patients had acute leukemia (AL), 21 chronic myeloid leukemia (CML), 2 non-Hodgkin Lymphoma (NHL) and 3 myelodysplastic syndrome (MDS). Fourteen patients were transplanted with good risk factors (first and second complete remission acute leukemia (n=8) and first chronic phase CML (n=6)). Twenty eight patients had advanced disease at transplant. Seven patients were previously given an autologous bone marrow transplant. GVHD prophylaxis consisted CsA alone (n=3) or associated with prednisone (n=32) and in 7 cases associated with methotrexate. Conditioning regimen varied according to the disease and the center. Twenty nine patients received total body irradiation and 37 received anti-thymocyte globulin as part of the preparatory regimen. Cord blood units came from European banks (n=15) or New-York cord blood bank (n=27). Two patients received an HLA identical unit and 40 an HLA mismatched unit with 1 HLA difference (8 cases), 2 HLA differences (21 cases), 3 HLA differences (10 cases), and 4 HLA differences in 1 case. The median number of nucleated cells infused was 1.7 10^7/kg (0.2-6).

Twelve patients had early deaths between day 14-48 and were censored for engraftment, 7 did not engraft. The median time for neutrophil recovery ($\geq$ 500/mm^3) was 35 days (13-57) and 176 days (30-180) for platelets engraftment ($\geq$20.000/mm^3). Neutrophil recovery at day 60 was 76$\pm$ 12%. Acute GVHD ($\geq$ grade II) was observed in 18 patients (grade II=5, grade III =3 and grade IV= 10). Grade III-IV was not influenced by the number of HLA disparities (p=0.58). Chronic GVHD was observed in 3 out of 12 patients at risk. One year-survival was 17$\pm$6%. Favorable factors for survival were cell dose ($\geq$1x10^7/kg) (p=0.0001) and good risk status at transplant (p= 0.02). All the 6 patients receiving less than 1x10^7/kg died. One year survival was 36$\pm$13% in good risk patients as compared to 7$\pm$5% in poor risk patients. Transplant-related mortality (TRM) at 100 days was also influenced by disease status (p=0.03) and cell dose (p=0.0001). A factor influencing adversely TRM was the absence of prednisone in GVHD prophylaxis (p=0.01). Thirty five patients died from relapse in 1 case, GVHD in 8 cases, interstitial pneumonitis in 5 cases, non engraftment in 8 cases, infection in 9 cases, CNS hemorrhage in 2 cases and, cardiac toxicity in 2 cases.

These results suggest that unrelated cord blood is an optional source of stem cells in adults patients with malignancies. However, the choice of units containing large number of cells or expanded cells and good disease status at transplants might improve results.

Cord blood transplants in hemoglobinopathies
Hemoglobinopathies are a very attractive indication for targeting populations for familial cord blood collection because families are well known and prenatal diagnosis is often performed. In addition, BMT from an HLA matched sibling offers 80-90% chance of success if performed early in life. We report the experience of Eurocord concerning 7 patients affected by thalassemia and 3 with sickle cell anemia (SCA) transplanted with CB from an HLA identical sibling (23). All 7 thalassemics were class I-II according to the Pesaro score; age was between 1-8 years, median NC infused was 3.3×10^7/kg (range 1.2-6.1). Conditioning regimens included BU (14-16 mg/kg) and CY(100-200 mg/kg); in 4 patients, thiotepa (6mg/kg) was added. GVHD prophylaxis consisted of CsA alone (n=5) or with MTX (n=2). Six patients received G-CSF at different times after transplant. Three patients with SCA were conditioned with BU 16mg/kg and CY 200 mg/kg. NC dose infused was 3.5×10^7/Kg, 3.5×10^7/Kg and 6.0×10^7/Kg respectively. CsA alone (n=2) and CsA with MTX (n=1) was administered for GVHD prophylaxis. G-CSF was added in 2 patients, GM-CSF in 1. All patients are currently alive and 5 patients are transfusion independent 3-38 months from CB transplant. Four are alive with thalassemia, one patient with SCA who did not engraft, is alive, transfusion independent, 1 year after a BMT from the same donor. Engraftment was observed in 6 out of 10 patients. One with thalassemia rejected 12 months later. Acute GVHD grade II was observed in only 1 case.

In class I-II thalassemia patients transplanted with BM from HLA matched siblings, the risk of rejection is low (5%); in SCA this risk is higher (12-18%). By contrast in the present experience concerning CBT in hemoglobinopathies only 5 out of 10 patients showed sustained engraftment. In patients with thalassemia, high marrow cell dose is considered of major importance to sustained engraftment. We can speculate that the reduced number of cells transplantable with a CB compared to BM might be crucial in these patients in association with the conditioning regimen. The small number of patients is obviously inadequate for drawing conclusion about CBT in hemoglobinopathies. At the present time, we can suggest that CBT be reserved for younger patients in order to increase the dose of cells infused. At the moment the use of CB from unrelated donors cannot be encouraged outside of a pilot study and in selected patients.

Cord blood transplantation in bone marrow failure syndromes
Between October 1988 and January 1998, 33 patients received a CBT for bone marrow failure syndrome. The median follow-up time was 27 months (1-112). Nineteen patients received a CBT from a related donor and 14 patients from an unrelated donor. In the related group, 13 patients had constitutional BMFS (9 Fanconi Anemia (FA), 2 Blackfan Diamond anemia (BDA), 1 Dyskeratosis Congenita (DC), 1 Amegakariocytic thrombocytopenia (AT)) and 6 acquired severe aplastic anemia) (SAA)). The median age was 7 years (3-12) and median weight 20 kg (13-45). The donor was HLA identical in 16 cases and HLA mismatched in 3 cases. GVHD prophylaxis consisted CsA alone (n=11) or associated with Mtx (n=6) or prednisone (n=2). Preparatory regimen consisted Cyclophosphamide alone (CY) (n=13) or with Busulfan (BU) (n=4) Thiotepa (n=1) or fludarabine (n=1). Irradiation containing regimen was administered to 10 patients (8 TLI and 2 TBI). Anti-T polyclonal or monoclonal antibody was added in 6 cases. Median number of nucleated cells infused was $4.0 \times 10^7/kg$ (0.9-11). In the unrelated group (n=14), 10 patients had constitutional BMFS (8 FA, 1 DC, 1 Kostmann's disease and 4 acquired SAA). The median age was 9 years (1-23) and median weight 33kg (8-68). The donor was HLA identical in 3 cases, and mismatched in 11 cases with 1 HLA disparity in 6 cases and 2 HLA disparities in 5 cases. GVHD prophylaxis consisted of CsA alone (n=5), with Mtx (n=2) or prednisone (n=7). Preparatory regimen consisted of CY alone (n=10) or associated with BU (n=2). Irradiation was administered in 9 patients (5 TLI and 4 TBI). Anti T polyclonal or monoclonal antibody was added in 13 cases. Median number of NC infused was $3.0 \times 10^7/kg$ (1-7).

In related CBT, the median time to neutrophil engraftment was 35 days (13-39) and to platelet recovery 45 days (14-138). Three patients did not engraft and 3 had early death. Neutrophil and platelet engraftment at day 60 were 81% and 72% respectively. Favorable factors influencing neutrophil recovery were age <7 years (p= 0.04), weight <24kg (p=0.01) and recipient negative CMV serology (p=0.02). Acute GVHD was observed in 3 patients and chronic GVHD in 2 patients. One year survival was 67 ±11%. Favorable factors affecting survival were age <7 years (p= 0.009), weight <24kg (p=0.003) and a negative CMV serology (p=0.04).

In the unrelated group, neutrophil recovery at day 60 was 36%. Acute GVHD was observed in 3 patients. One patient only is currently alive. Three patients died of non engraftment, 2 of liver veno-occlusive disease, 3 of acute respiratory distress syndrome, 4 of infection and 1 of hemolytic uremic syndrome.

It is interesting to see that despite the heterogeneity of the diagnosis, this group of patients which is at high risk of rejection because of transfusion immunization had a good engraftment of HLA identical cord blood cells despite the low number of cells infused. In mismatched related or unrelated CBT, survival was poor because of the poor status of the patients before transplant and the increased risk of rejection.

Cord blood transplantation in children with inborn errors
Fourteen children with inborn errors were transplanted between January 1994 and December 1996. The median age at transplantation was 1.7 years (0.2-11). Seven were transplanted with a related cord blood for Hurler's syndrome (n=3), leukocyte adhesion deficiency (n=1), Gunther's disease (n=1), bare lymphocyte syndrome (n=1) and severe combined immunodeficiency (n=1). In the group of seven patients receiving an unrelated cord blood, two patients had osteopetrosis, one inherited neuronal ceroid lipofuscinosis (INCL), one had familial erythrophagocytic lymphohistiocytosis (FEL), one adrenoleukodystrophy, one Langerhan's-cell histiocytosis (LCH), and one patient had severe combined immunodeficiency (SCID). The donor was an HLA identical sibling in 6 cases; a mismatched related donor in 1 case, an identical unrelated donor in 1 case and a mismatched unrelated donor in 6 cases (1 HLA difference in 5 cases and 2 HLA differences in 1 case). The conditioning regimen varied according to diagnosis and centers; it was Cy and Busulfan in 6 patients or associated with thiotepa (n=2), or VP16 (n=2). Two patients had Busulfan associated with Melphalan and 1 patient Cy alone. One patient with severe combined immunodeficiency was transplanted without conditioning. GVHD prophylaxis consisted of Mtx alone (n=1) or CsA alone (n=2) or associated with prednisone (n=6) or Mtx (n=4). In 1 patient with SCID, GVHD prophylaxis was not administered. The median number of nucleated cells infused was 7.25×10^7/kg (1.9-18). The overall survival at one year for all patients was 63%. It was 69% in related CBT and 57% in unrelated CBT. Two patients with Hurler's disease receiving a related CBT died of conditioning toxicity and fungal infection. In the unrelated group, 3 patients with FEL, osteopetrosis and LCH died of CMV disease, VOD, and relapse, respectively. Among 7 patients transplanted with a related cord blood, 1 patient with Hurler's syndrome had autologous reconstitution. In 7 unrelated CBT, 2 patients died early and one patient with INCL had graft failure 3 months after CBT. The Kaplan-Meyer estimate of neutrophil engraftment at day 60 was 83% and 62% for related and unrelated CBT respectively. Only 2 patients receiving an unrelated CBT with one HLA difference developed acute GVHD grade II and III. In 7 patients at risk, chronic GVHD was not observed

OTHER RESULTS

J. Kurtzberg et al reported a series of 25 patients who received an unrelated cord blood transplant provided by the New-York cord blood bank (24). All, except one, were children, 23 had a malignancy, 12 were in first or second complete remission, 7 were in relapse or in advanced stage of the disease, 2 had leukemia complicating Fanconi anemia and Kostmann's syndrome, 1 neuroblastoma and 1 common variable immunodeficiency disease-myelodysplastic syndrome. There were various degrees of HLA incompatibilities. The number of nucleated cells infused correlated with the rate of myeloid engraftment (p=0.002). GVHD was observed but it was mild. Twenty-two of these patients engrafted with a median time to reach >500/μl ANC of 22 days. However, all patients received G-CSF to accelerate engraftment. Twelve of the 25 patients had an event free survival rate of 48%. Seven of the 19 patients undergoing transplantation for malignant conditions survived, 6 of 12 patients transplanted in first or second CR survived but most had a short follow-up of less than one year. Only 1 of 8 patients who underwent CBT while in remission and survived for more than 100 days had a leukemic relapse.

J.Wagner et al (25) reported 18 patients who received an unrelated CBT from the New York cord blood bank. Most were children, 13 had a malignant disease, 5 patients only were in 1st or 2nd remission, the other had more advanced disease. Among 5 good risk patients, all were alive with a very short follow-up ranging from 170 to 317 days. The median number of NC was 4.1x10^7/kg (1.4 to 40) and of 13 patients surviving for more than 30 days, all engrafted with a median time to reach 500 ANC of 24 days.

Duke and Minneapolis Universities pooled their observations of 111 patients transplanted with unrelated cord blood from the New-York CB bank between August 1993 and August 1997 (26). The donor was HLA identical or had a single HLA difference in 51 cases, had 2 or 3 HLA differences in 58 cases and 4 HLA differences in a further 2 cases. The mean volume of cord blood collected was 84 ml (40-214) and the median number of NC infused was 3.5x10^7/kg (0.7-33.8). The probability of engraftment was 79% and this was unaffected by the number of HLA differences. The median time to reach≥ 500 ANC/μl was 23 days (12-59) and ≥50.000 platelets/μl was 2.4 months (1-8). In univariate analysis, the speed of engraftment was associated with the number of nucleated cells, the number of CD34$^+$ cells and the number of CFU-GM infused. The probability of Grade II-IV GVHD was 35% irrespective of HLA disparities. The frequency of chronic GVHD was low. With a median follow-up time of 1 year, the 2-year survival was 45%. The only factor predictive for survival was the number of cells infused.

P. Rubinstein et al have recently reported results of cord blood transplants provided by the New York cord blood bank, 493 patients transplanted in 93 centers were analyzed (27). By day 42, 81% of patients had engrafted. Median time to myeloid engraftment was 28 days. Engraftment speed correlated with cell dose. The incidence of transplant related events was related to the patient's underlying disease, age, WBC dose, HLA disparity and transplant center. Severe GVHD (Grade III-IV) occurred in 23% and chronic GVHD in 24% of evaluable patients. Relapse rate in acute leukemia was 8.5% within the first 100 days, 17% within 6 months and 26% by one year. Relapse rates correlated with diagnosis disease stage, and GVHD suggesting a GVL effect. Event free survival at 100 days post transplant was 49%.

DISCUSSION

Are there enough stem cells in a single cord blood for short and long term engraftment?

The first question about the general use of cord blood for allogeneic hematopoietic stem cell transplant has been the concern about the engraftment potential of a single cord blood unit in patients with all hematological conditions and all weights. We and others have shown that a high number of nucleated cells infused is a good prognostic factor for engraftment and survival (Figure 3). In our patients, the median number of NC found in related or unrelated transplanted units of CB was 11×10^8 NC (range: 0.13-58). We found that the number of NC infused/kg after thawing was a major factor for predicting recovery of neutrophil and platelet counts after transplantation. In unrelated CBT, patients who received less than 3.7×10^7 NC/kg had a median time to reach $\geq 500 \mu l$ ANC of 34 days (range: 14 to 48 days) and a median time to reach $\geq 20,000/\mu l$ platelets of 134 days (range: 30 to 180 days) while in patients who received more than the median cell dose, the median times were respectively 25 days (range: 10 to 56 days) for ANC and 47 days (range: 9 to 85 days) for platelets. In adults, we found that none of the patients who received less than 1×10^7 NC /kg survived. We have been looking at the outcome of patients who received less than 2×10^7 NC/kg and found that with this low cell dose, there was a 69% probability of reaching $\geq 500/\mu l$ ANC and 49% of reaching $\geq 20,000/\mu l$ platelets on day 60. A low number of infused nucleated cells infused is associated with both a delay of engraftment and an increased risk of non-engraftment. The number of CD34 cells present at collection and after thawing might also be a good indicator for engraftment, unfortunately, efforts at standardization of CD34 counts have failed and this is the reason why they were not included in our analysis. Of note, the number of cells infused is 1 log less than a standard allogeneic bone marrow transplant and 10 times less than a standard peripheral blood stem cell transplant. The number of cells infused is far below the recommended dose of bone marrow cells (28). This favors the hypothesis that cord blood cells have a selective qualitative advantage on adult bone marrow cells. We have also shown that other factors interfere with engraftment such as diagnosis and HLA differences. Patients with severe aplastic anemia or with hemoglobinopathies had less engraftment than patients with leukemia or inborn errors. This is, as for allogeneic bone marrow

90

transplantation, due to the addition of several factors including transfusion immunization and reduction of the conditioning myeloablative regimens used for transplantation in non malignant disorders. The role of HLA disparities is still unclear in related and unrelated situations, we did not find any correlation between the degree of HLA mismatch and granulocyte recovery. In contrast, in related cord blood transplant, we found a correlation between platelet recovery and HLA mismatch, one possible explanation can be due to the presence of histocompatibility antigens at the surface of platelets which are not tested by the current methods.

Figure 3. Non parametric estimation of the influence of number of nucleated cells infused on engraftment when accounting for age and weight in a multivariate analysis in 246 patients given a cord blood transplant.

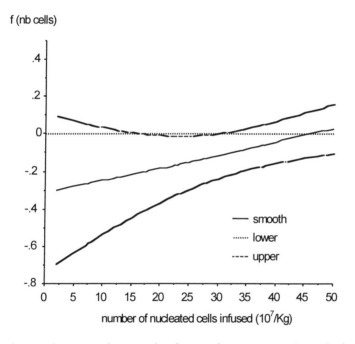

In order to improve the speed of engraftment, several methods can be investigated as the use of hematopoietic growth factors such as G-CSF, Kit L or Thrombopoietin. At this stage, the usefulness of these factors has not been demonstrated and deserves further investigation. Another approach could be to expand cord blood progenitors in vitro to improve short-term engraftment. This area of investigation seems particularly interesting, as in vitro studies have shown that expansion was increased in cord blood compared to bone marrow cells. The use of cytokines cocktails including TPO and FLT3 are particularly effective and preliminary clinical observations are encouraging. Another avenue of research is the possibility of using several cord blood units in order to increase the stem cell yield. This raises basic questions about the immunological reactivity of these cells between themselves and with the host. On the practical point of view, these findings are the basis for blood banks to collect as many cells as possible and to improve the technique of processing and volume reduction in order to have units available with high cellular counts. The other consequence is that, at this stage, we do not recommend transplant if the CBU, before thawing, contains less than 1×10^7 NC/kg.

Is GVHD reduced after cord blood transplantation?

One of the first concerns raised by the use of cord blood for allogeneic transplant was the possibility of inadvertent transplant of maternal cells. We, and other authors, have shown that, indeed, maternal cells were always present in cord blood but that their number was insufficient to induce GVHD (29). Their presence can be detected in the cord blood by high molecular resolution typing which shows a double population. For these reasons, the detection of maternal cells does not enter in the practice of cord blood banking. In addition, nobody has shown engraftment of maternal cells after cord blood transplantation, this suggests that either these cells are in small number or that they are inactive.

Immunologically immature CB cells might decrease the incidence and severity of acute GVHD even in a mismatched situation. At this time, there is no case-control study comparing the incidence of GVHD according to the stem cell source but there is some evidence that GVHD could be reduced after cord blood transplantation. In previously published CBT series, GVHD occurs but it is generally of lower incidence than expected for highly mismatched transplants without T cell depletion. In one study of unrelated bone marrow transplantation, grade III-IV GVHD was estimated at 21% in patients receiving a high resolution HLA matched unmanipulated unrelated bone marrow and 47% in patients receiving a mismatched unrelated bone marrow transplant (30). This must be compared to the incidence of 21% grade III-IV acute GVHD in unrelated mismatched CBT. In our study, we found that HLA incompatibilities were associated with acute GVHD in related transplants. In contrast, we did not find any correlation between the number of mismatches and GVHD in unrelated cord blood transplants. This could be due to the fact that we had only HLA DRB1 high resolution typing and that the other class I and class II antigens were not determined by high resolution typing. Minor histocompatibility differences might also play a role.

Is graft versus leukemia diminished after cord blood transplantation?

It is well known that T cells play a major role in eradicating leukemia mainly in chronic myeloid leukemia. This has been proven by the increased risk of relapse after T-cell depleted bone marrow transplantation and by the efficacy of donor lymphocyte infusions to treat relapse after allogeneic bone marrow transplantation. As cord blood lymphocytes are decreased in number and are immunologically immature, they might loose their GVL function. Experimental data suggest that indeed, there is some loss but, on the contrary, we have shown that NK cells and T cells in cord blood were inducible by allogeneic stimulation. In absence of comparative studies with other sources of stem cells and since the number of patients is limited and the follow-up is short, it is difficult to draw conclusions about CBT and GVL.

Is immune reconstitution delayed after cord blood transplantation?

The answer might be complex to analyze as there are many factors which interfere with the speed of immune reconstitution after allogeneic hematopoietic stem cell transplantation. They are the age of the patient, his serological status to Herpes group virus infections, the degree of HLA disparity, the conditioning regimen used and the occurrence of acute and chronic GVHD and its treatment. Preliminary results show that immune reconstitution seems similar to bone marrow transplantation in HLA identical sibling transplants.

What is the place of cord blood transplant compared to other sources of hematopoietic stem cells?

Current results show that cord blood has proven effective in treating children with malignancies and other disorders. There are not enough patients in other disease categories and in adults to perform a comparison with other stem cell sources. In children with acute leukemia, related and unrelated, matched or mismatched cord blood transplants give similar results. The main prognostic factor being the stage of the disease at time of transplantation. This cohort of patients compares favorably with other results of the literature (31-34) and a case-control study is currently being performed by the European Blood and Marrow Transplant group (EBMT). At this stage and in the absence of definitive answer, we recommend simultaneous searches of Bone Marrow Donor Registries and Cord Blood Banks. The final decision must take into account the degree of HLA identity, the availability of the donor, the speed of search, the urgency of the transplant, the number of cells present in the cord blood and, in the case of an unrelated bone marrow donor transplant, the donor age, sex, number of pregnancies and CMV status.

REFERENCES

1. Madrigal JA, Scott I, Arguello R, Szydlo R, Little AM, Goldman JM. Factors influencing the outcome of bone marrow transplants using unrelated donors. Immunological Reviews. Immunology of hematopoietic stem cell transplantation 1997;157:153- 166.
2. Speiser DE, Tiercy JM, Rufer N et al . High resolution HLA matching associated with decreased mortality after unrelated bone marrow transplantation. Blood 1996;10:4455-4462.
3. Petersdorf EW, Longton GM, Anasetti C et al. Definition of HLA-DQ as a transplantation antigen. Proc Natl Acad Sci. USA 1996;93:15358-63.
4. Petersdorf EW, Longton GM, Anasetti C et al. Association of HLA-C disparity with graft failure after marrow transplantation from unrelated donors. Blood 1997;89:1818-1823.
5. Hansen JA, Petersdorf E, Martin PJ, Anasetti C. Hematopoietic stem cell transplants from unrelated donors. Immunological Reviews. Immunology of hematopoietic stem cell transplantation. 1997;157: 141-151.
6. Broxmeyer HE, Gordon GW, Hangoc G et al. Human umbilical cord blood as a potential source of transplantable hematopoietic stem/progenitor cells. Proc Natl Acad Sci USA. 1989;86:3828-3832.
7. Broxmeyer HE, Hangoc G, Cooper S et al. Growth characteristics and expansion of human umbilical cord blood and estimation of its potential for transplantation in adults. Proc Natl Acad Sci USA. 1992;89:4109-4113.
8. Mayani H, Lansdorp PM. Thy-1 expression is linked to functional properties of primitive hematopoietic progenitors cells from human umbilical cord blood. Blood 1994;83:2410-2417.
9. Morrison SJ, Wandycz AM, Akashi K et al. The aging of hematopoietic stem cells. Nature Medicine 1996;2:1011-1016.
10. Vaziri H, Dragowska W, Allsop RC et al. Evidence for a mitotic clock in human hematopoietic stem cells: loss of telomeric DNA with age. Proc Natl Acad Sci USA 1994;91: 9857-9860.
11. Madrigal JA, Cohen SBA, Gluckman E, Charron DJ. Does cord blood transplantation result in lower graft versus host disease? It takes more than two to tango. Human Immunology 1997; 56:1-5.
12. Garderet L, Dulphy N, Douay C et al. The umbilical cord blood $\alpha\beta$ T cell repertoire: characteristics of a polyclonal and naive but completely formed repertoire. Blood 1998;91:340-346.
13. Cairo MS, Wagner JE. Placental and/or umbilical cord blood an alternative source of haemopoietic stem cells for transplantation. Blood 1997;90:4665-4678.
14. De La Selle V., Gluckman E, Bruley-Rosset M. Newborn blood can engraft adult mice without inducing graft versus host disease across non H-2 antigens. Blood 1996;87:3977-3983.

15. De La Selle V, Gluckman E, Bruley-Rosset M. Graft versus host disease and graft versus leukemia effect in mice grafted with newborn blood. Blood 1999; 92 (10): 3968-3975.
16. Rubinstein P, Rosenfield RD, Adamson JW, Stevens CE. Stored placental blood for unrelated bone marrow reconstitution. Blood 1993;81:1679-1690.
17. Rubinstein P, Dobrila L, Rosenfield RE et al. Processing and cryopreservation of placental/ umbilical cord blood for unrelated bone marrow reconstitution. Proc Natl Acad Sci USA 1995;92:10119-10122.
18. Gluckman E, Broxmeyer HE, Auerbach AD et al. Hematopoietic reconstitution in a patient with Fanconi 's anemia by means of umbilical cord blood from an HLA-identical sibling. New Engl J Med 1989;321:1174-1178.
19. Gluckman E, Rocha V, Boyer Chammard A et al. Outcome of cord blood transplantation from related and unrelated donors. New Engl. J. of Med 1997;337:373-381.
20. Rocha V, Chastang Cl, Souillet G et al for the Eurocord transplant group. Related cord blood transplants: the Eurocord experience of 78 transplants. Bone Marrow Transplantation 1998; 21 sup 3: S59-S62.
21. Gluckman E, Rocha V, Chastang C. European results of unrelated cord blood transplants. Bone Marrow Transplantation 1998;21 sup 3:S87-S91.
22. Locatelli F, Rocha V, Chastang C et al. Cord blood transplantation for children with acute leukemia. Bone Marrow Transplantation 1998;21 sup 3: S63-S65.
23. Miniero R, Rocha V, Saracco P et al on behalf of Eurocord. Cord blood transplantation in hemoglobinopathies. Bone Marrow Transplantation.1998;22 sup 1:S78-S79.
24. Kurtzberg J, Laughlin M, Graham L et al. Placental blood as a source of hematopoietic stem cells for transplantation into unrelated recipients. New England J of Medicine 1996;335:157-166.
25. Wagner JE, Rosenthal J, Sweetman R et al. Successful transplantation of HLA Matched and HLA mismatched umbilical cord blood from unrelated donors: analysis of engraftment and acute graft versus host disease. Blood 1996;88:795-802.
26. Wagner JE, DeFor T, Rubinstein P, Kurtzberg J Transplantation of unrelated donor umbilical cord blood: outcomes and analysis of risk factors. Blood 1997;90 suppl 1.p 398a Abstract#1767.
27. P. Rubinstein, Carrier C, Scaradavou A et al. Initial results of the placental/umbilical cord blood program for unrelated bone marrow reconstitution. (In Press).

28. Sierra J, Storer B, Hansen AJ, Bierke JW, Martin PJ, Petersdorf EW, Appelbaum FR, Bryant E, Chauncey TR, Sale G, Sanders JE, Storb R, Sullivan KM, Anasetti C: Transplantation of marrow cells from unrelated donors for treatment of high-risk acute leukemia: the effect of leukemic burden, donor HLA-matching, and marrow cell dose. Blood 1997;89:4226-4235.

29. Petit T, Dommergues M, Socié G et al. Detection of maternal cells in human fetal blood during the third trimester of pregnancy using allele specific PCR amplification. Brit J of Haematol. 1997;98:767-771.

30. Hansen JA, Gooley TA, Martin PJ et al. Bone marrow transplants from unrelated donors for patients with chronic myeloid leukemia. New Engl. J Med 1998;338: 962-968.

31. Hongeng S, Krance RA, Bowman LC et al Outcomes of transplantation with matched-sibling and unrelated donor bone marrow in children with leukemia. Lancet 1997;350:767-771.

32. Szydlo R, Goldman JM, Klein JP et al Results of allogeneic bone marrow transplants for leukemia using donors other than HLA identical siblings. J Clin. Oncol 1997;15:1767-1777.

33. Oakhill A, Pamphilon DH, Potter MN et al. Unrelated donor bone marrow transplantation for children with relapsed acute lymphoblastic leukaemia in second complete remission. Brit. J of Haematol 1996;94:574-578.

34. Aversa F, Tabilio A, Terenzi A et al. Successful engraftment of T-cell depleted haploidentical three loci incompatible transplants in leukemia patients by addition of recombinant human granulocyte colony stimulating factor mobilized peripheral blood progenitor cells to bone marrow inoculum. Blood 1994; 84: 3948-3955.

5
NON MYELOABLATIVE
"MINI TRANSPLANTS"

Sergio Giralt, M.D., Issa Khouri, M.D., and Richard Champlin, M.D.

University of Texas MD Anderson Cancer Center, Houston, TX, USA
Supported by Grant CA49639 and CA55164 from the National Cancer Institute

INTRODUCTION

High dose chemo-radiotherapy with allogeneic bone marrow transplantation (BMT) is an effective therapy for patients with hematologic malignancies (1,2). The curative potential of this procedure is mediated in part by an immune mediated graft-versus-leukemia effect (3-8). Direct evidence of this effect is the reinduction of remission obtained after infusions of donor lymphocytes in patients who have relapsed after an allogeneic progenitor cell transplant. (9-13) Responses are more frequent in patients with chronic myelogenous leukemia (CML), but have also been observed in patients with acute myelogenous leukemia (AML), chronic lymphocytic leukemia (CLL), myeloma and lymphoma relapsing after allogeneic BMT (14-16).

These observations suggest that graft-versus-leukemia may be sufficient for cure and that intense myeloablative therapy may not be needed. Thus, a strategy of inducing a graft versus leukemia effect by infusing allogeneic progenitor cells after standard dose non-ablative chemotherapy could be useful as treatment for susceptible malignancies in patients ineligible for high dose chemotherapy or total body irradiation (TBI). The hypothesis underlying this treatment strategy is that less intense preparative regimens would produce less inflammatory cytokines and therefore less regimen related toxicity and less GVHD (17-19).

NON MYELOABLATIVE CONDITIONING REGIMENS

Harnessing graft versus leukemia without myeloablative therapy will depend on developing conditioning regimens that are sufficiently immunosuppressive to allow durable engraftment, and yet have little non-hematologic toxicity. Likewise, in many cases, they will also need to be sufficiently active against the malignant disorder to provide time for the allogeneic cells to proliferate and thus exert their anti-tumor effect.

In humans, cyclophosphamide doses of 200 mg/kg have been associated with graft rejection rates of 30% in the sensitized aplastic anemia patient (20). In dogs total body irradiation doses (TBI) of 200-450 cGy allows for consistent durable engraftment of allogeneic matched related cells only if followed by post-transplant immune suppressive therapy (21,22).

The purine analogs fludarabine and 2-chlorodeoxyadenosine (2-CDA) have been shown to be active against a variety of hematologic malignances (23-25). These compounds are also immunosuppressive, effectively inhibiting the mixed lymphocyte reaction in-vitro (26,27). Both fludarabine and 2-CDA have been shown to inhibit the mechanisms of DNA repair and may therefore potentiate the antitumor effect of some alkylating agents, however, they have little extramedullary toxicity and have been well tolerated in elderly and debilitated patients. (27-30) Therefore, purine analog containing non-myeloablative chemotherapy would seem an appropriate way of exploring induction of graft-versus-leukemia without myeloablative therapy, a procedure that has been named "mini-transplant".

MINI-TRANSPLANTS FOR ACUTE MYELOID LEUKEMIA AND CHRONIC MYELOGENOUS LEUKEMIA

At M.D. Anderson, we performed a pilot trial of purine analog containing non-myeloablative therapy for patients with AML or CML considered ineligible for myeloablative therapy either because of age or medical condition, using the treatment schema depicted in Figure 1 (31,32). A total of 26 patients (AML:13, MDS:4, CML:9) have been treated. Patient characteristics are summarized in Table 1.

98

Figure 1: Treatment Schema for Mini-Transplants for AML and CML at M.D. Anderson Cancer Center

Mini Transplant for AML/MDS

Nonablative Preparative Regimen to Achieve Engraftment → **Allo PBPC or BMT** → **Short to Std GVHD Prophylaxis** → **DLI if Residual Disease**

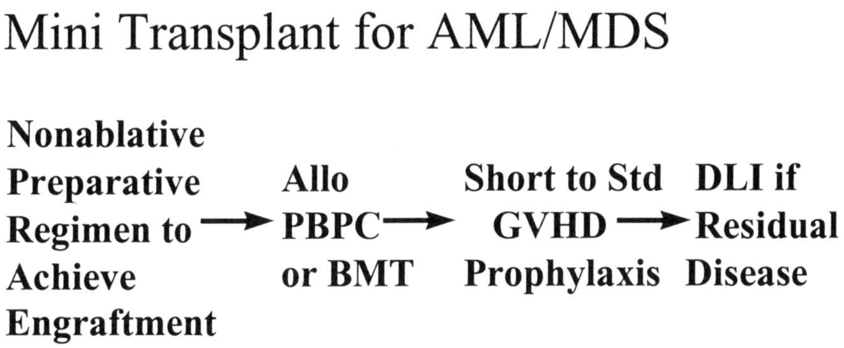

Table 1. Characteristics of Patients Undergoing Mini-transplant for AML and CML at M.D. Anderson Cancer Center.

N			26
Median age in years (range)			60 (28-72)
Diagnosis and Stage at BMT			
	AML		13
		First relapse untreated	2
		CR 2	2
		Refractory relapse or >CR 2	9
	MDS		
		Untreated	1
		First relapse untreated	
		Refractory relapse or >CR 2	
	CML		
		First Chronic Phase	5
		Transformed	4
Median time to transplant			490 days (77-3429)
Median # prior therapies			2 (1-3)
Preparative Regimen			
		FlagIda	17
		2CDA/AraC	9
Donor Type and Cell Source			
		Sib Full Match/1 Ag Mismatch	20/3
		6/6 MUD	2
		Syngeneic	1
		PBSC/BM	22/4
GVHD Prophylaxis (Twin excluded)			
		CSA or CSA/MP	19
		FK/MTX	6

Among the 17 patients with AML or MDS treated, 3 died before day 100 from infectious complications, but no other toxic deaths occurred. Three patients developed ≥ Grade 2 GVHD, all of them responding to therapy with either steroids alone or addition of ATG. Thirteen patients had neutrophil recovery a median of 10 days post transplant (range 9-18) and 11 achieved platelet transfusion independence a median of 12 days post transplant (range 8-78). Ten patients achieved complete remission (< 5% bone marrow blast with neutrophil recovery and platelet transfusion independence). Chimerism analysis of the 10 patients achieving complete remission on day 30 revealed that 7 of them had >80% donor cells either by cytogenetics or molecular techniques, 1 patient had autologous reconstitution and 2 patients were inevaluable for chimerism either because of technical difficulties or lack of difference in enzyme restriction pattern between donor and recipient (syngeneic transplant). At 3 months post transplant, 6 patients remained in remission, 4 of which had > 80% donor cells by similar studies, and by 1 year one of the 2 patients in remission remained 100% donor by molecular techniques and the other patient was inevaluable (syngeneic).

The median survival for patients achieving CR was 211 days with 3 patients remaining alive at 5, 22, and 23 months after transplant. Nine patients have relapsed, of which 2 were succesfully reinduced. One with a second mini-transplant and the other with a conventional syngeneic transplant using busulfan/cyclophosphamide conditioning. The median survival of the non-responding patients was 61 days, with none of them responding to subsequent salvage maneuvers. (Figure 2).

Figure 2: Overall Survival for patients with AML/MDS receiving Flag/Ida or 2CDA/AraC with allogeneic PBSC transplants according to response.

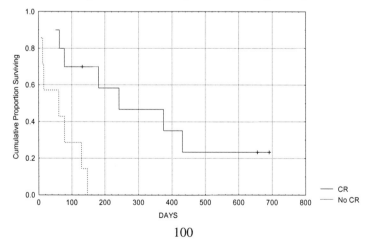

This initial experience permitted us to conclude that donor cell engraftment and remissions can be achieved in patients with advanced AML using purine analog containing non myeloablative chemotherapy followed by allogeneic peripheral blood stem cells. However, refractory patients relapse quickly and this strategy should be further explored in patients in remission but ineligible for conventional transplant techniques either because of age or medical condition.

Among the 9 patients with CML, 1 patient died from acute GVHD on day 43 and no other treatment related deaths have occurred. All patients had hematologic recovery of both neutrophil and platelets a median of 13 days post infusion, but 2 patients failed to have any evidence of donor cell engraftment (both recipients of matched unrelated donor cells). Bone marrow on day 30 revealed complete cytogenetic remission in 5 patients and major cytogenetic remission in another 3 with 1 patient having insufficient metaphases. Five of 7 evaluable patients had cytogenetic progression during the first 3 months after transplant, 1 patient remains in complete cytogenetic remission 6 months post transplant and the other relapsed 9 months post transplant. All 5 of the progressing patients had immune suppression withdrawn and received further infusion of donor lymphocyte with no responses reported to date.

These preliminary results suggest that the combination of fludarabine, idarubicin and ara-c although effective in achieving remissions may not be optimal for CML, although further study in chronic phases and longer follow-up will be needed.

Mini-transplants for Lymphoid Malignancies

The use of allogeneic transplantation is limited in patients with lymphoid malignancies such as chronic lymphocytic leukemia or lymphomas because they typically affect older patients. We have evaluated the induction of graft versus leukemia as primary therapy for patients with lymphoid malignancies who are considered poor candidates for conventional transplant techniques (32). Nine patients (CLL=5; lymphoma=4) have been treated of which eight were older than age 50. All patients, using one of 2 preparative regimens are summarized in Figure 3. Mixed chimerism was observed in 6 of 9 patients with a percentage of donor cells ranging from 50% to 100% one month post transplant. No regimen related deaths were observed, and 4 patients achieved complete remission, one after donor lymphocyte infusions.

Allogeneic transplants for multiple myeloma have been associated with a graft versus myeloma effect but have high regimen-related mortality (33-36).

Melphalan is an active drug in myeloma, and can be administered at a dose of 140 mg/m^2 without stem cell support (37). Combining melphalan at lower doses than traditionally used for autologous transplants with the purine analog fludarabine, could allow engraftment of allogeneic progenitor cells, and allow exploration of the graft versus myeloma effect without the toxicities of more intense myeloablative therapy.

Table 2. Patient and Treatment Characteristics for patients receiving Melphalan and purine analog combinations.

N		63
Median age, years (range)		49 (22-71)
Diagnosis		
	AML/MDS	27/8
	CML	16
	NHL/HD	5/3
	ALL	4
Time to BMT, days (range)		558 (69-6626)
Stage at BMT		
	Acute Leukemia	
	CR1/CR2	1 / 2
	Untreated first relapse	10
	Refractory or other	35
	CML	
	First Chronic Phase	2
	Accelerated	6
	Blast Crisis/CP2	3 / 4
Prior Regimens		2 (0-9)
Comorbid Conditions		
	Age>50	29
	Prior BMT	17
	Poor Organ Function	31
	PS 2	12
Donor Type		
	6/6 Sib	31
	5/6 Sib	2
	6/6 MUD	30
Preparative Regimen		
	Fludarabine/Melphalan	55
	2CDA/Melphalan	8

Other Mini Transplant Experience

Slavin et al. have recently reported the use of fludarabine in combination with busulfan 8 mg/kg and ATG as a less intensive preparative regimen for patients undergoing allogeneic transplant for hematologic malignancies. Twenty six patients (18 with either acute or chronic leukemia) were treated. Seventeen had complete donor cell engraftment, 9 were transiently chimeric, 4 patients died from complications of GVHD, and the overall disease free survival at 1 year was 81% (38).

At M.D. Anderson Cancer Center, we have been exploring the combination of the purine analogs fludarabine or 2CDA with melphalan for patients with advanced hematologic malignancies who were considered poor candidates for a conventional allogeneic progenitor cell transplant. (39) From 2/96 to 4/98 a total of 63 patients with a variety of hematologic malignancies have been treated. Patient and treatment characteristics are summarized in Table 2. All patients received FK506/methotrexate combinations for GVHD prophylaxis.

Fifty six patients had neutrophil recovery at a median of 14 days (range, 9-35), 40 patients recovered platelet transfusion independence at a median of 22 days (range 9-118). All engrafting patients except 1 had >80% donor cell engraftment by day 30, with one instance of autologous reconstitution and 1 case of secondary graft failure. In this group of patients, ineligible for conventional transplant, the 100 day mortality was 50% (31/63) with 4/8 patients in the 2CDA/melphalan arm dying from multiorgan failure. The overall survival for patients in CR1 or untreated first relapse was 68% at 1 year, versus 9% for patients with more advanced or refractory disease (Figure 3). We concluded that 2CDA/melphalan was too toxic, while fludarabine/melphalan combinations can allow engraftment of allogeneic progenitor cells including cells obtained from matched unrelated donors and that this strategy can produce long term disease control in patients with hematologic malignancies early in the course of their disease with acceptable risk and toxicity in patients ineligible for conventional myeloablative transplant therapies. Treatment related mortality, and disease recurrence limits the usefullness of this approach in this same patient population.

Figure 3: Overall Survival for patients with a variety of hematologic malignancies receiving melphalan in combination with purine analogs according to status at the time of BMT.

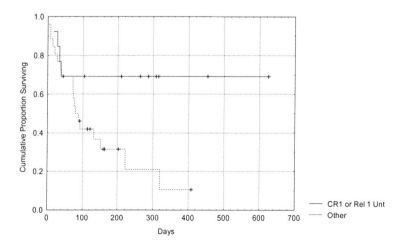

SUMMARY AND CONCLUSIONS

The efficacy of graft-vs.-leukemia induction to treat relapses after allogeneic progenitor cell transplant in a variety of hematologic malignancies suggest that it may be possible to use the graft versus leukemia as primary therapy for these malignancies without the need of myeloablative therapy. This type of strategy should be explored initially in patients considered ineligible for conventional myeloablative therapies either because of age or concurrent medical conditions.

GVHD remains a major obstacle that needs to be overcome. Although a potentially lower level of inflammatory cytokines may be present after non-myeloablative therapies, fatal GVHD still occurs. Methods to diminish GVHD after allogeneic transplant include selective T-cell depletion (39-43) and transduction of donor T-cells with Herpes simplex virus thymidine kinase which renders these cells sensitive to ganciclovir treatment (see chapter 16).

We and others have demonstrated that nonablative chemotherapy using fludarabine combinations is sufficiently immunosuppressive to allow engraftment of allogeneic blood progenitor cells. Patients could then receive graded doses of donor lymphocytes without rejection, to mediate GVL. Ideally, this therapy could be titrated to levels of residual malignant cells using sensitive detection techniques. This novel approach to therapy would reduce the toxicity of the transplant procedure, allow it to be administered more safely to debilitated patients and possibly extend the use of transplantation to older patients who are not presently eligible for BMT procedures. Other possible indications include treatment of non-malignant disorders and induction of tolerance for solid organ transplantation.

REFERENCES

1. Gale RP, Champlin RE. How does bone marrow transplantation cure leukemia? Lancet. 1984;2:28-30.
2. Bortin M, Horowitz M, Gale R, et al: Changing trends in allogeneic bone marrow transplantation for leukemia in the 1980's. JAMA, 1992; 268:607-612.
3. Weiden PL, Sullivan KM, Flournoy N, Storb R, Thomas ED, The Seattle Marrow Transplant Team. Antileukemic effect of chronic graft-versus-host disease: Contribution to improved survival after allogeneic marrow transplantation. NEJM. 1981;304:1529-1533.

4. Horowitz MM, Gale RP, Sondel PM, et al. Graft-versus-leukemia reactions after bone marrow transplantation. Blood. 1990;75:555-562.
5. Sullivan KM, Storb R, Buckner CD, et al. Graft-versus-host disease as adoptive immunotherapy in patients with advanced hematologic neoplasms. N Engl J Med. 1989;320:828-834.
6. Sullivan KM, Weiden PL, Storb R, et al. Influence of acute and chronic graft-versus-host disease on relapse and survival after bone marrow transplantation from HLA-identical siblings as treatment of acute and chronic leukemia. Blood. 1989;73:1720-1728.
7. Goldman JM, Gale RP, Bortin MM, et al. Bone marrow transplantation for chronic myelogenous leukemia in chronic phase: increased risk of relapse associated with T-cell depletion.. Ann Intern Med. 1988;108:806-814.
8. Gale RP, Horowitz MM, Ash RC, et al. Identical-twin bone marrow transplants for leukemia. Ann Intern Med. 1994;120:646-652.
9. Kolb HJ, Schattenberg A, Goldman JM, et al. Graft-vs-leukemia effect of donor lymphocyte transfusions in marrow grafted patients.. Blood. 1995;86:2041-2050.
10. Van Rhee F, Lin F, Cullis JO, et al. Relapse of chronic myeloid leukemia after allogeneic bone marrow transplant: The case for giving donor leukocyte transfusions before the onset of hematologic relapse. Blood. 1994;83:3377-3383.
11. Mackinnon S, Papadopoulos EB, Carabasi MH, et al. Adoptive immunotherapy evaluating escalating doses of donor leukeocytes for relapse of chronic myeloid leukemia after bone marrow transplantation: separation of graft-versus-leukemia responses from graft-versus-host disease.. Blood. 1995;86:1261-1268.
12. Cullis JO, Jiang YZ, Schwarer AP, Hughes TP, Barrett AJ, Goldman JM. Donor leukocyte infusions for chronic myeloid leukemia in relapse after allogeneic bone marrow transplantation. Blood. 1992;79:1379-1381.
13. Drobyski WR, Keever CA, Roth MS, et al. Salvage immunotherapy using donor leukocyte infusions as treatment for relapsed chronic myelogenous leukemia after allogeneic bone marrow transplantation: Efficacy and toxicity of a defined T-cell dose. Blood. 1993;82:2310-2318.
14. Tricot G, Vesole DH, Jagannath S, Hilton J, Munshi N, Barlogie B. Graft-versus-myeloma effect: Proof of principle. Blood. 1996;87:1196-1198.
15. Rondón G, Giralt S, Huh Y, et al. Graft-versus-leukemia effect after allogeneic bone marrow transplantation for chronic lymphocytic leukemia. Bone Marrow Transplantation. 1996;18:669-672.
16. Collins R, Shpilberg O, Drobyski W, et al: Donor leukocyte infusions in 140 patients with relapsed malignancy after allogeneic bone marrow transplant. J Clin Oncol, 1997; 15:433-444.

17. Ferrara JL, Deeg HJ. Mechanisms of disease: Graft-versus-host disease. N Engl J Med. 1991;324:667-674.

18. Holler E, Kolb H, Moller A, et al: Increased serum levels of tumor necrosis factor α precede major complications of bone marrow transplantation. Blood, 1990; 7:1011-1016.

19. Hill G, Crawford J, Cooke K, Brinson Y, Pan L, Ferrrara J: Total body irradiation and acute graft versus host disease: The role of gastrointestinal damage and inflammatory cytokines. Blood, 1997; 90:3204-3213.

20. Van Bekkum D: Conditioning regimens for marrow grafting. Semin Hematol, 1984; 21:81-90.

21. Yu C, Storb R, Mathey B, et al: DLA-identical bone marrow grafts after low dose total body irradiation: Effects of high dose corticosteroids and cyclosporine on engraftment. Blood, 1995; 86:4376-4381.

22. Storb R, Yu C, Wagner J, et al: Stable mixed hematopoietic chimerism in DLA-identical littermate dogs given sublethal total body irradiation before and pharmacological immunosuppression after marrow transplantation. Blood, 1997; 89:3048-3054.

23. Keating MJ, O'Brien S, Robertson LE, et al. The expanding role of fludarabine in hematologic malignancies. Leuk Lymphoma. 1994;14 Suppl. 2:11-6.

24. Keating M, Kantarjian H, Talpaz M, et al: Fludarabine: A new agent with major activity against chronic lymphocytic leukemia. Blood, 1989; 74:19-25.

25. Redman J, Cabanillas F, Velasquez W, et al: Phase II trial of fludarabine phosphate in lymphoma: an effective new agent in low grade lymphoma. J Clin Oncol, 1992; 10:790-794.

26. Goodman E, Fiedor P, Fein S, et al: Fludarabine phosphate and 2 chlorodeoxyadenosine:Immuno-suppressive DNA synthesis inhibitors with potential application in islet allo-xenotransplantation. Transplantation Proc, 1995; 27:3293-3294.

27. Plunkett W, Sanders P: Metabolism and action of purine nucleoside analogs. Pharmacol Ther, 1991; 49:239-245.

28. Gandhi V, Estey E, Keating MJ, Plunkett W. Fludarabine potentiates metabolism of cytarabine in patients with acute myelogenous leukemia during therapy. J Clin Oncol. 1993;11:116-124.

29. Li L, Glassman A, Keating M, Stros M, Plunkett W, Yang L: Fludarabine triphosphate inhibits nucleotide excision repair of cisplatin-induced DNA adducts in vitro. Cancer Res 1997; 57:1487-1494.

30. Estey E, Plunkett W, Gandhi V, Rios MB, Kantarjian H, Keating MJ. Fludarabine and arabinosylcytosine therapy of refractory and relapsed acute myelogenous leukemia. Leuk Lymphoma. 1993;9:343-350.

31. Giralt S, Estey E, Van Besien K, et al. Engraftment of allogeneic hematopoietic progenitor cells with purine analog containing chemotherapy: harnessing graft-vs-leukemia without myeloablative therapy.. Blood 1997; 89(12): 4531-4536.
32. Giralt S, Gajewski J, Khouri I, et al: Induction of graft-vs-leukemia as primary treatment of chronic myelogenous leukemia: Blood 1997; 90:418a.
33. Khouri I, Keating MJ, Przepiorka D, et al. Engraftment and induction of GVL with fludarabine-based non-ablative preparative regimen in patients with chronic lymphocytic leukemia.. Blood. 1996;88(suppl 1):301a.
34. Bensinger W, Buckner C, Clift R, et al: A phase I study of busulfan and cyclophosphamide in preparation for allogeneic marrow transplant for patients with multiple myeloma. J Clin Oncol 1992; 10:1492-1497.
35. Bjorkstrand B, Ljungman P, Svensson H, et al: Allogeneic bone marrow transplantation versus autologous stem cell transplantation in multiple myeloma: A retrospective case-matched study from the European Group for Blood and Marrow Transplantation. Blood 1996; 88: 4711-4718.
36. Lokhorst H, Schattenberg A, Cornelissen J, Thomas L, Verdonck L: Donor leukocyte infusions are effective in relapsed multiple myeloma after allogeneic bone marrow transplantation. Blood 1997; 90:4206-4211.
37. Lokhurst K, Meuwissen O, Verdonck L, Dekker A, High risk multiple myeloma treated with high dose melphalan. J Clin Oncol 1992; 10: 47-51.
38. Slavin S, Nagler A, Naparstek E, et al: Nonmyeloablative stem cell transplantation and cell therapy as an alternative to conventional bone marrow transplantation with lethal cytoreduction for the treatment of malignant and nonmalignant hematologic diseases. Blood 1998; 91:756-763.
39. Giralt S, Cohen A, Mehra R, et al: Preliminary results of fludarabine/melphalan or 2CDA/melphalan as preparative regimens for allogeneic progenitor cell transplantation in poor candidates for conventional myeloablative conditioning. Blood 1997; 90:417a.
40. Champlin R, Ho W, Gajewski J, et al. Selective depletion of CD8+ T lymphocytes for prevention of graft-versus-host disease after allogeneic bone marrow transplantation. Blood. 1990;76:418-423.
41. Nimer SD, Giorgi J, Gajewski JL, et al. Selective depletion of CD8+ cells for prevention of graft-versus-host disease after bone marrow transplantation: A randomized controlled trial. Transplantation. 1994;57:82-87.
42. Giralt S, Hester J, Huh Y, et al. CD8+ depleted donor lymphocyte infusion as treatment for relapsed chronic myelogenous leukemia after allogeneic bone marrow transplantation: graft vs leukemia without graft vs. host disease.. Blood. 1995;86:4337-4343.

43. Alyea E, Soiffer R, Canning C, et al: Toxicity and efficacy of defined doses of CD4+ donor lymphocytes for treatment of relapse after allogeneic bone marrow transplant. Blood 1998; 91:3671-3680.
44. Bordignon C, Bonini C, Verzeletti S, et al. Transfer of the HSV-tk gene into donor peripheral blood lymphocytes for in vivo modulation of donor anti-tumor immunity after allogeneic bone marrow transplantation. Hum Gene Ther. 1995;6:813-819.

6

ALLOGENEIC HEMATOPOIETIC STEM CELL TRANSPLANTATION IN RECIPIENTS OF CELLULAR OR SOLID ORGAN ALLOGRAFTS

Norma S. Kenyon, Maria Chatzipetrou, Andreas Tzakis,
Joshua Miller,
Rodolfo Alejandro, and Camillo Ricordi

Diabetes Research Institute, Departments of Medicine and Surgery, University of Miami School of Medicine and Miami VA Medical Center, Miami, FL, USA

Transplantation of solid organs and cells (e.g., islets) has been made possible because of immunosuppressive agents. Cyclosporin A (CsA) or FK506 is often given in combination with other agents, such as polyclonal or monoclonal antibody based induction therapy, steroids, and/or mycophenolate mofetil (MMF). Immunosuppression must be administered throughout the recipient's life, and while one year graft survival rates for solid organ transplants are excellent, the survival of transplanted organs drops dramatically over time (1). There are several adverse consequences associated with the use of chronic, generalized anti-rejection agents, including increased incidence of infection and malignancy, stunting of normal growth and development, diabetogenicity, nephrotoxicity, and osteoporosis (2-8).

For these reasons, it has long been a goal of the organ transplant community to develop protocols that would allow for the induction of donor specific tolerance, obviating the requirement for life-long immunosuppression. Over the years, various approaches to the induction of tolerance have proven successful in several rodent transplant models. Attempts to translate these findings to pre-clinical models (e.g. dogs and non-human primates), however, have met with inconsistent results (9).

Bone marrow transplantation into cytoablated recipients to create a state of hematopoietic chimerism is a well established approach to the induction of donor specific tolerance to subsequent cellular or solid organ allografts in many experimental models (9,10). Fully allogeneic chimeras, in which immune cells are entirely of donor origin, are problematic, in that engraftment is difficult to obtain when protocols such as T cell depletion of the marrow prior to transplant are utilized to prevent the occurrence of lethal graft versus host disease (GVHD) (10). If engraftment does occur, the animals are relatively immunoincompetent due to lack of MHC compatible, host antigen presenting cells (APC) to present antigen to donor T cells that have been educated in the host thymus (10). These problems can be avoided via the production of mixed allogeneic chimeras, which do not suffer from lethal GVHD, are immunocompetent, and are also tolerant of subsequent cellular or solid organ allografts from animals of the same strain as the bone marrow donor (10). Application of this approach to the field of human transplantation has been hampered by the requirement for cytoreductive treatment of the recipient, a measure that is not advantageous for individuals who are not suffering from malignancy. Recent demonstration of bone marrow engraftment in noncytoablated animals, via multiple infusions of large numbers of donor bone marrow cells (11), has provided the impetus to explore this approach in humans. In addition, and independent of the issue of chimerism, administration of donor antigen (in the form of hematopoietic cells, e.g., bone marrow, blood, splenocytes) at the time of transplantation has long been studied as a means to induce acceptance of grafted tissues in both animals and humans (12,13).

ATTEMPTS TO INDUCE TOLERANCE VIA HEMATOPOIETIC STEM CELL TRANSPLANTATION: RODENT AND PRE-CLINICAL MODELS

The majority of the data available on the use of bone marrow transplantation to enhance the acceptance of solid organ or cellular allografts has been generated in rodent models (Table 1).

In 1945, Owen was the first to find that dizygotic cattle twins possess red blood cells that could only have come from the twin sibling via vascular anastomosis in the placenta (14). Medawar and Billingham, in their attempts to distinguish identical from dizygotic cattle twins by exchanging skin grafts, were surprised by the survival of the vast majority of the grafts. They quoted Owen's work as an explanation for their finding and published their data in 1951 (15). In 1953, Billingham, Brent, and Medawar reported on studies with the first model of neonatal tolerance: mice inoculated in utero with donor cells did not reject donor strain skin grafts transplanted 6 to 8 weeks after birth (16). Thus began studies of hematologic chimerism and tolerance.

Table 1. Donor bone marrow infusion in rodents.

Host Conditioning with Cytoablation
1. Total body irradiation (TBI) (30,31,33,39,40)
   a) plus cyclophosphamide (cyP) (37,50)
   b) plus cyclosporine (51,52)
   c) plus antilymphocyte globulin (ALG) (37)
   d) plus monoclonal antibodies (32,60,61)
   e) plus FK-506 (53,54)
2. Lymphoid irradiation (46,47,48,49),

Host Conditioning without Cytoablation
1. monoclonal antibodies (41)
2. FK-506 (55)
3. Antilymphocyte serum (ALS) plus thymectomy (56,57)
4. Antilymphocyte serum (ALS) without thymectomy (58,59)
5. CTLA4Ig (63)

Donor bone marrow modulation
1. T cell depletion (35,43,44,45)
2. Intrathymic inoculation of DBMC (65,66)

Proposed central (thymus) and peripheral mechanisms of graft acceptance include clonal deletion in the thymus, T-cell ignorance or anergy, deletion of reactive T cells in the periphery, and suppression (9). Tolerance in bone marrow chimeras has generally been considered to be promoted by central mechanisms. It has been demonstrated that donor bone marrow cells migrate into the recipient's thymus and induce deletion of potentially donor reactive T cells via activation induced apoptosis (17). Experiments in mice (18) and rats (19) have demonstrated that tolerance in neonatal chimeric animals was induced centrally within the thymus. Similar results were obtained in a study of adult mice, where it was shown that only euthymic, mixed allogeneic bone marrow chimeras lost their tolerance upon depletion of donor antigen (20). Intrathymic clonal deletion has also been demonstrated in xenogeneic (rat → mouse) bone marrow chimeras (21). Other mechanisms that maintain tolerance in bone marrow transplant models, such as anergy and suppression have been suggested (22,23). Qin et al, demonstrated anergy in vivo, via induction of tolerance of adult mice to skin grafts, given after treating the recipient with CD4 and CD8 specific monoclonal antibodies plus donor bone marrow infusion (24). Recently, the same team (25) reported that the pathway to tolerance in murine bone marrow transplant models depends on the dose of bone marrow cells; while high dose marrow infusion (> 4×10^5 cells) created tolerance by central and peripheral deletion, low dose bone marrow infusion (< 4×10^5 cells) was associated with the development of suppression. This suppression was dependent on $CD4^+$ T cells and could be passed onto naive T cells as if infectious (25). A "veto" mechanism has been suggested for bone marrow cell engraftment (26). Any cell that can cause inactivation, anergy or death of a T cell upon its recognition by that T cell is a veto cell. Martin et al (27), reported that host effectors responsible for rejection could be inactivated through a veto mechanism in a marrow transplanted rodent model, and that not only $CD8^+$ (28), but also $CD4^+$ cells have this specific activity.

Creation of hematologic chimerism in adulthood requires conditioning of the host in order to impair its immune system and make "space" for engraftment for the donor cells (29). Total body (TBI) or lymphoid irradiation (TLI), cytoablative pharmacologic agents, thymectomy, antilymphocyte globulin (ALG) and monoclonal antibodies, or a combination of the above, have been used in order to facilitate bone marrow engraftment and are discussed in detail below (9,29).

The first allogeneic bone marrow chimeras were achieved in rodents forty years ago (30). A fully allogeneic chimera is the outcome of transplantation of allogeneic bone marrow into a lethally irradiated recipient (A→B) (31), so all the bone marrow derived cells are of donor origin. Transplantation of both syngeneic and allogeneic bone marrow into a lethally irradiated host (A + B→A) (31), or allogeneic bone marrow in a sublethally irradiated recipient (32) results in a mixed allogeneic chimera, first described by Singer, et. al. (33). Fully allogeneic chimeras are prone to graft versus host disease (GVHD) and are relatively immunoincompetent (34); primary immune responses, such as antibody production or antiviral reaction are impaired because antigen presenting cells (APC) of the host are absent (34). This can be avoided by using mixed allogeneic chimeras that do not develop GVHD and are immunocompetent (10,35). Furthermore, because the toxicity caused by lethal conditioning of the recipient represents a major limitation to a possible clinical application, production of mixed chimeric rodent models, obtained via sublethal conditioning, have been attempted (32, 36,37). Stable xenogeneic chimerism (rat → mouse) has been achieved by rat bone marrow transplantation into lethally irradiated mouse recipients. These chimeric mice were tolerant to donor rat skin and islet xenografts but reactive to third party rat and mouse grafts (38,39). It has been shown that 750 cGy is the minimal dose of total body irradiation (TBI) that allows for engraftment of rat bone marrow in mice (40). MHC-disparate bone marrow usually requires higher doses of TBI than MHC-congenic combinations. In order to avoid fully allogeneic bone marrow, one group reported a study in which transplantation of syngeneic bone marrow, that expressed a single donor class I MHC antigen, induced long term survival of a fully allogeneic cardiac graft (41).

In addition to recipient conditioning, depletion of T cells from donor bone marrow has been used to reduce the ability of donor marrow to attack the host and cause GVHD (42). Whereas this approach eliminates the risk of GVHD, it actually increases the incidence of rejection, so larger numbers of bone marrow cells or higher doses of irradiation of the recipient are necessary. Bone marrow does not cause GVHD in mixed allogeneic chimeras because they maintain their immunocompetence (43). Stable mixed chimeric mouse models (B10 mouse + B10.BR mouse → B10 mouse) that resulted from TCD bone marrow transplantation and conditioning with TBI (950 cGy) were specifically tolerant to donor skin grafts (35,44). Also, transplantation of TCD syngeneic mouse plus xenogeneic rat bone marrow into lethally conditioned mice resulted in mixed xenogeneic chimerism (45).

An alternative to total body irradiation is nonmyeloablative total lymphoid irradiation (TLI) (major lymph nodes, thymus and spleen), a less aggressive method for conditioning of the recipient before bone marrow infusion to induce mixed chimerism and tolerance (46,47,48). Even a short course of TLI (sTLI), followed by selective elimination of residual donor-specific alloreactive host T cells, prior to fully mismatched bone marrow transplantation, results in stable mixed chimeras, free of GVHD and capable of long-lasting acceptance of heterotopic heart muscle in mice (49).

Cytoreductive chemotherapeutic or immunosuppressive agents have also been used to create space in the recipient microenviroment. Cyclophosphamide (CyP) has been successfully used in combination with sublethal irradiation in mice to induce multilineage chimerism, and donor specific tolerance (50) and to reduce the minimum dose of irradiation required for engraftment (37). Cyclosporine (CyA) has been included in conditioning protocols in rodents to facilitate marrow engraftment, as it is an anti-T cell agent, but development of GVHD after its withdrawal has been observed in mouse chimeric models (51,52). It has been reported that FK-506 treatment of syngeneic bone marrow transplanted mice results in delay (53) but not inhibition (54) in T cell maturation. Despite the inhibition of activation-induced T cell apoptosis by FK-506, the drug does not affect thymic negative selection (54), that as has been mentioned earlier, is considered a major mechanism for tolerance induction in bone marrow chimeras. In experiments in fully allogeneic rats (Brown Norway → Lewis) cell suspensions of bone marrow, spleen, thymus and lymph node as well as, heart, kidney, and intestinal grafts were rejected without treatment, whereas a 2-week course of treatment with FK-506 prolonged graft survival to 100 days (55).

Monaco, Wood, and their colleagues initially demonstrated tolerance in mice, without myeloablative conditioning of the recipient. Cryopreserved bone marrow cells were transplanted a few days to 3 weeks after the primary allograft, with combination of ALS and thymectomy. Their experiment resulted in tolerance for skin grafts from F1 offsprings to parents (56), and subsequently, with a higher dose of bone marrow cells donor-specific tolerance was achieved with (57) or without thymectomy in non- F1 models (58,59). Mice treated with anti-CD4 and anti-CD8 specific monoclonal antibodies (mAbs) and bone marrow cells have been chimeric and tolerant to MHC-congenic skin grafts (55). ALG (37) and monoclonal antibodies (32,60,61) have been used in combination with nonlethal irradiation alone or with thymic irradiation for transplantation with MHC-disparate allogeneic or xenogeneic bone marrow resulting in prolonged acceptance of donor skin grafts. Interestingly, the importance of a functional Fas ligand has been recently addressed in an adult mouse model of ATG and donor bone marrow treatment (62). In this experiment, the survival of skin allografts in mice given bone marrow from C3H-gld mice, that have a FasL defect, was not prolonged beyond that of the controls (treated only with ATG).

Interaction of T cell receptor and antigen in the cleft of the MHC molecule, as well as secondary signals from surface molecules, such as CD28 and B7, are responsible for the T cell activation that causes rejection of allografts. A non-myeloablative protocol, using CTLA4-Ig, a protein that blocks the CD28:B7 pathway, and donor bone marrow, induced prolonged survival of murine cardiac allografts, donor-specific unresponsiveness to secondary skin grafts and evidence of hematopoietic chimerism in recipients with long-term graft survival (63). Because of persistence of donor cells in the peripheral lymph nodes and skin of the recipient, a functional role of hematopoietic chimerism could be assumed in this model, since CTLA4-Ig alone without bone marrow augmentation was not effective in inducing tolerance (64)

Transplantation of syngeneic bone marrow in combination with intrathymic inoculation of allogeneic bone marrow cells has successfully been used for tolerance and prevention of chronic rejection of cardiac (65) and renal allografts (66) without cytoablation, despite an absence of chimerism.

An additional impetus to continue to explore approaches to transplantation tolerance via the establishment of chimerism is the potential for prevention of recurrent diabetes in recipients of islet cell transplants. Establishment of chimerism could, theoretically, prevent both rejection and recurrence of autoimmunity in transplanted allogeneic islets. Studies in NOD mice have yielded evidence to support the concept that autoimmune diabetes is a disease that can be prevented by transplantation of bone marrow from diabetes resistant donors into irradiated NOD mice (67). Data has been published which demonstrates that mixed allogeneic chimerism, achieved with sublethal irradiation, can also prevent the occurrence of diabetes in NOD mice (68). Recently published data from Mathieu and Waer suggests that a minimum of 5%, and as much as 25%, chimerism may be essential to prevent the development of diabetes in cases where diabetes prone marrow is part of the hematopoietic system (69).

Attempts to reproduce the results generated in rodents have been undertaken in pre-clinical models such as dogs and non-human primates. In general the results in these models have not been as promising as those obtained in rodent models. The availability of novel immunointervention agents, such as anti-CD154, may allow for enhanced success in these models in the future. Tables 2 and 3 summarize studies done in these pre-clinical models.

Table 2.   Donor bone marrow infusion in dogs.

HOST CONDITIONING

1.   Total body irradiation (TB1) (70,71,72)
         a.   Plus immunosuppression (73,74,75)
         b.   Plus Ia-positive cells (76)
         c.   Plus donor lymphoid cells (77,78,79,80)
         d.   Plus granulocyte colony-stimulating factor (G-CSF) (81,82)
         e.   Plus anti-CD44 (83)
2.   Antilymphocyte serum (ALS) (84,85)
         a.   Antilymphocyte serum (ALS) plus cyclosporine (86,87,88,89,90)
         -   Plus prednisone (Pr) and azathioprine (Aza) (91)
         -   Plus rapamycin (Rapa) (92)
         b. Antilymphocyte serum (ALS) plus azathioprine (Aza) (93)
3.   Class II Dim donor bone marrow plus CsA (94)
4.   Monoclonal antibody plus CsA (95,96)

DONOR CONDITIONING
T cell depletion (97,98)

Table 3. Donor bone marrow infusion in non-human primates.

HOST CONDITIONING

1.   Total body irradiation (TB1) (99)
2.   Antithymocyte globulin (ATG) (100,101,102)
       a.   Antithymocyte globulin (ATG) plus cyclosporine (103)

DONOR CONDITIONING

1.   T-cell depleted (TCD) bone marrow into irradiated recipient (104,105)
2.   DR depleted bone marrow (106)
       a.   DR depleted bone narrow into ATG-treated recipient (107
       b.   DR and CD3 depleted bone marrow (108)

ATTEMPTS TO INDUCE TOLERANCE VIA HEMATOPOIETIC STEM CELL TRANSPLANTATION: HUMAN TRIALS

Based on studies performed in rodents, Monaco and colleagues performed a clinical simultaneous bone marrow / kidney transplant (109). A cadaveric renal allograft recipient was immunosuppressed with prednisone and azathioprine, plus induction therapy with anti-lymphocyte serum (ALS) for the first 14 days post-transplant, and infused with 11 billion donor bone marrow cells on post operative day (POD) 25 (109). The patient eventually expired from peritonitis but did not experience clinical rejection episodes during the 8 months of follow-up. Minimal evidence of rejection was observed at autopsy (109). In his discussion of the results, Monaco acknowledged the experience gained from pre-transplant blood transfusion studies, which highlighted the importance of the number and timing of infusions in obtaining a successful outcome (109). In subsequent clinical studies, Barber and colleagues assessed the impact of donor bone marrow infusion on the survival of allogeneic kidneys. Patients were treated with CsA, prednisone, azathioprine, and Minnesota ALG on POD 1-11, and donor bone marrow was infused on POD 18; CsA was not given on the day of BMC infusion (110,111). Although one year graft survival was improved in recipients of marrow, no significant difference in the number of rejection episodes, estimated renal plasma flow, glomerular filtration rate, or urine protein were observed (110). Subsequent reports of microchimerism in long-term human transplant recipients who had discontinued immunosuppression, yet did not reject their grafts (112,113), led the group to reanalyze their patients with regards to the presence of chimerism (111). It was later observed that recipients

116

of donor marrow, with demonstrable chimerism, were 91.3% rejection-free as compared to controls, with 85.7% of the control patients experiencing at least one episode of rejection (111).

Studies of long term human transplant recipients who had discontinued their immunosuppressive medications, yet had not rejected their kidney or liver allografts, have revealed the presence of multilineage microchimerism, with repopulation of host tissues with donor derived dendritic cells 27-29 years posttransplant (112,113). The concept of infusing donor bone marrow at the time of solid organ or cellular transplant, to enhance the potential for the establishment and maintenance of chimerism, which might lead to donor specific tolerance, was therefore proposed, followed by the initiation of clinical trials (114). Starzl and his colleagues reported the results obtained from a trial including 36 organ allograft recipients of 3 x 10^8/kg whole vertebral body marrow cells (VBMC) obtained from the organ donor (114). The levels of chimerism in recipients of VBMC were 1000 fold higher than the control group, and a positive correlation between a functioning graft and the ability to detect donor derived cells (PCR based methodology) in the peripheral blood was observed (114). Over 50% of the VBMC recipients were MLR hyporesponsive to donor cells, as compared to 12.5% in the control group (115). At 3 years follow-up, a significantly lower incidence of late, acute cellular rejection was observed for anti-donor MLR hyporesponsive recipients of VBMC as compared to patients who received VBMC but retained anti-donor reactivity (116).

Results emerging from clinical trials at the University of Miami Medical School strongly support a graft promoting effect of donor bone marrow infusion on allograft survival. From July of 1994 through July of 1997, 417 recipients of various cadaveric solid organ allografts were infused with bone marrow cells derived from the vertebral bodies of the organ donor (Table 4). Fifteen of these solid organ recipients also received islet allografts (Table 4). In addition, several living-related kidney (117) and 3 living-related liver allografts (118) have been performed. The source of donor hematopoietic cells has been iliac crest aspirate (117) and mobilized peripheral blood (118) for the kidney and liver transplant patients, respectively. Results from immunofluorescent labeling and flow cytometric analysis of these various cell sources are shown in Table 5. Calculation of the number of CD34$^+$ stem cells (SC) and CD3$^+$ T cells infused per billion CD45$^+$ cells reveals that vertebral body marrow > iliac crest marrow > mobilized peripheral blood (MPB) with regards to the CD34$^+$ SC content (Table 6). With regards to T cell content, iliac crest (IC) marrow contains the smallest number and vertebral body marrow (VBM) contains slightly more (Table 6). MPB, on the other hand, has almost 4 and 6 times more T cells than VBM and IC marrow, respectively (Table 6).

Table 4. Solid Organ/Bone Marrow Recipients As of 7/23/97

Liver Alone	266
Multivisceral	23
Liver / Kidney	13
Liver/ Kidney / Islets	1
Liver / Islets	5
Liver / Heart	1
Small Bowel	5
Kidney Alone	72
Kidney / Pancreas	22
Kidney / Islet	9
Total	***417***

In the absence of cytoablation, the variables of cell dose, timing of infusion, and type of induction therapy play a key role in the enhancement of allograft acceptance.   The results from initial clinical trials of liver/bone marrow transplantation at the University of Miami revealed that, while one donor bone marrow infusion at the time of allogeneic liver transplant (primary transplant) resulted in an increase in the incidence of acute rejection (n=9), two (n=26) or more (n=37) delayed infusions (beginning at day 5 post-transplant) resulted in a significant decrease in the incidence of rejection and in significant improvement in graft and patient survival (119,120). As the cell dose and number of infusions were increased, however, an increase in the incidence of graft versus host disease (GVHD), which was not a concern with one infusion, was observed (120). Significant improvement in graft survival continues to hold at 3 years follow-up, and a significant decrease in the incidence of acute rejection episodes and major bacterial infection has been observed (C Ricordi and A. Tzakis, manuscript in preparation).

With regards to chimerism, studies in liver transplant recipients have demonstrated that microchimerism occurs at higher levels in recipients of donor marrow (very low levels can occur with liver transplantation alone) as compared to controls. The data is being analyzed to determine if any correlation exists between the occurrence of chimerism and graft rejection/acceptance. In addition to the recipients of cadaveric livers, 3 living-related liver transplants have been done (118). One complete HLA mismatch, one haploidentical, and one HLA identical transplant were performed (118). In the absence of cytoablation, and despite the high content of $CD3^{+}$ T cells (Tables 5,6), GVHD (successfully resolved) was only observed in the recipient of mismatched liver/marrow (118).

Table 5. Composition of Donor Hematopoietic Stem Cell Sources[1]

Percentage Positive[5]

	N	CD45	CD34	HLA-DR	CD3	CD4	CD8	CD19	CD14	CD33	CD15
VBM[2]	20-27	85.2 (7.7)	3.2 (1.5)	10.7 (5.0)	6.7 (2.7)	4.2 (2.7)	5.1 (3.5)	6.6 (4.0)	2.7 (2.0)	58.8 (20.1)	56.3 (9.5)
IC[3]	17-20	84.9 (15.3)	1.1 (0.7)	7.5 (3.7)	4.5 (1.6)	2.9 (1.8)	2.5 (1.2)	4.3 (4.1)	3.8 (2.7)	68.5 (23.2)	60.6 (17.5)
MPB[4]	1-3	82.0 (13.0)	0.7 (0.2)	28.5 (19.6)	26.3 (4.2)	19.2 (1.3)	15.7 (11.1)	23.8 (2.9)	24.3 (5.4)	34.0 (12.6)	13.7

1.   *Results from flow cytometric analysis of the total cell population (total gate)*
2.   *Vertebral body marrow, RBC lysed*
3.   *Iliac crest aspirate, RBC lysed*
4.   *Mobilized peripheral blood, unlysed*
5.   *Mean ± (SD)*

With regards to kidney/bone marrow recipients, stem cells of donor origin have been documented in the peripheral blood and bone marrow of these patients, and a correlation between the degree of stem cell engraftment and total cell dose/number of infusions has been observed (121). A decrease in chimerism has been observed in conjunction with rejection episodes (117,121,122). Interestingly, recipients of iliac crest marrow and living-related kidney transplants achieve higher levels of chimerism, thus highlighting the role of MHC compatibility in engraftment (117,122). A clear decrease in the incidence of chronic rejection has been observed for kidney/bone marrow recipients as compared to patients who receive kidneys alone (117). For both kidney and liver transplant patients, the levels of chimerism at one year post-transplant are on the order of 1%, a level that may not be adequate for the induction and maintenance of donor specific tolerance.

With regards to recipients of combined solid organ/islet allografts, donor bone marrow infusion on POD 5 and 11 did not result in enhancement of islet survival, despite continued function of the transplanted organ (R. Alejandro and C. Ricordi, manuscript in preparation). It has been postulated that loss of the islets could be due to the occurrence of subclinical GVHD. Since the liver is a primary target of GVHD, production of proinflammatory mediators, such as cytokines and nitric oxide, could lead to islet damage, as beta cells are known to be highly sensitive to these molecules (123). An additional possibility is that, while infusion of donor marrow on POD 0 increases the incidence of rejection in liver transplant recipients, POD 0 infusion may actually be critical for islet cell recipients, as islets do not contain a substantial component of hematopoietic cells. Evidence in support of a graft promoting effect of DBMC infusion, administered on POD 0, 5, 10, 15, and 20, on islet allograft survival has been obtained in a canine model of islet/bone marrow transplantation (124). Ongoing studies in non-human primate models also suggest that POD 5 and 11 infusion may not be optimal for islet cell transplantation (N. Kenyon and C. Ricordi, unpublished data). In addition to issues of timing, the nature of graft promoting cells is being investigated. Preliminary data in a canine model suggests that, similar to data obtained in rodent models, $CD8^+$ cells may play a key role in enhancing islet allograft survival (N. Kenyon and C. Ricordi, unpublished). In this regard, this field may face the same issues that challenge traditional applications of bone marrow transplantation, namely that elimination of $CD8^+$ cells clearly prevents GVHD but also results in a lack of engraftment.

The results of recent studies clearly support a graft promoting effect of donor hematopoietic cell infusion on the survival of transplanted allogeneic cells or organs. The levels of chimerism achieved, however, are low and may be inadequate to induce a state of donor specific tolerance. Identification of approaches to 1) increase the levels of engraftment and chimerism in the mismatched setting and 2) employ bone marrow cells as a stimulus to induce donor specific tolerance (e.g., in the presence of costimulatory blockade), are clearly critical to the eventual success and broad based application of bone marrow transplantation in the fields of solid organ and cellular allotransplantation.

Table 6. Number of [1]Stem Cells and [2]T Cells Infused per [3]Billion CD45 Positive Cells

	STEM CELLS	T CELLS
VBM	32×10^6	67×10^6
IC	11×10^6	45×10^6
MPB	7×10^6	263×10^6

1.   Defined as CD34 + Cells
2.   Defined as CD3 + Cells
3.   For the purposes of this calculation, the percentage of CD45 + Cells in VBM, IC, and MPB were considered to be equal. Actual % of CD45 + Cells was 85.2, 84.9, and 82.0 for VBM, IC, and MPB, respectively (see table 3).

REFERENCES

1. Nagano H and Tilney NL. Chronic allograft failure: the clinical problem. The Amer J of the Med Sci 1997; 313(5):305-309.
2. Gaya SB, Rees AJ, Lechler RI, Williams G, Mason PD: Malignant disease in patients with long-term renal transplants.   Transplantation 1995; 59(12):1705-1709.
3. Balistreri WF, Bucuvalas JC, Ryckman FC: The effect of immunosuppression on growth and development. Liver Transl Surg 1995; 1 (suppl 5):64-73.
4. Andoh TF, Burdmann EA, and Bennett WM: Nephrotoxicity of immunosuppressive drugs: experimental and clinical observations. Sem in Nephrol 1997; 17(1):34-45.
5. Boudreaux JP, McHugh L, Canafax DM, Ascher N, Sutherland DE, Payne W, Simmons RL, Najarian JS, Fryd DS: The impact of cyclosporine and combination immunosuppression on the incidence of posttransplant diabetes in renal allograft recipients. Transplantation 1987; 44(3):376-381.
6. Teuscher AU, Seaquist ER, Robertson DP: Diminished insulin secretory reserve in diabetic pancreas transplant and nondiabetic kidney transplant recipients. Diabetes 1994; 43(4):593-598.
7. Christiansen E, Andersen HB, Rasmussen K, Christensen NJ, Olgaard K, Kirkegaard P, Tronier B, Volund A, Damsbo P, Burcharth F, et al: Pancreatic beta-cell function and glucose metabolism in human segmental

pancreas and kidney transplantation. Am J Physiol 1993; 264(3):E441-E449.

8. Schmaldienst S and Horl WH: Bacterial infections after renal transplantation. Nephron 1997; 75:140-153.

9. Charlton B, Auchincloss Jr, H, Fathman CG: Mechanisms of transplantation tolerance. Ann Rev Immunol 1994; 12:707-734.

10. Kostecke RA, Ildstad ST: Chimerism and the facilitating cell. Transplant Rev 1995; 9:97-110.

11. Stewart FM, Crittenden RB, Lowry PA, Pearson-White S, Quesenberry PJ: Long-term engraftment of normal and post-5-fluorouracil murine marrow into normal nonmyeloablated mice. Blood 1993; 81:2566-2571.

12. Blumberg N, Heal JM: Effects of transfusion on immune function. Cancer recurrence and infection. Arch Pathol Lab Med 1994; 118:371-379.

13. Brennan DC, Mohanakumar T, Flye W: Donor-specific transfusion and donor bone marrow infusion in renal transplantation tolerance: a review of efficacy and mechanisms. Amer J of Kidney Dis 1995; 26(5):701-715.

14. Owen RD: Immunogenic consequences of vascular anastomosis between bovine twins. Science 1945; 102: 400-401.

15. Anderson D, Billingham RE, Lampkin GH, Medawar PB, Williams HLI: Heredity 1951; 5: 379-397.

16. Billingham RE, Brent L, Medawar P: Actively acquired tolerance of foreign cells. Nature 1953; 172: 603-606.

17. Kappler JW, Roehm N, Marrack P: T cell tolerance by clonal elimination in the thymus. Cell 1987; 49: 273-280.

18. Wood PJ, Streilein JW: Ontogeny of acquired immunological tolerance to H-2 alloantigens. Eur J Immunol 1982; 12: 188-194.

19. Cuttler AJ, Bell EB: Neonatally tolerant rats actively eliminate donor-specific lymphocytes despite persistent chimerism. Eur J Immunol 1996; 26: 320-328.

20. Khan A, Tomita Y, Sykes M: Thymic dependence of loss of tolerance in mixed allogeneic bone marrow chimeras after depletion of donor antigen. Transplantation 1996; 62(3): 380-387.

21. Nikolic B, Lei H, Pearson DA, Sergio JJ, Swenson KG, Sykes M. Role of intrathymic rat class II+ cells in maintaining deletional tolerance in xenogeneic rat → mouse bone marrow chimeras. Transplantation 1998; 65: 1216-1224.

22. Tutschka PJ, Ki PF, Beschorner WE, Hess AD, Santos GW. Suppressor cells in the transplantation tolerance. II. Maturation of suppressor cells in the bone marrow chimera. Transplantation 1981; 32: 321-325.

23. Roser BJ: Cellular mechanisms in neonatal and adult tolerance. Immunol Rev 1989; 107:179-202.

24. Qin S, Cobbold SP, Benjamin R, Waldman H. Imduction of classical transplantation tolerance in the adult. J Exp Med 1990; 169: 779-794.

25. Bemelman F, Honey K, Adams E, Cobbold S, Waldmann H. Bone marrow transplantation induces either clonal deletion or infectious tolerance depending on the dose. J Immunol 1998; 160: 2645-2648.
26. Wood ML, Orosz CG, Gottschalk R, Monaco AP: The effect of injection of donor bone marrow on the frequency of donor-reactive CTL in antilymphocyte serum-treated, grafted mice. Transplantation 1992; 54: 665-671.
27. Martin P: Prevention of allogeneic marrow graft rejection by donor T cells that do not recognize recipient alloantigens: potential role of a veto mechanism. Blood 1996; 88(3): 962-969.
28. Sambhara SR, Miller RG: Programmed cell death of T cells signaled by the T cell receptor and the a 3 domain of class I MHC: Science 1991; 252:1424-1427.
29. Jankowski RA, Ildstad ST: Chimerism and tolerance: from freemartin cattle and neonatal mice to humans. Hum Immunol 1997; 52: 155-161.
30. Trentin JJ: Mortality and skin transplantability in X-irradiated mice receiving isologous, homologous or heterologous bone marrow. Proc Soc Exp Biol Med 1957; 92: 688-693.
31. Ildstad ST, Sachs DH: Reconstitution with syngeneic plus allogeneic or xenogeneic bone marrow leads to specific acceptance of allografts or xenografts. Nature 1984; 307:168-170.
32. Sharabi Y, Sachs DH: Mixed chimerism and permanent specific transplantation tolerance induced by a nonlethal preparative regimen. J Exp Med 1989; 169: 493-502.
33. Singer A, Hathcock KS, Hodes RJ: Self recognition in allogeneic radiation bone marrow chimeras. A radiation-resistant host element dictates the self specificity and immune response gene phenotype of T-helper cells. J Exp Med 1981; 153; 1286-1301.
34. Ildstad S, Wren S, Bluestone J, Barbieri S, Stephany D, Sachs D: Effect of selective T cell depletion of host and/or donor bone marrow on hemtopoietic repopulation, tolerance, and graft-vs-host disease in mixed allogeneic chimeras (B10 + B10.D2→ B10). J Immunol 1986, 136:28-33.
35. Ruedi E, Sykes M, Ildstad S, Chester C, Althage A, Hengartner H, Sachs S, Zinkernagel R: Antiviral T cell competence and restriction specificity of mixed aloogeneic (P1+ P2→ P1) irradiation chimeras. Cell Immunol 1989; 121: 185-195.
36. McCarthy SA, Griffith IJ, Gambel P, Francescutti LH, Wegman TG: Characterization of host lymphoid cells in antibody-facilitated bone marrow chimeras. Transplantation 1985; 40: 12-17.
37. Colson Y, Li H, Boggs SS, Patrene KD, Johnson PC, Ildstad ST: Durable mixed allogeneic chimerism and tolerance by a nonlethal radiation-based cytoreductive approach. J Immunol 1996; 157: 2820-2829.

38. Ildstad ST, Wren SM, Boggs SS, Hronakes ML, Vecchini F, van den Brink MRM: Cross-species bone marrow transplantation: evidence for tolerance induction, stem cell engraftment, and maturation of T-lymphocytes in a xenogeneic stromal enviroment (rat (mouse). J Exp Med 1991; 174: 467-478.

39. Zeng YJ, Ricordi C, Tzakis A, Rilo HLR, Caroll PB, Starzl TE, Ildstad ST: Long term survival of donor-specific pancreatic islet xenografts in fully xenogeneic chimeras (WF rat → B10 mouse). Transplantation 1992; 53:277-283.

40. Abou El-Ezz AY, Boggs SS, Johnson PC, Li H, Patrene KD, Istkowitz MS, Kaufman CL, Ildstad ST: A minimal conditioning approach to achieve stable multilineage mouse plus rat chimerism. Transplant Immunol 1995; 3: 98-106.

41. Wong W, Morris,PJ, Wood K: Syngeneic bone marrow expressing a single donor class I MHC molecule permits acceptance of a fully allogeneic cardiac allograft. Transplantation 1996; 632(10): 1462-1468.

42. Vallera DA, Blazar BR: T cell depletion for graft- versus-host disease prophylaxis. A perspective on engraftment in mice and humans. Transplantation 1989; 47: 751-760.

43. Sykes M, Eisenthal A, Sachs DH: Mechanism of protection from graft-vs.-host disease in murine mixed allogeneic chimeras: I. Development of a null cell population supprressive of CML responses and derived from the syngeneic bone marrow compartment. J Immunol 1988; 140: 2903-2911.

44. Ildstad ST, Wren SM, Oh E, Hronakes ML: Mixed allogeneic reconstitution (A+B→A) to induce donor-specific transplantation tolerance: permanent acceptance of simultaneous skin grafts. Transplantation 1991; 51:1262-1267.

45. Ildstad ST, Boggs SS, Vecchini F, Wren SM, Hronakes ML, Johnson PG, Van den Brink MRM: Mixed xenogeneic chimeras (rat + mouse → rat): evidence for rat stem cell engraftment, strain-specific transplantation tolerance, and skin-specific antigens. Transplantation 1992; 53: 815-822.

46. Slavin S, Strober S, Fuks Z, Kaplan HS: Induction of specific tissue transplantation tolerance using fractionated total lymphoid irradiation in adult mice: long-term survival of allogeneic bone marrow and skin grafts. J Exp Med 1977; 146:34-48.

47. Zan-Bar I, Slavin S, Strober S: Induction and mechanism of tolerance to bovine serum albumin in mice given total lymphoid irradiation (TLI). J Immunol 1978; 121: 1400-1404.

48. Slavin S, Reitz B, Bieber CP, Kaplan HS, Strober S: Transplantation tolerance in adult rats using total lymphoid irradiation: permanent survival of skin, heart, and marrow alllografts. J Exp Med 1978; 147:700-707.

49. Prigozhina TB, Gurevitch O, Zhu J, Slavin S: Permanent and specific transplantation tolerance induced by a nonmyeloablative treatment to a wide variety of allontigeneic tissues. Transplantation 1997; 63:1394-1399.

50. Colson YL, Wren SM, Schuchert MJ, Patrene KD, Johnson PC, Boggs SS, Ildstad ST: A nonlethal conditioning approach to achieve durable multilineage mixed chimerism and tolerance across major, minor, and hematopoietic histocompatibility barriers. J Immunol 1995; 155: 4179-4188.

51. Bryson JS, Jennings CD, Caywood BE, Kaplan AM: Induction of a syngeneic graft-versus-host disease-like syndrome in DBA/2 mice. Transplantation 1989; 48: 1042-1047.

52. Bryson JS, Caywood BE, Kaplan AM: Relationship of cyclosporine A-mediated inhibition of clonal deletion and development of syngeneic graft-versus-host disease. J Immunol 1991; 147: 391-397.

53. Woo J, Ildstad ST, Thompson AW: FK 506 inhibits the differentiation of developing thymocytes but not negative selection of T cell receptor Vβ5$^+$ and Vβ11$^+$ T lymphocytes in vivo. Transplant Immunol 1994; 2: 11-21.

54. Woo J, Thomson AW, Ildstad ST: Effects of FK 506 on chimerism and the induction of donor-specific unresponsiveness following fully allogeneic bone marrow transplantation in mice. Transplant Immunol 1995; 3: 86-90.

55. Murace N, Starzl TE, Tanabe M, Fujisaki S, Miyazawa H, Ye Q, Delaney CP, Fung JJ, Demetris AJ: Variable chimerism, graft-versus-host disease, and tolerance after different kinds of cell and whole organ transplantation from Lewis to Brown Norway rats. Transplantation 1995; 60: 158-171.

56. Monaco AP, Wood ML, Russel PS: Studies on heterologous antilymphocyte serum in mice. III. Immunologic tolerance and chimerism produced across the H-2 locus with adult thymectomy and anti-lymphocyte serum. Ann NY Acad Sci 1966; 129: 190-206.

57. Monaco AP, Wood ML: Studies on heterologous antilymphocyte serum in mice. VII. Optimal cellular antigen for induction of immunologic tolerance with antilymphocyte serum. Transplant Proc 1970; 2: 489-496.

58. Wood ML, Monaco AP, Gozzo JJ, Liegeois A: Use of homozygous allogeneic bone marrow for induction of tolerance with antilymphocyte serum: dose and timing. Transplant Proc 1971; 3: 676-679.

59. Wood ML, Monaco AP: The effect of timing of skin grafts on subsequent survival in ALS-treated, marrow-infused mice. Transplantation 1977; 23: 78-86.

60. Sharabi Y, Aksentijevich I, Sundt TM III, Sachs DH, Sykes M: Specific tolerance induction across a xenogeneic barrier: production of mixed rat/mouse lymphohematopoietic chimeras using a nonlethal preparative regimen. J Exp Med 1990; 172: 195-202.

61. de Vries-van der Zwan A, Besseling C, de Waal LP, Boog CJ: Specific tolerance induction and transplantation: a single-day protocol. Blood 1997; 89: 2596-2601.

62. George JF, Sweeney SD, Kirklin JK, Simpson EM, Goldstein DR, Thomas JM: An essential role for Fas ligand in transplantation tolerance induced by donor bone marrow. Nat Med 1998; 4: 333-335.

63. Pearson TC, Alexander DZ, Hendrix R, Elwood ET, Lisnley PS, Winn KJ, Larsen CP: CTLA4-Ig plus bone marrow induces long term allograft survival and donor specific unresponsiveness in the murine model. Transplantation 1996; 61; 997-1004.

64. Lin H, Bolling SF, Linsley PS, Wei RQ, Gordon D, Thompson CB, Turka LA: Long-term acceptance of major histocompatibility complex mismatched cardiac allografts induced by CTLA4-Ig plus donor specific transfusion. J Exp Med 1993; 178: 1801-1806.

65. Orloff MS, DeMara EM, Coppage ML, Leong N, Fallon MA, Sickel J, Zuo XJ, Prehn J, Jordan SC: Prevention of chronic rejection and graft arteriosclerosis by tolerance induction. Transplantation 1995; 59: 282-288.

66. Blom D, Morrissey N, Mesonero C, Zuo XJ, Jordan S, Fisher T, Bronsther O, Orloff MS: Tolerance induction by intrathymic inoculation presents chronic renal allograft rejection. Transplantation 1998; 65:272-275.

67. LaFace DW, Peck AB: Reciprocal allogeneic bone marrow transplantation between NOD mice and diabetes – nonsusceptible mice associated with transfer and prevention of autoimmune diabetes. Diabetes 1989; 38:894.

68. Li H, Kaufman CL, Boggs SS, Johnson PC, Patrene KD, Ildstad ST: Mixed allogeneic chimerism induced by a sublethal approach prevents autoimmune diabetes and reverses insulitis in nonobese diabetic (NOD) mice. J Immunol 1996; 156(1):380-388.

69. Mathieu C, Casteels K, Bouillon R, Waer M: Protection against autoimmune diabetes in mixed bone chimeras. J Immunol 1997; 158:1453-1457.

70. Storb R, Raff RF, Appelbaum FR, Deeg HJ, Graham TC, Schuening FG, Sale G, Bryant E, Seidel K: Fractionated versus-dose total body irradiation at low and high dose rates to condition canine littermates for DLA-Identical marrow grafts. Blood 1994; 83(11):3384-3389.

71. Storb R, Raff RF, Deeg HJ, Graham TC, Schuening FG, Shulman H, Bryant E: DLA-Identical marrow grafts after low-dose total-body irradiation. Transplantation 1995; 59(10): 1481-1502.

72. Storb R, Raff R, Deeg HJ, Graham T, Appelbaum FR, Scheuning FG, Shulman H, Seidel K, Leisenring W: Dose rate-dependent sparing of the gastrointestinal tract by fractionated total body irradiation in dogs given marrow autografts. Physics 1998; 40(4): 961-966.

73. Yu C, Storb R, Deeg HJ, Graham TC, Scheuning FG, Huss R, Seidel K, Fitzsimmons WE: Tacrolimus (FK506) and methotrexate regimens to prevent graft-versus-host disease after unrelated dog leukocyte antigen (DLA) nonidentical marrow transplantation. Bone Marrow Transplantation 1996; 17(4):649-653.

74. Storb R, Yu C, Wagner JL, Deeg HJ, Nash RA, Kiem HP, Leisenring W, Shulman H: Stable mixed hematopoietic chimerism in DLA-identical littermate dogs given sublethal total body irradiation before and pharmacological immunosuppression after marrow transplantation. Blood 1997; 89(8):3048-54.

75. Yu C, Seidel K, Nash RA, Deeg HJ, Sandmaier BM, Barsoukov A, Santos E, Storb R: Synergism between mycophenolate mofetil and cyclosporine in preventing graft-versus-host disease among lethally irradiated dogs given DLA-nonidentical unrelated marrow grafts. Blood 1998; 91(7):2581-2587.

76. Berenson RJ, Bensinger WI, Kalamasz D, Schuening F, Deeg HJ, Graham T, Storb R: Engraftment of dogs with Ia-positive marrow cells isolated by Avidin-Biotin immunoadsorption. Blood 1987; 69(5):1363-1367.

77. Storb R, Epstein RB, Ragde H, Thomas ED: Marrow grafts by combined marrow and leukocyte infusions in unrelated dogs selected by histocompatibility typing. Transplantation 1979; 6:587-593.

78. Deeg HJ, Storb R, Weiden PL, et al: Abrogation of resistance to and enhancement in DLA-nonidentical unrelated marrow grafts in lethally irradiated dogs by thoracic duct lymphocytes. Blood 1979; 53:552-557.

79. Storb R, Deeg HJ: Failure of allogeneic canine marrow grafts after total body irradiation. Allogeneic 'resistance' versus transfusion-induced sensitization. Transplantation 1986; 42:571-580.

80. Schwarzinger I, Raff RF, Flowers M, Niederwieser D, Graham T, Shulman H, Appelbaum FR, Scheuning F, Storb R: Recipient-specific donor cytotoxic T lymphocytes enhance engraftment of unrelated, DLA non-identical canine marrow. Bone Marrow Transplantation 1994; 13:303-309.

81. De Revel T, Appelbaum FR, Storb R, Scheuning F, Nash R, Deeg HJ, McNiece I, Andrews R,, Graham T: Effects of granulocyte colony-stimulating factor and stem cell factor, alone and in combination, on the mobilization of peripheral blood cells that engraft lethally irradiated dogs. Blood 1994; 83(12):3795-3799.

82. Storb R, Raff RF, Appelbaum FR, Deeg HJ, Graham T, Scheuning FG, Shulman H, Yu C, Bryant E, Burnett R, Seidel K: DLA-identical bone marrow grafts after low-dose total body irradiation: The effect of canine recombinant hematopoietic growth factors. Blood 1994; 84(10):3558-3566.

83. Sandmaier BM, Storb R, Bennett KL, Appelbaum FR, Santos EB: Epitope specificity of CD44 for monoclonal antibody-dependent facilitation of marrow engraftment in a canine model. Blood 1998; 91(9):3494-3502.

84. Caridis T, Liegeois A, Barrett I, Monaco AP: Enhanced survival of canine real allografts of ALS-treated dogs given bone marrow. Transplantation Proc 1973; 5:671-673.
85. Hartner WC, De Fazio SR, Maki T, Markees TG, Monaco AP, Gozzo JJ: Prolongation of renal allograft survival in antilymphocyte serum-treated dogs by postoperative injection of density-gradient-fractionated donor bone marrow. Transplantation 1986; 42:593-597.
86. Hartner WC, De Fazio SR, Markees TG, Maki T, Monaco AP, Gozzo JJ: Specific tolerance to canine renal allografts following treatment with fractionated bone marrow and antilymphocyte serum. Transplantation Proc 1987; 19:476-477.
87. Hartner WC, De Fazio SR, Markees TG, Khouri WA, Maki T, Monaco AP, Gozzo JJ: Effect of cyclosporin A supplementation and on renal allograft survival in ALS plus bone marrow treated dogs. Transplantation Proc 1989; 21(1):959-960.
88. Hartner WC, Markees TC, De Fazio SR, et al: the effect of antilymphocyte serum, fractionated donor bone marrow, and cyclosporine on renal allograft survival in mongrel dogs. Transplantation 1991; 52:784-789.
89. Hartner WC, Shaffer D, Markees TG, De Fazio SR, Monaco AP, Gozzo JJ: Effect of cyclosporine A treatment on induction of donor specific unresponsiveness in mongrel dogs following a short course of ALS and donor bone marrow infusion. Transplantation Proc 1991; 23:477-479.
90. Hartner WC, Markees TG, De Fazio SR, Shaffer D, Van der Werf WJ, Gilchrist B, Yatko C, Monaco AP, Gozzo JJ: Effect of early administration of donor bone marrow cells on renal allograft survival in dogs treated with antilymphocyte serum and cyclosporine. Transplantation 1995; 59(1):131-154.
91. Mathews KA, Holmberg DL, Johnston K, Miller CM, Binnington AG, Maxie G, Atilola M, Smith G: Renal allograft survival in outbred mongrel dogs using rabbit anti-dog thymocyte serum in combination with immunosuppressive drug therapy with or without donor bone marrow. Veterinary Surgery 1994; 23:347-357.
92. Hartner WC, Van der Werf WJ, Lodge JP, Gilchrist B, De Fazio SR, Markees TG, Yatko C, Monaco AP, Gozzo JJ: Effect of rapamycin on renal allograft survival in canine recipients treated with antilymphocyte serum, donor bone marrow, and cyclosporine. Transplantation 1995; 60(11):1347-1350.
93. Yamamoto M: Prolongation of canine renal allograft survival in combined therapy with rabbit-anti-dog antilymphocytic serum, azathioprine and the allotransplantation of the donor's bone marrow. Tohoku J. Exp Med. 1970; 101:333-338.

94. Kenyon NS, Selvaggi G, Fernandez L, Xu XM, Knapp J, Montelongo J, McMannis J, Russel TR, Alejandro R, Ricordi: Infusion of class II DIM donor bone marrow enhances islet allograft survival in low-dose CyA treated dogs. Transplantation Proc 1997; 29(4):2189.

95. Brendel MD, Kong SS, Schachner RD, Qian T, Selvaggi G, Alejandro R, Mintz DH, Ricordi C, Federlin K, Bretzel RG: The influence of donor specific vertebral body derived bone marrow cell infusion on canine islet allograft survival without irradiation conditioning of the recipient. Exp & Clin Endocrine & Diabetes 1995; 103(2):129-132.

96. Brendel MD, Kong SS, Schachner RD, Qian T, Selvaggi G, Alejandro R, Mintz DH, Ricordi C: Canine islet allograft survival after donor specific vertebral body derived bone marrow cell transplantation without irradiation conditioning of the recipient. Transplantation Proc 1995; 27(6):3174.

97. Schumm M, Gunther W, Kolb HJ, Rieber P, Buttner M, Voss C, Kremmer E, Reitmeier P, Thierfelder S, Wilmanns W: Prevention of graft-versus-host disease in DLA-haplotype mismatched dogs and hemopoietic engraftment of CD6-depleted marrow with and without cG-CSF treatment after transplantation. Tissue Antigens 1994; 43:170-178.

98. Kolb HJ, Gunther W, Schumm M, Holler E, Wilmanns W, Thierfelder S: Adoptive immunotherapy in canine chimeras. Transplantation 1997; 63(3):430-436.

99. Wagemaker G, Vriesendorp HM, and van Bekkum DW: Successful bone marrow transplantation across major histocompatibility barriers in Rhesus monkeys. Transplantation Proc 1981; 13(1):875-880.

100. Thomas FT, Carver FM, Foil MB, Pryor WH, Larkin EW, Hall WR, Haisch CE, Thomas JM: Long-term incompatible kidney survival in outbred higher primates without chronic immunosuppression. Ann. Surg 1983; 370-378.

101. Thomas J, Carver M, Cunningham P, Park K, Gonder J, Thomas F: Promotion of incompatible allograft acceptance in rhesus monkeys given posttransplant antithymocyte globulin and donor bone marrow: Transplantation 1987; 43(3):332-338.

102. Thomas JM, Carver FM, Foil MB, Hall WR, Adams C, Fahrenbruch GB, Thomas FT: Renal allograft tolerance induced with ATG and donor bone marrow in outbred rhesus monkeys. Transplantation 1993; 36(1):104-106. .

103. Thomas JM, Carver M, Cunningham P, Sash C, Park K, Thomas F: Promotion of incompatible allograft acceptance in rhesus monkeys given posttransplant antithymocyte globulin and donor bone marrow II. Effects of adjuvant immunosuppressive drugs. Transplantation 1989; 47:209-215. .

129

104. Moses RD, Orr DS, Bacher JD, Sachs DH, Clark RE, Gress RE: Cardiac allograft survival across major histocompatibility complex barriers in the rhesus monkey following T Lymphocyte-depleted autologous marrow transplantation. II. Prolonged allograft survival with extensive marrow T cell depletion. Transplantation 1989; 47(3):435-444.

105. Moses RD, Sharrow SO, Stephany DA, Orr KS, Gress RE: Cardiac allograft survival across major histocompatibility complex barriers in the rhesus monkey following T Lymphocyte-depleted autologous marrow transplantation. Transplantation 1989; 48:774-781.

106. Thomas JM, Carver FM, Kasten-Jolly J, Haisch CE, Rebellato LM, Gross U, Vore SJ, Thomas FT: Further studies of veto activity in rhesus monkey bone marrow in relation to allograft tolerance and chimerism. Transplantation 1994; 57:101-115.

107. Thomas JM, Verbanac KM, Smith JP, Kasten-Jolly J, Gross U, Reballato LM, Haisch CE, Carver FM, Thomas FT: The facilitating effect of one-DR antigen sharing in renal allograft tolerance induced by donor bone marrow in rhesus monkeys: Transplantation 1995; 59:245-255.

108. Thomas JM, Neville DM, Contreras JL, Eckhoff DE, Meng G, Lobashevsky AL, Wang PX, Huang ZQ, Verbanac KM, Haisch CE, Thomas FT: Preclinical studies of allograft tolerance in rhesus monkeys. Transplantation 1997; 64:124-135.

109. Monaco AP, Clark AW, Wood ML, Sahyoun AI, Codish SD, Brown RW: Possible active enhancement of a human cadaver renal allograft with antilymphocyte serum (ALS) and donor bone marrow: case report of an initial attempt. Surgery 1976; 79(4):384-392.

110. Barber WH, Mankin JA, Laskow DA, Deierhoi MH, Julian BA, Curtis JJ, Diethelm AG: Long-term results of a controlled prospective study with transfusion of donor-specific bone marrow in 57 cadaveric renal allograft recipients. Transplantation 1991; 51(1):70-75.

111. McDaniel DO, Naftilan J, Hulvey K, Shaneyfelt S, Lemons JA, Logoo-Deenadayalan S, Hudson S, Diethelm AG, Barber WH: Peripheral blood chimerism in renal allograft recipients transfused with donor bone marrow. Transplantation 1994; 57(6):852-856.

112. Starzl TE, Demetris AJ, Noriko M, Ildstad ST, Ricordi C, Trucco M: Cell migration, chimerism and graft acceptance. Lancet 1992; 339:1579-2582.

113. Starzl TE, Demetris AJ, Trucco M, Ricordi C, Murase N, Thomson AW: The role of cell migration and chimerism in organ transplant acceptance and tolerance induction. Transplant Science 1993; 3:47-50.

114. Fontes P, Rao A, Demetris AJ, Zeevi A, Trucco M, Carroll P, Rybka W, Ricordi C, Dodson F, Shapiro R, Tzakis AG, Todo S, Abu-Elmagd K, Jordan M, Fung JJ, Starzl TE: Bone marrow augmentation of donor-cell chimerism in kidney, liver, heart, and pancreas islet transplantation. Lancet 1994; 344(8916): 151-155.

115. Zeevi A, Pavlick M, Lombardozzi S, Banas R, Pappo O, Rao AS, Fontes P, Demetris J, Shapiro R, Forrest D, Trucco M, Carroll P, Pham S, Fung JJ, Strazl TE: Immune status of recipients following bone marrow-augmented solid organ transplantation. Transplantation 1995; 59(4):616-620.

116. Zeevi A, Pavlick M, Banas R, Bentlejewski C, Spichty K, Rao AS, Fontes A, Lyengar A, Shapiro R, Dodson F, Jordan M, Pham S, Keenan R, Griffith B, Corry R, Egidi F, Fung JJ, Starzl TE: Three years of follow-up of bone marrow-augmented organ transplant recipients: The impact of donor-specific immune modulation. Transplant Proc 1997; 29:1205-1206.

117. Gaetano C, Garcia-Morales R, Burke GW, Roth D, Esquenazi V, Tzakis AG, Miller J: Donor bone marrow, chimerism, histocompatibility and renal allograft rejection. Transplant Proc 1998: in press.

118. Tsaroucha A, Ricordi C, Noto TA, Kenyon NS, Garcia-Morales R, Nery J, Miller J, and Tzakis A: Donor peripheral stem cell infusion in recipients of living related liver allografts. Transplantation 1997; 64(2):362-364.

119. Ricordi C, Karatzas T, Selvaggi G, Nery J, Webb M, Fernandez H, Ruiz P, Kong SS, Esquenazi V, Miller J, Schiff E, Tzakis AG: Multiple bone marrow infusions to enhance acceptance of allografts from the same donor. Ann N Y Acad Sci 1995; 70:345-350.

120. Ricordi C, Karatzas T, Nery J, Webb M, Selvaggi G, Fernandez L, Khan FA, Ruiz P, Schiff E, Olson L, Fernandez H, Bean J, Esquenazi V, Miller J, Tzakis AG: High dose donor bone marrow infusions to enhance allograft survival: The effect of timing. Transplantation 1997; 63:7-11.

121. Garcia-Morales R, Esquenazi V, Zucker K, Gomez C, Fuller L, Carreno M, Cirocco R, Alamo A, Karatzas T, Burke II GW, Ciancio G, Temple D, Fernandez H, Ricordi C, Tzakis AG, Miller J: An assessment of the effects of cadaver donor bone marrow on kidney allograft recipient blood cell chimerism by a novel technique combining PCR and flow cytometry (PCR-Flow). Transplantation 1996; 62:1149-1160.

122. Garcia-Morales R, Carreno M, Mathew J, Cirocco R, Zucker K, Ciancio G, Burke G, Roth D, Temple D, Fuller L, Esquenazi V, Eskind L, Kenyon NS, Ricordi C, Tzakis AG, Miller J: Continuing observations on the regulatory effects of donor-specific bone marrow cell infusions and chimerism in kidney transplant recipients. Transplantation 1998; 5(7):956-965.

123. McDaniel ML, Kwon G, Hill JR, Marshall CA, Corbett J: Cytokines and nitric oxide in islet inflammation and diabetes. Proc Soc Exp Biol Med 1996; 211(1):24-32.

124. Kenyon NS, Selvaggi G, Fernandez L, Xiu XM, Knapp J, Montelongo J, McMannis J, Russell TR, Alejandro R, and Ricordi C: Infusion of class II dim donor bone marrow enhances islet allograft survival in low dose CsA treated dogs. Txpl Proc 1997; 29:2189.

7

ALLOGENEIC PERIPHERAL BLOOD PROGENITOR CELL TRANSPLANTATION IN SOLID TUMORS

Naoto T. Ueno, Gabriel N. Hortobagyi, Richard E. Champlin

Department of Blood and Marrow Transplantation, University of Texas M. D. Anderson Cancer Center, Houston, TX 77030

INTRODUCTION

High-dose chemotherapy and autologous transplantation is used as treatment for selected solid tumors, such as breast and ovarian cancer. This approach produces high complete response rates but relapse of the malignancies remains the major problem. This is generally due to incomplete eradication of the disease by high-dose chemotherapy. In addition, autologous transplantation may be contaminated by malignant cells that may contribute to systemic relapse. Allogeneic peripheral blood progenitor cells (PBPC) or bone marrow transplantation has been associated with an immune graft-*vs*-malignancy effect against leukemias and lymphomas. However, it is uncertain whether a similar graft-*vs*-malignancy effect will occur against solid tumors. Preliminary trials of allogeneic transplantation have been performed in patients with various solid tumors with the goal of inducing graft-*vs*-malignancy effects. In this chapter, we will review the rationale and our recent experience of allogeneic transplantation for metastatic breast cancer.

BACKGROUND

The number of autologous transplants performed annually has exceeded the number of allogeneic transplantations since 1990. Breast cancer is now the most common disease treated with autologous transplantation (1). Other chemotherapy-responsive solid tumors, such as ovarian cancer (2, 3), testicular/germ cell carcinomas (4, 5), and small cell carcinoma of the lung (6) are being actively studied in the adult population. Although high-dose chemotherapy for these solid tumors achieves a high response rate, long-term progression-free survival remains disappointing. The major cause of treatment failure is recurrent malignancy, primarily related to incomplete eradication of the disease. In addition, reinfusion of the autologous marrow or PBPC contaminated with tumor cells may contribute to relapse (7-9).

Allogeneic transplantation eliminates the risk of reinfusing autologous malignant cells and has the potential to induce an immune graft-*vs*-malignancy effect in combination with the cytoreduction from high-dose chemotherapy. Graft-*vs*-malignancy effects are well documented in allogeneic transplantation for leukemias, non-Hodgkin lymphomas, and myeloma (10-22). The evidence supporting the concept of graft-*vs*-malignancy effects includes a lower rate of relapse in patients with graft-*vs*-host disease (GVHD) and a higher rate of relapse in patients who had identical twin donors (23, 24). In addition, T lymphocyte-depleted allogeneic transplantation is associated with a higher risk of relapse (25, 26). This indicates that T lymphocytes or natural killer cells participate in mediating graft-*vs*-malignancy effects and that allogeneic targets (i.e., polymorphic minor histocompatibility antigens) are involved. The most direct evidence of graft-*vs*-malignancy is the reinduction of remission by donor lymphocyte infusion in patients who had relapsed after allogeneic transplantation (10-15).

The target antigens of graft-*vs*-malignancy effects are unknown. This process could involve broadly expressed major and minor histocompatibility antigens overlapping with GVHD. Many patients with chronic myelogenous leukemia (CML) have achieved complete remission after donor lymphocyte infusion without developing GVHD (10-14) suggesting that the target antigens of GHVD and graft-*vs*-malignancy may differ. Patients with CML responding to donor lymphocyte infusion generally have elimination of both malignant and donor host derived cells consistent with a hematopoietic but not leukemia specific target. Graft-vs.-malignancy effects could target tissue-specific polymorphic antigens. Hematopoietic lineage restricted minor histocompatibility antigens have been identified. However, it is unknown whether polymorphic antigens present in epithelial tissue, which are not involved in GVHD, serve as targets for graft-*vs*-malignancy effects.

Recently, we explored the graft-*vs*-malignancy effects in breast cancer at the University of Texas M. D. Anderson Cancer Center, and have initiated pilot studies to assess the feasibility of this approach in melanoma and colon cancer. Other transplant centers are also evaluating the potential of allogeneic transplantation for a variety of solid tumors (Table 1). Only limited data is available for most diagnoses. In this chapter, we focus on allogeneic transplantation in metastatic breast cancer, the disease in which the most data is available (27-30).

Table 1   Experience of allogeneic transplantation in solid tumors

Disease type	No. of cases	Institution	Conditioning regimen	Reference
Breast carcinoma	16	MDACC	CBT	[27]
	4	University of Colorado	Busulfan/melphalan	Personal communication from Dr. Elizabeth Shpall
	1	University of Innsbruck	Cyclophosphamide/ carboplatin/thiotepa	[28]
	1	Roger William Cancer Center Rhode Island Blood Center	NA	[29]
	1	University of Geneva	FC	[30]
Colon carcinoma	1	MDACC	CB	Personal communication
Melanoma	4	NHLBI	FC	Personal communication from Dr. John Barrett
	2	MDACC	CBT	Personal communication from Dr. Sergio Giralt
Renal cell carcinoma	2 *	NHLBI	FC	Personal communication with Dr. John Barrett

Abbreviations: CB =cyclophosphamide/BCNU; CBT = cyclophosphamide /BCNU/thiotepa; FC = fludarabine/cyclophosphamide; GVT = graft-*vs*-tumor; MDACC = M. D. Anderson Cancer Center; NA = not available; NLHBI = National Heart, Lung, and Blood Institute; No.= number; pts = patients
* One patient underwent one-antigen HLA mismatch allogeneic transplantation.

ALLOGENEIC TRANSPLANTATION IN BREAST CANCER

Background and rationale

High-dose chemotherapy with autologous PBPC or bone marrow transplantation produces a high response rate in patients with metastatic breast cancer. The most effective high-dose chemotherapy regimens include combinations of alkylating agents and related drugs including cyclophosphamide, ifosfamide, melphalan, thiotepa, carmustine (BCNU), cisplatin or carboplatin. The dose of these agents can be increased approximately threefold over the standard when followed by autologous transplantation to restore hematopoiesis. Most remissions are transient, median time to progression is 1.5 years, and 5-year progression-free survival rates are in the 10% to 20% range (31-35). There continues to be controversy regarding the benefit of high-dose chemotherapy for breast cancer. Patient selection bias complicates analysis of progression-free survival in phase II trials (36). Two randomized studies have favored high-dose chemotherapy over standard chemotherapy (31, 32) and several large prospective randomized studies are currently ongoing.

Over the past decade, considerable data indicate that patients with advanced metastatic breast cancer have multiple immunologic defects, e.g., decreased antigen presentation by dendritic cells (37, 38), dormant cytotoxic T lymphocytes (39), reduced interleukin (IL)-2 levels and IL-2 receptors on lymphocytes (40, 41), decreased natural killer cell activity (39, 42), and lack of MHC class I/II molecular on breast cancer cells (43). Mucin or fas expressed by malignant cells may inhibit antitumor immune responses (44, 45). These defects probably allow breast cancer cells to escape immunosurveillance, and could explain why single-agent immunotherapy, such as IL-2 or interferon-alpha, has generally been unsuccessful in breast cancer. Additionally, these immunotherapies were primarily studied in patients with advanced, bulky disease for whom clinical impact of immunotherapy may be difficult to observe (46-48).

On the other hand, there are considerable data to indicate that cytotoxic T lymphocytes and natural killer cells can lyse breast cancer cells in a MHC restricted and non-restricted manner (49-56). Mazumder *et al.* showed that with IL-2-induced autologous graft-*vs*-host disease (57), a post-transplant graft-*vs*-

breast cancer effect could be detected *in vitro* (49, 57-60).

A number of innovative approaches have been studied to improve the long-term outcome of autologous transplantation in metastatic breast cancer, including modification of the high-dose chemotherapy conditioning regimen, ex-vivo purging of the marrow, or introducing post-transplantation immunomodulation (61). Biologic or immunologic therapies are attractive strategies to address minimal residual breast cancer persisting after high-dose chemotherapy. Interleukin-2 after autologous transplantation is under evaluation (62, 63) and the effects of a GVHD-like syndrome induced by cyclosporine withdrawal and interferon-gamma treatment are also being studied (64, 65).

We hypothesized that allogeneic cells may be more capable to induce graft-*vs*-malignancy effects than autologous lymphocytes. Allogeneic cells contain normal lymphocytes and functional antigen presenting dendritic cells. Allogeneic T lymphocytes may recognize abnormally expressed or polymorphic tissue-specific antigens present on the tumor. An additional advantage of allogeneic cells is the lack of contamination by occult breast cancer. We initiated a study in 1995 to assess the feasibility of allogeneic PBPC transplantation to induce graft-*vs*-malignancy effects from a human leukocyte antigen (HLA)-identical related donor in patients with metastatic breast cancer focusing on poor prognosis patients with liver or bone marrow involvement, a group with less than 5% progression-free survival after high-dose chemotherapy with autologous transplantation.

Evaluation, Conditioning Regimen, GVHD Prophylaxis, and Supportive Care

Sixteen patients with metastatic breast cancer underwent allogeneic PBPC transplantation between September 1995 and February 1998. Eligibility criteria included histological confirmation of invasive carcinoma of the breast involving the liver or more than 20% of the bone marrow or both. The patients' disease had to be either responding or stable on standard-dose chemotherapy, and they had to have a related, HLA-identical donor, be no more than 55 years of age, have a Zubrod performance status of 0 or 1, and have adequate organ function. Patients with active central nervous system involvement were not eligible.

High-dose chemotherapy consisted of cyclophosphamide, carmustine, and thiotepa (the CBT regimen), including cyclophosphamide, 2,000 mg/m² intravenously (IV) over 24 hours on days –5, –4, –3 (total dose: 6,000 mg/m²); carmustine, 150 mg/m² IV over 40 minutes on days –7, –6, –5 (total dose: 450 mg/m²); and thiotepa, 240 mg/m² IV over 4 hours daily on days –7, –6, –5 (total dose: 720 mg/m²). Mesna, 500 mg/m², was given IV 1/2 hour before the first dose of cyclophosphamide, then 2,000 mg/m² as a continuous infusion over 24 hours for 3 days. Filgrastim was administered subcutaneously daily from day 1 through the first day that the absolute neutrophil count reached >1,000/mm³ and for a maximum of 28 days. Patients received allogeneic PBPC from HLA-identical siblings, minimum of 4 X 10⁶ CD34+ cells/kg were collected. No positive selection or T-cell depletion procedures were performed. The PBPC were cryopreserved by programmed freezing in 5% dimethylsulfoxide (DMSO) before the preparative regimen was started. On the day of transplantation, the PBPC were thawed and infused.

GVHD prophylaxis consisted of cyclosporine and methylprednisolone in the first two patients (patients no. 1 and no. 2) (66). The other 14 patients were treated with tacrolimus (FK506) and micro-methotrexate based upon improved control of acute GVHD with that regimen (67). Tacrolimus was continued for 6 months after transplantation. The dosage was then tapered by 20% every 2 weeks until it was discontinued by 8 months after transplantation. Patients who developed grade 2 or greater acute GVHD were treated with methylprednisolone, 2 mg/kg/day in divided doses and tapered as tolerated. Infection prophylaxis consisted of acyclovir and fluconazole plus oral quinolones or a nonabsorbable antibiotic during neutropenia. After granulocyte level recovered to > 1.0 X 10⁹/L, patients who tested positive for CMV or who received PBPC from a seropositive donor received prophylactic ganciclovir until day 100 (68, 69). Patients were treated prophylactically for *Pneumocystis carinii* with trimethoprim/sulfamethoxazole or aerosolized pentamidine for 1 year after PBPC transplantation (70, 71). Intravenous immunoglobulin (0.2 gm/kg) was administered weekly for 100 days and then monthly for 1 year (72). Those with chronic GVHD continued to receive prophylactic antibiotics. Irradiated blood products were administered to maintain a hemoglobin level of more than 8 g/dL and a platelet count of more than 20 X 10⁹/L.

Immunosuppressive therapy for patients with residual or recurrent breast cancer was rapidly tapered. If GVHD was not present, additional donor lymphocytes were infused (starting at 0.5 x 10^8 mononuclear cells/kg). The original donor underwent leukapheresis, without G-CSF or other therapy, to collect mononuclear cells.

Patient Characteristics

All 16 patients were women, with a median age of 42 years (range, 29 to 55) (patient no. 1 to 16). Patient characteristics are summarized in Table 2. All patients had metastatic disease involving the liver and/or bone marrow. Eleven patients had recurrent disease, and five initially presented with metastatic disease. Nine patients had bone marrow involvement. Eight patients had liver involvement, and one had both. The median number of metastatic sites was 2.5 (range, 1 to 5). The estrogen-receptor assay was negative in four patients, positive in nine patients, and unavailable in three patients. All patients received induction standard-dose chemotherapy with FAC (5-fluorouracil, cyclophosphamide, adriamycin) and/or a paclitaxel-containing regimen.

Table 2. Patient characteristics of 16 female patients receiving allogeneic transplantation in metastatic breast cancer

Pt no.	Disease	Age	Stage at Dx	BM	Liver	No. of distant metastatic sites	ER	Surgery	Neo-adjuvant or adjuvant CT	Prior hormonal Rx	Prior XRT	Rx for metastatic disease
1	Breast*	37	II	+	-	5	NA	MRM	FAC	None	-	Pac
2	Breast	55	II	+	-	4	-	Lumpectomy	None	None	+	Pac
3	Breast	42	IV	+	-	3	NA	None	None	None	-	FAC/Pac
4	Breast	46	II	-	+	2	+	MRM	FAC	None	-	Pac
5	Breast	37	I	-	+	2	+	MRM	CMF	Tamoxifen	-	FAC/Pac/PC
6	Breast	41	IIIA	+	-	3	-	MRM	FAC	None	-	Pac
7	Breast	51	IV	-	+	1	-	Simple mastectomy	None	None	-	FAC
8	Breast	42	IV	-	+	4	NA	None	None	None	-	FAC
9	Breast	46	II	+	+	3	+	MRM	CMF	Tamoxifen / Megace	-	FAC
10	Breast	29	IV	-	+	1	-	Lumpectomy	None	None	-	FAC/Pac
11	Breast	40	IIIB	-	+	3	+	MRM	FAC	None	+	Pac
12	Breast	31	I	+	-	3	+	RM	None	Tamoxifen	+	Tam/FAC/Pac
13	Breast	39	II	+	-	2	+	MRM	FAC	Tamoxifen	+	Docetaxel
14	Breast	50	II	+	-	2	+	MRM	FAC/MTX-Velban	Tamoxifen	+	FAC/Pac
15	Breast	47	IV	+	-	2	+	MRM	None	None	-	FAC/Pac/Vinorelbine
16	Breast	52	II	-	+	2	+	MRM	CMF	None	-	FAC

Table 2 (continuing)

* Refractory anemia with excess blasts in 1989

Abbreviations: BM, bone marrow; CMF, cyclophosphamide, methotrexate, 5-

fluorouracil; Dx, diagnosis; ER, estrogen receptor assay; FAC, 5-fluorouracil, adriamycin, cyclophosphamide; MRM, modified radical mastectomy; NA, not available; No, number; Pac, paclitaxel; PC, paclitaxel, cisplatin; Rx, therapy; XRT, radiation therapy.

Engraftment and GVHD
All 16 patients achieved complete hematopoietic engraftment. Their median time to reach an absolute granulocyte count of 1.0×10^9/L was 11 days (range, 6 to 17) and to a platelet count > 20×10^9/L, 13 days (range, 8 to 24).

Acute GVHD grade 2 developed in eight patients (Table 3). Six patients had stage 3 skin GVHD. The other two patients had stage 3 gastrointestinal and stage 1 skin GVHD, and stage 4 gastrointestinal GVHD. All patients responded to methylprednisolone therapy. Four patients developed chronic GVHD, which was controlled by further immunosuppressive therapy. However, one patient (no. 8) eventually developed progressive chronic GVHD involving the liver.

Table 3. GVHD in patients with metastatic breast cancer who underwent allogeneic transplantation

	No. of pts
Acute GVHD	
Overall	8
Skin	6
Liver	0
Gastrointestinal	2
Chronic GVHD	
Overall	4
Limited	3
Extended	1

Toxicity and Infections
Data on toxicity and infections are summarized in Table 4. Grade 2-3 toxicities developed in eight patients. One patient (no. 2) with myelodysplastic syndrome in addition to breast cancer died on day 53 of a systemic *Candida krusei* infection causing multiple-organ failure. Another patient (no. 9) died on day 106 of bacterial sepsis and GVHD. This patient also had grade 2 hepatotoxicity and grade 3 renal toxicity. Patient no. 11 died on day 80 of disseminated fungal

infection. Other patients had transient grade 2 mucositis and grade 2 diarrhea.

Table 4. Clinical Toxicity in patients with metastatic breast cancer who underwent allogeneic transplantation

Toxicity	No. of patients
Treatment-related death	3
Grade II-IV toxicity	
Cardiac	2
Renal	1
Hepatic	1
Mucositis	4
Gastrointestinal (diarrhea)	1
Nausea/vomiting	2
Infection	
Bacterial	7
Fungal	2
CMV pneumonia	0
CMV viremia	3
HSV	1
Parainfluenza type 3	1

Abbreviations: CMV, cytomegalovirus; HSV, herpes simplex virus; No, number.

Anti-tumor Effects

Antitumor responses before and after allogeneic transplantation are listed in Table 5. Before transplantation, one patient was in complete remission (CR), seven had partial response, and eight had stable disease after standard-dose chemotherapy. After high-dose CBT chemotherapy and allogeneic transplantation, one patient remained in CR, five patients had further 50% reduction in tumor volume (partial remission; PR), eight had stable disease, and one had progressive disease.

Table 5 Outcome of allogeneic transplantation in metastatic breast cancer

	Pre-BMT Response	Duration of F/U in days	Response to BMT	Date of progression	Progression site	Death	Duration of survival	Immunomodulation after BMT	Response to immunomodulation
1	SD	363	PR	231	bone	Yes	363	None	
2	PR	53	PR	NA	ED	Yes	53	None	
3	PR	690	SD	290	Bone	No	690 +	DLI x 1	No
4	CR	810	CR	342	liver/bone	No	810 +	DLI x 2	No (1st), NA (2nd)
5	SD	815	SD	244	Liver	No	815 +	FK506	Yes (regression in the liver)
6	PR	741	SD	None	NED	No	741 +	None	BM became negative over a year
7	SD	512	SD	350	liver	Yes	512	None	
8	SD	445	PR	96	bone	Yes	445	Steroid	Yes (regression in the liver)
9	SD	106	SD	NA	ED	Yes	108	None	
10	SD	268	PR	124	liver	Yes	268	FK506	No
11	PR	80	NA	NA	ED	Yes	80	None	
12	PR	307	SD	91	BM	No	307 +	FK506	NA
13	SD	300	SD	300	bone	No	300 +	T/C	
14	SD	180	PD	114	liver	No	180 +	FK506	NA
15	PR	138	SD	None	NA	No	138 +	T/C	
16	PR	105	PR	None	NA	No	105 +	T/C	

Abbreviations: ED, early death; DLI, donor lymphocyte infusion.

The median follow up time is 307 days (range, 53 to 815). Nine patients were alive at a median of 307 days (range, 105 to 815) after transplantation (Figure 1). Four patients had progressive disease in the bone on days 96, 231, 290, and 300. Four patients had progression in the liver on days 114, 124, 244 and 350. One patient progressed in both liver and bone disease on day 342, and one patient had increasing bone marrow disease on day 91. Median, progression-free survival was 106 days (range, 53 to 741).

Figure 1. Overall survival since allogeneic transplantation for metastatic breast cancer in 16 patients.

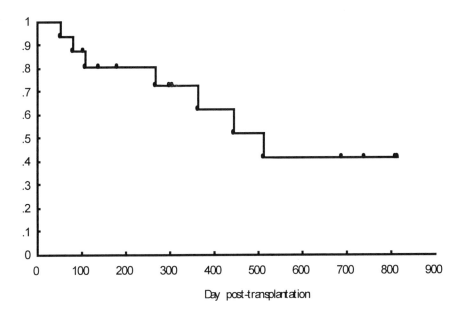

Day post-transplantation

Fig 2   Progression-free survival since allogeneic transplantation for metastatic breast cancer in 16 patients.

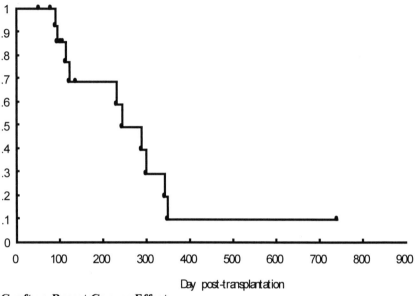

Day post-transplantation

Graft-vs-Breast Cancer Effects

Five patients with disease progression had their immunosuppressive therapy reduced and two received donor lymphocyte infusion to enhance graft-*vs*-malignancy effects. Regression of the tumor was seen in two patients who had metastatic liver lesions in association with the development or exacerbation of acute cutaneous GVHD after methylprednisolone (patient no. 8) or after tacrolimus was withdrawn (patient no. 5).   Patient no. 10 had tacrolimus discontinued on day 126 without development of GVHD. Twenty-eight days (day 154) later, her disease progressed in her liver. Two patients (no. 3 and 4) who received donor lymphocyte infusion showed neither regression of the tumor nor development of GVHD.

Two Case Reports

Patient no. 8 was a 42-year-old woman with metastatic breast cancer involving the liver (Figure 3A) and bone. She developed skin GVHD (stage 3) on day 28, which responded initially to methylprednisolone, 1 mg/kg; but later became steroid dependent. On day 96, she was found to have progressive disease and new bone pain in her left hip, associated on bone scan with a new lesion. Metastatic liver lesions had regressed after high-dose chemotherapy, as verified by abdominal CT scan on day 98, but had perivascular enhancement consistent with persistent metastasis (Figure 3B). At that time she was receiving methylprednisolone, 0.5 mg/kg/day, and oral tacrolimus to maintain a full therapeutic level (5-15 mg/ml). The methylprednisolone dose was reduced with the goal of enhancing graft-*vs*-breast cancer effects, and exacerbation of skin GVHD occurred. On day 132, her abdominal CT scan revealed a complete resolution of the metastatic liver disease (Figure 3C) and stable bone disease. The patient's left hip pain resolved and she no longer required analgesics. Her skin GVHD was eventually controlled by adding mycophenolate mofetil on day 154, and her steroids were tapered off successfully on day 173. On day 185, her bone scan revealed improvement, but the patient was found to have a recurrence of disease in her liver. She eventually developed chronic GVHD involving the liver, and survived 445 days post-transplantation.

Patient no. 5 was a 37-year-old woman with metastatic breast cancer predominantly involving the liver and bone; she had progressive disease in the liver on day 248. Tacrolimus was discontinued. On day 263, cutaneous chronic GVHD developed (36%). Low-dose tacrolimus and methylprednisolone were administered, and they controlled the rash. Her restaging workup on day 292, 44 days after tacrolimus was discontinued, showed regression of the metastatic liver lesions. She intermittently developed a transient rash consistent with chronic GVHD, which was controlled by corticosteroid therapy. On day 605, her disease progressed again in the liver. This patient remains alive 815 days after transplantation.

Fig 3   Abdominal CT scan (A) before transplantation; small metastatic lesions seen on the right hepatic lobe; (B) day 98, regression of the tumor, but extensive perivascular enhancement consistent with metastasis is noted; (C) day 132, complete resolution of the metastatic site.

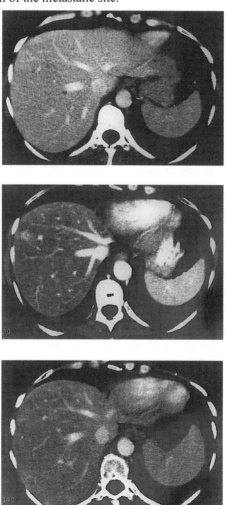

Discussion

The purpose of this initial study in metastatic breast cancer was to assess the feasibility of allogeneic transplantation. The goal was also to improve remission duration by inducing a graft-*vs*-malignancy effect against metastatic breast cancer in addition to the cytoreduction from high-dose chemotherapy.

Our results suggest that allogeneic transplantation is a feasible procedure for the treatment of metastatic breast cancer. We used the same preparative regimen employed for autologous transplantation in breast cancer at our center. Regimen-related toxicities, GVHD, and infections occurred at similar rates to those seen with allogeneic transplantation for hematologic malignancies. All patients had durable engraftment. Given the anticipated risks of allogeneic transplantation, eligibility was limited to patients with metastatic cancer who had a very poor prognosis. The overall response rate after high-dose chemotherapy and allogeneic transplantation was 40%; only one patient remained in complete remission. The relatively poor initial tumor response rate to high-dose chemotherapy was likely due to poor prognostic factors; e.g., high number sites of metastatic disease, also reflected in the poor response to induction standard-dose chemotherapy before transplantation.

If allogeneic graft-*vs*-malignancy effects were to occur, it would be expected to produce additional cytoreduction in the same time frame as GVHD develops, and would act to prevent or delay progression of the malignancy. The regression of metastatic breast cancer in the liver associated with GVHD after the withdrawal of immunosuppressive therapy suggests the possible existence of a graft-*vs*-breast cancer effect. Additionally, one patient has had slow clearance of metastatic bone marrow involvement and remains disease-free over one year after transplantation. These preliminary observations need to be confirmed in additional studies demonstrating improved progression-free survival with allogeneic transplantation. A graft-vs-malignancy effect in metastatic breast cancer in the liver was also reported by Eibl *et al* in a patient who underwent allogeneic bone marrow transplantation (28). These investigators reported regression of the tumor in the liver at the same time acute GVHD developed. The existence of a graft-*vs*-breast cancer effect can be most directly proved by showing tumor regression after donor lymphocyte infusion. It is important to address the potential antigens for a putative graft-*vs*-breast cancer effect.

However, polymorphism in relevant minor histocompatibility antigens as well as heterogenicity in tumor sensitivity to immunologic effects may limit the benefit only to a fraction of patients.

Insufficient data exist to determine whether allogeneic transplantation will improve progression-free survival compared with autologous transplantation or alternative therapies. To assess whether the putative graft-*vs*-malignancy effects will improve the progression-free survival, allogeneic transplantation should be prospectively compared with autologous transplants in patients receiving identical chemotherapy. The use of allogeneic transplantation can be justified only if the benefits outweigh the increased risk of treatment-related morbidity and mortality. When allogeneic transplantation was performed among patients with advanced chronic myelogenous leukemia in blast crisis, the long-term disease-free survival was less than 10%. However, once its feasibility was confirmed, its use was expanded to CML in chronic phase, resulting in a significant improvement in progression-free survival. Similarly, allogeneic transplantation is most effective in lymphoma and acute leukemia patients with less-advanced disease. If allogeneic transplantation in breast cancer is to be useful, it will likely be in patients who have chemosensitive disease with low tumor bulk. We have recently modified our eligibility criteria for allogeneic transplantation to study metastatic breast cancer patients who have partially responded to pre-transplantation chemotherapy or those who have minimum residual or recurrent disease after autologous transplantation. Allogeneic hematopoietic transplantation should only be performed in the context of clinical trials designed to address the major outstanding issues.

Acknowledgments
The authors wish to thank Dr. Sergio Giralt, Dr. John Barrett and Dr. Elizabeth J. Shpall to provide their experience. We thank Mr. Walter Pagel (Department Scientific Publication) for critically reviewing the manuscript.

REFERENCE

1. Antman K, Rowling PA, Vaughan WP, Pelz CJ, Fay JW, Fields KK, Freytes CO, Gale RP, Hillner BE, Holland HK. High-dose chemotherapy with autologous hematopoietic stem-cell support for breast cancer in North America. J Clin Oncol 1997; 15: 1870-1879.

2. Stiff PJ, Bayer R, Kerger C, Potkul RK, Malhotra D, Peace DJ, Smith D, Fisher SG. High-dose chemotherapy with autologous transplantation for persistent/relapsed ovarian cancer: a multivariate analysis of survival for 100 consecutively treated patients. J Clin Oncol 1997; 15: 1309-1317.

3. Legros M, Dauplat J, Fleury J, Cure H, Suzanne F, Chassagne J, Bay JO, Sol C, Canis M, Condat P, Choufi B, Tavernier F, Glenat C, Chollet P, Plagne R. High-dose chemotherapy with hematopoietic rescue in patients with stage III to IV ovarian cancer: long-term results. J Clin Oncol 1997; 15: 1302-1308.

4. Lotz JP, Andre T, Donsimoni R, Firmin C, Bouleuc C, Bonnak H, Merad Z, Esteso A, Gerota J, Izrael V. High dose chemotherapy with ifosfamide, carboplatin, and etoposide combined with autologous bone marrow transplantation for the treatment of poor-prognosis germ cell tumors and metastatic trophoblastic disease in adults. Cancer 1995; 75: 874-885.

5. Droz JP, Pico JL, Kramar A. Role of autologous bone marrow transplantation in germ-cell cancer. Urol Clin North Am 1993; 20: 161-171.

6. Lazarus HM. Autologous bone marrow transplantation for the treatment of lung cancer. Semin Oncol 1993; 20(5 Suppl 6): 72-79.

7. Kennedy MJ, Beveridge RA, Rowley SD, Gordon GB, Abeloff MD, Davidson NE. High-dose chemotherapy with reinfusion of purged autologous bone marrow following dose-intense induction as initial therapy for metastatic breast cancer. J Natl Cancer Inst 1991; 83: 920-926.

8. Rill DR, Santana VM, Roberts WM, Nilson T, Bowman LC, Krance RA, Heslop HE, Moen RC, Ihle JN, Brenner MK. Direct demonstration that autologous bone marrow transplantation for solid tumors can return a multiplicity of tumorigenic cells. Blood 1994; 84: 380-383.

9. Fields KK, Elfenbein GJ, Trudeau WL, Perkins JB, Janssen wE, Moscinski LC. Clinical significance of bone marrow metastases as detected using the polymerase chain reaction in patients with breast cancer undergoing high-dose chemotherapy and autologous transplantation. J Clin Oncol 1996; 14: 1868-1876.

10. Mackinnon S, Papadopoulos EB, Carabasi MH, Reich L, Collins NH, Boulad F, Castro MH, Childs BH, Gillio AP, Kernan NA, et al. Adoptive immunotherapy evaluating escalating doses of donor leukocytes for relapse of chronic myeloid leukemia after bone marrow transplantation: separation of graft-versus-leukemia responses from graft-versus-host disease. Blood

1995; 86: 1261-1268.

11. Giralt S, Hester J, Huh Y, Hirsch GC, Rondon G, Seong D, Lee M, Gajewski J, Van BK, Khouri I, et al. CD8-depleted donor lymphocyte infusion as treatment for relapsed chronic myelogenous leukemia after allogeneic bone marrow transplantation. Blood 1995; 86: 4337-4343.

12. Kolb HJ, Schattenberg A, Goldman JM, Hertenstein B, Jacobsen N, Arcese W, Ljungman P, Ferrant A, Verdonck L, Niederwieser D, et al. Graft-versus-leukemia effect of donor lymphocyte transfusions in marrow grafted patients. European Group for Blood and Marrow Transplantation Working Party Chronic Leukemia. Blood 1995; 86: 2041-2050.

13. Kumar L. Donor leucocyte infusions for relapse in chronic myelogenous leukaemia. Lancet 1994; 344: 1101-1102.

14. Porter DL, Roth MS, McGarigle C, Ferrara JL, Antin JH. Induction of graft-versus-host disease as immunotherapy for relapsed chronic myeloid leukemia. N Engl J Med 1994; 330: 100-106.

15. Lokhorst HM, Schattenberg A, Cornelissen JJ, Thomas LL, Verdonck LF. Donor leukocyte infusions are effective in relapsed multiple myeloma after allogeneic bone marrow transplantation. Blood 1997; 90: 4206-4211.

16. Mehta J. Graft-versus-leukemia reactions in clinical bone marrow transplantation. Leuk Lymphoma 1993; 10: 427-432.

17. Drobyski WR, Keever CA, Roth MS, Koethe S, Hanson G, McFadden P, Gottschall JL, Ash RC, van TP, Horowitz MM, et al. Salvage immunotherapy using donor leukocyte infusions as treatment for relapsed chronic myelogenous leukemia after allogeneic bone marrow transplantation: efficacy and toxicity of a defined T-cell dose. Blood 1993; 82: 2310-2318.

18. Bar BM, Schattenberg A, Mensink EJ, Geurts VKA, Smetsers TF, Knops GH, Linders EH, De WT. Donor leukocyte infusions for chronic myeloid leukemia relapsed after allogeneic bone marrow transplantation. J Clin Oncol 1993; 11: 513-519.

19. Brenner MK, Heslop HE. Graft versus leukaemia effects after marrow transplantation in man. Baillieres Clin Haematol 1991; 4: 727-749.

20. van Besien KW, Mehra RC, Giralt SA, Kantarjian HM, Pugh WC, Khouri IF, Moon Y, Williams P, Andersson BS, Przepiorka D, McCarthy PL, Gajewski JL, Deisseroth AB, Cabanillas FF, Champlin R. Allogeneic bone marrow transplantation for poor-prognosis lymphoma: response, toxicity

and survival depend on disease histology. Am J Med 1996; 100: 299-307.

21. van Besien KW, Khouri IF, Giralt SA, McCarthy P, Mehra R, Andersson BS, Przepiorka D, Gajewski JL, Bellare N, Nath R, et al. Allogeneic bone marrow transplantation for refractory and recurrent low-grade lymphoma: the case for aggressive management. J Clin Oncol 1995; 13: 1096-1102.
22. Jones RJ, Ambinder RF, Piantadosi S, Santos GW. Evidence of a graft-versus-lymphoma effect associated with allogeneic bone marrow transplantation. Blood 1991; 77: 649-653.
23. Gale RP, Champlin RE. How does bone-marrow transplantation cure leukaemia? Lancet 1984; 2: 28-30.
24. Sullivan KM, Weiden PL, Storb R, Witherspoon RP, Fefer A, Fisher L, Buckner CD, Anasetti C, Appelbaum FR, Badger C, et al. Influence of acute and chronic graft-versus-host disease on relapse and survival after bone marrow transplantation from HLA-identical siblings as treatment of acute and chronic leukemia (published erratum appears in Blood 1989 Aug 15; 74(3):1180). Blood 1989; 73: 1720-1728.
25. Champlin RE. T-cell depletion for bone marrow transplantation: effects on graft rejection, graft-versus-host disease, graft-versus-leukemia, and survival. (Review) (81 refs). Cancer Treatment & Research 1990; 50: 99-111.
26. Goldman JM, Gale RP, Horowitz MM, Biggs JC, Champlin RE, Gluckman E, Hoffmann RG, Jacobsen SJ, Marmont AM, McGlave PB, et al. Bone marrow transplantation for chronic myelogenous leukemia in chronic phase. Increased risk for relapse associated with T-cell depletion. Ann Intern Med 1988; 108: 806-814.
27. Ueno NT, Rondon G, Mirza NQ, Geisler DK, Anderlini P, Giralt SA, Andersson BS, Claxton DF, Gajewski JL, Khouri IF, Körbling M, Mehra RC, Przepiorka D, Rahman Z, Samuels BI, van Besien K, Hortobagyi G, Champlin RE. Allogeneic peripheral blood progenitor cell transplantation for poor-risk patients with metastatic breast cancer. J Clin Oncol 1998; 16: 986-993.
28. Eibl B, Schwaighofer H, Nachbaur D, Marth C, Gachter A, Knapp R, Bock G, Gassner C, Schiller L, Peterson F, Niederwieser D. Evidence for a graft-versus-tumor effect in a patient treated with marrow ablative chemotherapy and allogeneic bone marrow transplantation for breast cancer. Blood 1996; 88: 1501-1508.

29. Oblon DJ, Paul S, Oblon MB, Yankee R. Allogeneic peripheral blood stem cell transplants: preliminary results. Blood 1994; 84, Suppl 1: 94a:366.

30. Carella AM, Frassoni F, Di Stefano F, Celesti R, Corsetti MT, Lerma E, Celesti L, Dejana A, Gualandi F, Van Lint MT, Bacigalupo A. Engraftment of allogeneic stem cells after nonmyeloablative chemotherapy with fludarabine-containing regime. Proc Amer Soc Clin Oncol 1998; 17: 131a (503).

31. Peters WP, Jones RB, Vredenburdgh J, Shpall EJ, Hussein A, Elkordy M, Rubin P, Ross M, Affronti ML, Moore S, Barry D. Large prospective randomized trial of high-dose combination alkylating agents (CPB) with autologous cellular support (ABMS) as consolidation for complete remission after intensive doxorubicin-based induction therapy (AFM). Breast Cancer Res Treat 1996; 37: 35 (11).

32. Bezwoda WR, Seymour L, Dansey RD. High-dose chemotherapy with hematopoietic rescue as primary treatment for metastatic breast cancer: a randomized trial. J Clin Oncol 1995; 13: 2483-2489.

33. Dunphy FR, Spitzer G, Buzdar AU, Hortobagyi GN, Horwitz LJ, Yau JC, Spinolo JA, Jagannath S, Holmes F, Wallerstein RO, et al. Treatment of estrogen receptor-negative or hormonally refractory breast cancer with double high-dose chemotherapy intensification and bone marrow support. J Clin Oncol 1990; 8: 1207-1216.

34. Dunphy FR, Spitzer G, Fornoff JE, Yau JC, Huan SD, Dicke KA, Buzdar AU, Hortobagyi GN. Factors predicting long-term survival for metastatic breast cancer patients treated with high-dose chemotherapy and bone marrow support (published erratum appears in Cancer 1994 Jul 15; 74(2):773). Cancer 1994; 73: 2157-2167.

35. Ayash LJ, Wheeler C, Fairclough D, Schwartz G, Reich E, Warren D, Schnipper L, Antman K, Frei Er, Elias A. Prognostic factors for prolonged progression-free survival with high-dose chemotherapy with autologous stem-cell support for advanced breast cancer. J Clin Oncol 1995; 13: 2043-2049.

36. Rahman ZU, Frye DK, Buzdar AU, Smith TL, Asmar L, Champlin RE, Hortobagyi GN. Impact of selection process on response rate and long-term survival of potential high-dose chemotherapy candidates treated with standard-dose doxorubicin-containing chemotherapy in patients with metastatic breast. J Clin Oncol 1997; 15: 3171-3177.

37. Gabrilovich DI, Kavanaugh D, Corak J, Nadaf-Rahrov S, Cunningham T, Carbone DP. Defective function of dendritic cells in patients with breast cancer can be overcome by generation of these cells from precursors, a new approach to cancer immunotherapy (Meeting abstract). Proc Annu Meet Am Soc Clin Oncol 1996; 15: A1040.
38. Savary CA, Graiutti ML, Melichar B, Przepiorka D, Freedman RS, Cowart RE, Chen DM, Anaissie EJ, Woodside DG, McIntyre BW, Pierson DL, Pellis NR, Rex JH. Multidimensional flow-cytometric analysis of dendritic cells in peripheral blood of normal donors and cancer patients. Cancer Immunol Immunother 1997; in press:.
39. Yamasaki S, Kan N, Mise K, Harada T, Ichinose Y, Moriguchi Y, Kodama H, Satoh K, Ohgaki K, Tobe T. Cellular interaction against autologous tumor cells between IL-2-cultured lymphocytes and fresh peripheral blood lymphocytes in patients with breast cancer given immuno-chemotherapy. Biotherapy 1993; 6: 63-71.
40. Hakim AA. Peripheral blood lymphocytes from patients with cancer lack interleukin-2 receptors. Cancer 1988; 61: 689-701.
41. Arduino S, Tessarolo M, Bellino R, Colombatto S, Leo L, Wierdis T, Lanza A. Reduced IL-2 level concentration in patients with breast cancer as a possible risk factor for relapse. European Journal of Gynaecological Oncology 1996; 17: 535-537.
42. Konjevic G, Spuzic I. Stage dependence of NK cell activity and its modulation by interleukin 2 in patients with breast cancer. Neoplasma 1993; 40: 81-85.
43. Cordon-Cardo C, Fuks Z, Drobnjak M, Moreno C, Eisenbach L, Feldman M. Expression of HLA-A,B,C antigens on primary and metastatic tumor cell populations of human carcinomas. Cancer Res 1991; 51: 6372-6380.
44. Gimmi CD, Morrison BW, Mainprice BA, Gribben JG, Boussiotis VA, Freeman GJ, Park SY, Watanabe M, Gong J, Hayes DF, Kufe DW, Nadler LM. Breast cancer-associated antigen, DF3/MUC1, induces apoptosis of activated human T cells. Nature Med 1996; 2: 1367-1370.
45. Nagata S, Golstein P. The Fas death factor. Science 1995; 267: 1449-1456.
46. Sparano JA, Fisher RI, Weiss GR, Margolin K, Aronson FR, Hawkins MJ, Atkins MB, Dutcher JP, Gaynor ER, Boldt DH, et al. Phase II trials of high-dose interleukin-2 and lymphokine-activated killer cells in advanced breast carcinoma and carcinoma of the lung, ovary, and pancreas and other

tumors. J Immunother Emphasis Tumor Immunol 1994; 16: 216-223.

47. Budd GT, Osgood B, Barna B, Boyett JM, Finke J, Medendorp SV, Murthy S, Novak C, Sergi J, Tubbs R, et al. Phase I clinical trial of interleukin 2 and alpha-interferon: toxicity and immunologic effects. Cancer Res 1989; 49: 6432-6436.

48. Israel L, Cour V, Pihan I, Morere JF, Breau JL, Franks CR, Palmer P, Loriaux E. Some theoretical and practical limitations of interleukin-2. Ten cases of advanced breast cancer treated with continuous infusion of IL-2. Cancer Treat Rev 1989; 16 (Suppl A): 169-171.

49. Mazumder A, Grimm EA, Zhang HZ, Rosenberg SA. Lysis of fresh human solid tumors by autologous lymphocytes activated in vitro with lectins. Cancer Res 1982; 42: 913-918.

50. Rayner AA, Grimm EA, Lotze MT, Wilson DJ, Rosenberg SA. Lymphokine-activated killer (LAK) cell phenomenon. IV. Lysis by LAK cell clones of fresh human tumor cells from autologous and multiple allogeneic tumors. J Natl Cancer Inst 1985; 75: 67-75.

51. Grimm EA, Wilson DJ. The human lymphokine-activated killer cell system. V. Purified recombinant interleukin 2 activates cytotoxic lymphocytes which lyse both natural killer-resistant autologous and allogeneic tumors and trinitrophenyl-modified autologous peripheral blood lymphocytes. Cell Immunol 1985; 94: 568-578.

52. Jerome KR, Barnd DL, Bendt KM, Boyer CM, Taylor PJ, McKenzie IF, Bast RJ, Finn OJ. Cytotoxic T-lymphocytes derived from patients with breast adenocarcinoma recognize an epitope present on the protein core of a mucin molecule preferentially expressed by malignant cells. Cancer Res 1991; 51: 2908-2916.

53. Celis E, Tsai V, Crimi C, De MR, Wentworth PA, Chesnut RW, Grey HM, Sette A, Serra HM. Induction of anti-tumor cytotoxic T lymphocytes in normal humans using primary cultures and synthetic peptide epitopes. Proc Natl Acad Sci U S A 1994; 91: 2105-2109.

54. Baxevanis CN, Dedoussis GV, Papadopoulos NG, Missitzis I, Stathopoulos GP, Papamichail M. Tumor specific cytolysis by tumor infiltrating lymphocytes in breast cancer. Cancer 1994; 74: 1275-1282.

55. Linehan DC, Goedegebuure PS, Peoples GE, Rogers SO, Eberlein TJ. Tumor-specific and HLA-A2-restricted cytolysis by tumor-associated lymphocytes in human metastatic breast cancer. J Immunol 1995; 155: 4486-4491.

56. Chakravarty PK, Sinha DK. Inhibition of mammary tumorigenesis in virgin rats by adoptive transfer of splenocytes from parous donors. Cancer Immunol Immunother 1991; 33: 263-266.

57. Mazumder A, Verma U, Areman E, Rajagopal C, Cahill R, Swain S. Peripheral blood stem cell (PBSC) transplantation in breast cancer patients with interleukin-2 (IL-2) activated PBSC leads to visceral graft vs host disease (GVHD) (Meeting abstract). Proc Annu Meet Am Soc Clin Oncol 1994; 13: A91.

58. Areman EM, Mazumder A, Kotula PL, Verma UN, Rajagopal C, Hancock S, Guevarra C, Djahanmir M, Sacher RA, Meehan KR. Hematopoietic potential of IL-2-cultured peripheral blood stem cells from breast cancer patients. Bone Marrow Transplantation 1996; 18: 521-525.

59. Mazumder A, Grimm EA, Rosenberg SA. Lysis of fresh human solid tumor cells by autologous lymphocytes activated in vitro by allosensitization. Cancer Immunol Immunother 1983; 15: 1-10.

60. Verma UN, Bagg A, Brown E, Mazumder A. Interleukin-2 activation of human bone marrow in long-term cultures: an effective strategy for purging and generation of anti-tumor cytotoxic effectors. Bone Marrow Transplantation 1994; 13: 115-123.

61. Shpall EJ, Jones RB, Bearman S. High-dose therapy with autologous bone marrow transplantation for the treatment of solid tumors. Curr Opin Oncol 1994; 6: 135-138.

62. Verma UN, Charak BS, Rajagopal C, Mazumder A. Interleukin-2 in bone marrow transplantation. (99 Refs). Cancer Treatment & Research 1995; 76: 315-336.

63. Verma UN, Meehan KR, Mazumder A. Post-bone marrow transplant use of immunotherapy. (158 Refs). (Review). Cancer Treatment & Research 1997; 77: 27-55.

64. Kennedy MJ, Vogelsang GB, Beveridge RA, Farmer ER, Altomonte V, Huelskamp AM, Davidson NE. Phase I trial of intravenous cyclosporine to induce graft-versus-host disease in women undergoing autologous bone marrow transplantation for breast cancer. J Clin Oncol 1993; 11: 478-484.

65. Kennedy MJ, Jones RJ. Autologous graft-versus-host disease: immunotherapy of breast cancer after bone marrow transplantation. Breast Cancer Res Treat 1993; 26(Suppl): S31-40. Review.

66. Forman SJ, Blume KG, Krance RA, Miner PJ, Metter GE, Hill LR, O'Donnell MR, Nademanee AP, Snyder DS. A prospective randomized study of acute graft-v-host disease in 107 patients with leukemia: methotrexate/prednisone v cyclosporine A/prednisone. Transplant Proc 1987; 19: 2605-2607.

67. Przepiorka D, Ippoliti C, Khouri I, Woo M, Mehra R, Bherz DL, Giralt S, Gajewski J, Fischer H, Fritsche H, Deisseroth AB, Cleary K, Champlin R, van Besien K, Andersson B, Maher R, Fitzsimmons W. Tacrolimus and minidose methotrexate for prevention of acute graft-versus-host diseasee after matched unrelated donor marrow transplantation. Blood 1996; 88: 4383-4389.

68. Przepiorka D, Ippoliti C, Panina A, Goodrich J, Giralt S, van Besien K, Mehra R, Deisseroth AB, Andersson B, Luna M, et al. Ganciclovir three times per week is not adequate to prevent cytomegalovirus reactivation after T cell-depleted marrow transplantation. Bone Marrow Transplant 1994; 13: 461-464.

69. Goodrich JM, Bowden RA, Fisher L, Keller C, Schoch G, Meyers JD. Ganciclovir prophylaxis to prevent cytomegalovirus disease after allogeneic marrow transplant. Ann Intern Med 1993; 118: 173-178.

70. Masur H. Prevention and treatment of pneumocystis pneumonia (published erratum appears in N Engl J Med 1993 Apr 15; 328(15):1136). N Engl J Med 1992; 327: 1853-1860.

71. Przepiorka D, Selvaggi K, Rosenzweig PQ, Borochovitz D, Taylor D. Aerosolized pentamidine for prevention of Pneumocystis pneumonia after allogeneic marrow transplantation. Bone Marrow Transplant 1991; 7: 324-325.

72. Winston DJ, Ho WG, Bartoni K, Champlin RE. Intravenous immunoglobulin and CMV-seronegative blood products for prevention of CMV infection and disease in bone marrow transplant recipients. Bone Marrow Transplant 1993; 12: 283-288.

8
HEMATOPOIETIC STEM CELL TRANSPLANTATION OF MULTIPLE SCLEROSIS, RHEUMATOID ARTHRITIS, AND SYSTEMIC LUPUS ERYTHEMATOSUS

Richard K Burt, M.D., Ann Traynor, M.D.
Northwestern University Medical Center, Chicago, IL 60611

William Burns, M.D.
Medical College of Wisconsin, Milwaukee, WI. 53226

RATIONALE

The standard treatment for autoimmune diseases is immune modulation or suppression. For patients with severe autoimmune diseases, some studies suggest a benefit of intensifying immunosuppression to the point of myelosuppression or myeloablation (1-12). In this setting reconstitution of a new hematopoietic and immune system is facilitated by infusion of hematopoietic progenitor cells (CD34$^+$ cells) which expand and differentiate into T and B cells, macrophages, and monocytes.

Anecdotal case reports of patients with hematologic diseases and coincidental autoimmune disorders suggest that durable remissions or cure of the autoimmune disease may occur after hematopoietic stem cell transplantation (HSCT) (13-21). In general, remissions are more durable with allogeneic compared to autologous transplants. However, some patients receiving autologous marrow enter and maintain remission. These case reports suffer from publication bias, since it is unlikely that an autoimmune process which fails to improve after HSCT would be reported. Preliminary data suggests that if autologous marrow is to be used for hematopoietic rescue, the hematopoeitic stem cell product should be purged of lymphocytes before re-infusion. Animal autoimmune diseases also remit after hematopoietic stem cell transplantation (22-34). There are two broad categories of autoimmune diseases in animals: those arising spontaneously and those induced by environmental exposure.

Spontaneous-onset animal autoimmune diseases

In general, spontaneous-occurring animal autoimmune illnesses are restricted to inbred strains. They may arise from single or limited genetic defects in the hematopoietic stem cell compartment. Examples of spontaneous-occurring autoimmune diseases are: a systemic lupus erythematosus-like syndrome in NZB/NZW F1 (B/W) and MRL/lpr mice (35-37); a scleroderma-like illness in Tsk mice (38,39) and UCD L200 chickens (40, 41); an inflammatory bowel disease in cotton top tamarin monkeys (42); and an islet cell inflammatory disease similar to type I diabetes mellitus in NOD mice (43, 44) In most cases, the exact genetic defect(s) causing spontaneous autoimmunity remains enigmatic but probably involves alterations in normal apoptotic, proliferative, and/or signal transduction pathways arising from the stem cell compartment. Spontaneous onset autoimmune diseases require an allogeneic transplant from an unaffected strain for cure (45,46).

Environmentally-induced animal autoimmune diseases

Autoimmune disorders that arise after environmental exposure may occur in a variety of outbred species and appear to be due to priming (i.e. activation) of normal but previously unstimulated (i.e. unresponsive) lymphocytes. The lymphocytic repertoire of animals that develop an environmentally-induced autoimmune disease is capable of recognizing self antigens, but remains unresponsive unless immunized to self protein or otherwise activated by environmental stimuli. In general, induced animal autoimmune diseases appear to arise from interaction of multiple genetic loci with environmental triggers. Those induced by immunization include: adjuvant-induced arthritis (AIA) (47); collagen induced arthritis (CIA) (47,48); experimental autoimmune myasthenia gravis (EAMG) (49, 50); experimental autoimmune encephalomyelitis (EAE) (51, 52); and experimental autoimmune myositis (53). In these diseases, injection of tissue-specific protein in complete Freund's adjuvant initiates disease in susceptible species.

Environmentally induced animal autoimmune diseases are arrested by either allogeneic, syngeneic, or autologous HSCT. Following autologous HSCT, the inflammatory synovitis of adjuvant induced arthritis (AIA) resolves (54, 55). After syngeneic HSCT in animals with EAMG, anti-acetylcholine receptor antibodies disappear and weakness reverses (56), while in EAE, neurologic progression is stopped (28-34). We and other investigators have already reported amelioration, improvement, and/or cure of clinical symptoms in EAE following syngeneic or autologous bone marrow transplantation (28-34). These experiments were performed in SJL/J mice as well as Lewis and Buffalo rats with similar beneficial effects.

158

Human autoimmune diseases

A variety of trials utilizing autologous HSCT for autoimmune diseases have been initiated by our group and others (table 1) (1-12). Early results suggest that autologous lymphocyte depleted HSCT is able to induce remission in otherwise treatment refractory disease, although durability of remission is as yet unknown.

Table 1 Results of autologous hematopoietic stem cell transplantation (HSCT) for autoimmune disease

Author (Reference)	Disease (Number of patients)	Outcome
Fassas (1)	MS (15)	Improved mean disability score
Burt (2)	MS (3)	No progression
Burt (6)	MS, SLE, RA (10)	All patients stabilized or improved
Joske (3)	RA (1)	Improved
Tyndall (5)	Scleroderma (1)	Improved
Burt (4)	SLE (1)	Improved
Brooks (9)	RA (8)	200 mg/kg cyclophosphamide 3/4 improved (2 at 6 months).
McSweeney (7)	Scleroderma (5)	No progression
Wulffraat (8)	JRA (5)	All in remission
Huhn (12)	ITP (4)	1 relapse, 3 responding
Burt (10)	SLE, RA (6)	All 4 SLE in remission, 1 RA relapsed, 1 RA improved beyond one year
Burt (11)	MS, SLE, RA (17)	2 patients with RA relapsed, all others improved

Why autologous transplantation?

As mentioned earlier, some animal autoimmune diseases are genetically inherited stem cell disorders and can only be cured by an allogeneic transplant. Most case reports of patients being transplanted for a hematologic or malignant disease who also had a coincidental autoimmune disease have demonstrated a high relapse rate for autologous (but none lymphocyte depleted) transplants. In contrast durable remissions with very few relapses have been reported after an allogeneic transplant. It is, however, premature to initiate allogeneic transplants for autoimmune diseases until results have been obtained with the less morbid autologous stem cell source. The major disadvantage of an allogeneic transplant is graft versus host disease (GVHD). Some centers have considered mini-transplant allogeneic protocols for autoimmune diseases. A mini-transplant is nothing more than low dose conditioning which does not alter the risk of GVHD. The morbidity and mortality of allogeneic transplants arises predominately from GVHD rather than the conditioning regimen. The incidence of severe acute GVHD (grade III and IV) is 20% while that of extensive chronic GVHD is approximately 40%. We and others are experimenting with methods to better control GVHD such as insertion of a suicide gene within donor lymphocytes. However, this approach to control GVHD is as of yet unproven. We believe advances that are proven to consistently prevent or abort GVHD in patients with hematologic malignancies are necessary before considering allogeneic transplantation for autoimmune disorders, if it is proven that the relapse rate after autologous transplantation is too high.

Why Phase I/II studies?
Blinded randomized studies in which BMT is a treatment arm are virtually impossible given the treatment-related experiences of the patient, including transient pancytopenia requiring blood product transfusions, requirement for antibiotics and growth factors, and physical changes including alopecia, nausea, xerostomia and other side-effects often encountered with high dose chemotherapy and/or total body irradiation, and nursing care and physician awareness concerning considerations for pre and post transplant patients. Enthusiasm for a randomized study with a control group monitored in parallel with the treatment group is tempered by the difficulties involved in recruiting patients with extremely serious diseases who approach such studies with the expectation that the transplant treatment arm offers them the best chance to arrest or cure their disease. This has been true in studies involving leukemias with the result that most such studies have settled for the allogeneic HSCT arm offered not on the basis of randomization but on the availability of a marrow donor (biological randomization). Even when the HSCT arm is a less dangerous autologous transplant with true randomization, it has been difficult to accrue patients because many of them have perhaps unrealistic but nevertheless strongly held views favoring the efficacy of the transplant treatment arm. Another consideration has been the possible need to include a transplant option for patients entered into the study and randomized to the non-transplant arm and who have progression of their disease during the study period. The ethical considerations and financial and other obligations to such patients would be considerable, difficult to predict, and place unacceptable obligations on the institutions participating in the study. Because of these considerations, we have opted for a non-randomized, non-blinded Phase I/II study without a concomitantly followed control group, with evaluation of efficacy (treatment failure/progression) as the primary goal for all three disease, MS, SLE, and RA.

This is, however, problematic for autoimmune diseases that rely heavily on the subjective evaluation of the patient and examining physician for assessment of improvement. The "gold standard" to define treatment success or failure in MS is based on the Extended disability status score (EDSS) which is dependent on physician interpretation of neurologic score. American College of Rheumatology (ACR) criteria in RA for improvement are heavily dependent on physician assessment of tender and swollen joint count and patient and physician assessment of disease activity via a visual analog scale. Blinded studies where there is no difference between treatment and placebo groups yet both show improvement are in confirmation of the concept of "expectation bias". This "expectation bias" by both the patient and physician may also explain differences in efficacy of open versus blinded trials. The ability of an open trial to create bias has been documented in both multiple sclerosis and RA. Noseworthy et. al. designed a multi-arm immunosuppressive treatment trial for MS (57). Evaluations were conducted by neurologists who were either blinded or unblinded to the treatment. The unblinded neurologists demonstrated statistically significant improvement for one treatment group over placebo, while neurologists blinded for therapy found no difference in outcome for all groups including patients treated with placebo. The anti-CD4 monoclonal antibody experience for RA is another example of "expectation bias" (58). Between 1989 and 1995, eight open trials showed benefit of anti-CD4 monoclonal antibody in treating RA, while three blinded placebo control studies showed no benefit. Even when performed by the same investigators, there is a difference between the outcome of open and blinded trials. When using more than a 50% improvement in tender and swollen joints, Moreland et. al. reported a significant improvement for anti-CD4 antibody in the open trial but in the blinded study no significant improvement of treated versus control group was present. As Pocock stated: "There is a potential danger that evaluators will error towards recording more favorable responses on the new treatment: after all most trials are conducted on the hope that a new treatment will appear superior and that it is only human nature to anticipate such superiority." (59)

Therefore, we are presented with a dilemma in performing phase I/II studies in autoimmune diseases in which response is defined by physician and patient assessment instead of objective tests. Without a control arm, we will be subject to the "expectation bias" experienced in other phase I/II studies. As we have already mentioned, because of the impractical aspects of a control arm for transplantation and because to date very few transplants for autoimmune disease have been done, a blinded and placebo controlled study is not practical. However, in an effort to diminish "expectation bias", we considered having patients on the MS and RA studies evaluated by both a treating and non-treating physician at each time point. The non-treating physician could even be at a different institution from the transplantation centers. However, because of the invasive and extensive nature of the procedure, both the patient and non-treating physician would still be aware of the transplant and subject to "expectation bias". Therefore, although constrained by tradition to the physician and patient evaluation of disease, we will emphasize more recent objective assessment parameters. For MS this includes MRI, 9 hole peg test, and timed ambulation. For RA, evaluation will include sed rate, CRP (C reactive protein), and hand and knee joint radiographs.

AUTOLOGOUS HEMATOPOIETIC STEM CELL TRANSPLANTATION

Mechanism of action

The mechanism of remission following autologous hematopoietic stem cell transplantation is unknown. The immune system may be fundamentally unaltered and an autologous transplant may be nothing more than dose-intense immunosuppression. At the other extreme, the disease-mediating effector cells may be entirely destroyed, although this is unlikely since we have shown that flow cytometric analysis of the post transplant immune system suggests that some memory cells ($CD45RO^+$) survive and only after 3-6 months do naive ($CD45RA^+$) lymphocytes appear (6). Alternatively, an autologous transplant may shift the balance between immunity and tolerance through as yet undefined mechanisms. Theoretically, this may include: clonal exhaustion, veto cells, suppressor cells, other autoregulatory cells, immune indifference, idiotypic T or B cell networks, cytokine alterations, changes in receptor avidity, or changes in T or B cell repertoire or function.

Selection of stem cell transplantation candidates

Extensive animal and limited clinical data suggest that patients with autoimmune disease may benefit from high-dose therapy and HSCT. However, this therapy carries a substantial risk of toxicity and even mortality and many patients with autoimmune disease will respond to less aggressive interventions. The risk-benefit ratio of this approach is most likely to be favorable in patients with features predicting a poor response to conventional therapies. The general approach is to identify candidates failing currently available therapies yet transplant early in the disease's course before irreversible damage to affected organs occurs.

CLINICAL RESULTS OF OUR RECENTLY COMPLETED PHASE I STUDY OF AUTOLOGOUS HEMATOPOIETIC STEM CELL TRANSPLANTATION IN MULTIPLE SCLEROSIS

Since immunosuppression is an effective but often temporary treatment of MS, we hypothesized in an editorial published in Bone Marrow Transplantation in 1995 that BMT might be useful in MS (60). In October of 1996, we initiated a

U.S. FDA approved Phase I Study of hematopoietic stem cell transplantation for patients with multiple sclerosis. We recently reported our Phase I results for our initial 6 patients with severe, rapidly progressive MS and have now completed this study (total of ten patients) (2,6). The reasoning that went into the development of that protocol is recounted .

Selection of Immunosuppressive (Transplant) Regimen

Most pre-transplant regimens are employed for their antitumor effects and therefore often include alkylating agents. For patients with multiple sclerosis, we were not interested in anti-tumor efficacy but rather intense immunosuppression capable of penetrating into the CNS. The regimen most immunosuppressive and with the best chance of affecting the CNS lesions would be one incorporating TBI. We were concerned about possible toxicities that might occur following irradiation of CNS lesions and sought evidence related to this. We were encouraged that in our animal models, TBI based conditioning did not cause exacerbation of disease. Other relevant information was the use of total lymphoid irradiation (TLI) for treatment of MS (61). In this procedure the spinal cord receives much of the radiation and there would presumably be some spinal MS lesions present in the radiation field. Again, no untoward toxicities were noted and in fact the patients receiving TLI doses that produced the most profound lymphopenia had the most improvement (transient) in their MS symptoms. For these reasons we felt we could employ a TBI-containing regimen. Other groups in the USA have proposed using busulphan and cyclophosphamide while European groups have agreed on BEAM (BCNU, etoposide, adriamycin and melphalan) (1). However, busulphan is less immunosuppressive than TBI and the BEAM regimen would not be expected to penetrate the CNS as reliably as TBI. We, therefore, selected a cyclophosphamide and TBI containing regimen.

Type of Transplant

Autologous transplant has a mortality of 1-3% in breast cancer patients and up to 10-15% in patients with lymphomas and other malignancies. The latter patients usually have been heavily treated before transplant and the accumulation of treatment toxicities is thought to play a role in their increased transplant-related mortality. Survival in MS correlates inversely with the level of disability. Less than 6% of patients with an unrestricted activity level are dead within 10 years, but there is increased mortality for patients with increasing disability. We felt that the increased mortality in MS patients with increasing disability and functional impairments along with their increasing morbidities justified the relatively low expected risk of mortality from autologous BMT. Since allogeneic transplantation carries a much higher mortality due primarily to graft versus host disease (GVHD), we reasoned that it should be tried only if clinical benefits achieved with autologous transplants were not realized or were of short duration. Furthermore, we reasoned that we could deplete the collected stem cells of T cells and thus achieve a very high level of immuno-ablation with less risk in the autologous setting.

Method of Harvesting Stem Cells
Initially we planned to harvest bone marrow by multiple marrow aspirations with the patient under anesthesia. We achieved inadequate harvests in our first 3 patients for reasons that are unclear. We modified our protocol to mobilize stem cells with granulocyte-colony stimulating factor (G-CSF) and collected stem cells by apheresis, with subsequent bone marrow harvest performed only if needed to supplement the peripheral blood stem cells (PBSC). We chose G-CSF over GM-CSF because of the latter's known maturing and activating influence on dendritic cells involved in antigen presentation. We want to minimize the potential of immunizing the new immune system with CNS antigens. In our Phase I study we used the CellPro CEPRATE column that positively selects for cells bearing the CD34 antigen. Using this procedure we routinely achieved > 2-log depletion of T cells with good recovery of the CD34+ cells.

Patient Selection
We anticipated the best results from immune ablation and hematopoietic stem cell (HSC) rescue would occur in younger patients with a short duration of progressive disease and low burden of neurologic deficits. Since gadolinium enhancement on MRI indicates blood brain barrier break-down at areas of acute inflammation, we also anticipated that patients with gadolinium enhancing lesions on MRI would be more likely to respond than patients with nonenhancing plaques which may represent areas of axonal degeneration and glial scarring. To prevent inherent bias in outcome due to spontaneous fluctuation of disease, we did not consider patients with relapsing-remitting disease to be candidates for BMT in this study. Since a variable relapse and progression rate with spontaneous remissions could limit the determination of treatment efficacy (a secondary endpoint in this Phase I study), we chose patients with progressive disease, severe impairments, and marked deterioration in their baseline neurologic function during the 12 months prior to enrollment. We also terminated all immunosuppressive and immunomodulatory medications prior to transplantation. After extensive discussions with neurologists consulting or directly involved in the study (Drs. Lori Lobeck and Cass Terry at MCW, Dr. Bruce Cohen at NU, and Dr. Henry McFarland at the NIH, NINDS and Dr. Jerry Wolinsky at UT in Houston), we decided on the following neurological eligibility criteria:
1) An established clinical diagnosis of MS.
2) A Kurtzke EDSS score (Appendix VII) of 5.0 to 8.0 at the time of pre-transplant evaluation and an increase in score by 1.5 points over the past 12 months in patients with an EDSS of 5.5 or less at the start of the evaluation period, or an increase of 1 point in patients with an EDSS score of 6 or greater at the start of the evaluation period.

3) Failure to stabilize active clinical progression with intravenous methylprednisolone given for a minimum of 3 days at 1 gram per day.

4) While not mandatory, selecting patients with evidence of active disease as reflected by blood brain barrier disruption on MRI (gadolinium enhancement) in either the spinal cord or brain was stressed.

5) Two neurologists, Drs. McFarland (NIH) and Wolinsky (UT), function as an Outside Panel and as the final arbiters of patient selection. After evaluation at NU or MCW, the evaluations and MRIs were sent to the Outside Panel who had to be satisfied that the criteria were met.

Monitoring

On post-transplant visits patients were seen and evaluated by the same neurologists who evaluated the patient prior to transplant at the respective institution. Patients were also seen at these visits by Transplant physicians for evaluation of transplant-related toxicities or problems. MRIs with and without gadolinium were also obtained. These visits were at 1, 3, 6, 12, 18, and 24 months and then yearly.

Results

Ten patients have been enrolled. One is currently undergoing transplant while nine are now 7-30 months post-transplant. Nine patients had secondary progressive MS and one had primary progressive disease. All had rapid, cumulative impairment/disability during the year prior to transplant and had failed steroid and other immunomodulatory therapies. One patient's disease flared while being mobilized with G-CSF. All patients received cyclophosphamide (60 mg/kg) daily for 2 days, followed by TBI administered 150 cGy twice per day for 4 days. One gram of methylprednisolone was given on the same days as TBI. This pre-transplant regimen was well tolerated without MS-specific toxicities. Stem cells were infused the day after TBI ended. Median time to absolute neutrophil counts > 500/ul and platelet counts > 20,000/ul occurred on day 10 and 14 post transplant, respectively. Since transplant, no patients have received any immunosuppressive or immunomodulatory medications. Seven patients are more than 1 year post transplant and, to date, all patients have had stabilization of their disease.

Table 2 Phase I Study Results - Hematopoietic stem cell transplantation for MS. EDSS and NRS are neurologic functional scales. EDSS ranges from O (normal) to 10 (dead), while NRS ranges from O (dead) to 100 (normal).

Patient	Months after BMT	No. of Relapses	EDSS pre-BMT and most recent	NRS pre-BMT and most recent
1	30	0	8.5/8.5	15/16
2	30	0	8.0/8.0	30/29
3	26	0	8.0/8.0	34/37
4	18	0	6.5/6.0	49/63
5	17	0	7.0/6.5	29/38
6	17	0	6.0/6.0	51/61
7	13	0	7.0/	67
8	7	0	8.0/	33
9	7	0	8.5/8.5	17/24
10	in house	N/A	N/A	N/A

How do these results compare to those achieved by the latest immunomodulatory treatment? Recently, the European Study Group on Interferon-1β in Secondary Progressive MS reported their findings (62). Their patient population resembled ours in diagnosis (secondary progressive). We required more rapid progression of disease in the prior year as they required either > 2 relapses or > 1 point increase in EDSS in the preceding 2 years. Our patients had higher EDSS scores prior to treatment. Of course, it is impossible to compare the results of the 2 studies statistically since ours is a small Phase I study and their study was a pivotal Phase III study of 718 patients. Their patients were followed for at least 2 years and up to 3 years. Nonetheless, we note that they had confirmed progression of 38.9% in the treatment group (vs 49.7% in the placebo group). Also of note, 53.6% of the treated patients received steroids during the 2 to 3 year period. In our admittedly very small study with median follow-up of only 1 year, it is encouraging that disease has been at least stabilized in all patients, no significant deterioration has been observed, there has been some improvement in patients transplanted with lower baseline EDSS scores, no enhancing lesions have been observed on MRIs, and no patients have received steroids or immunomodulatory drugs.

Our preliminary conclusions from this Phase I study are:
1) The use of PBSC is preferable to bone marrow as a source of stem cells for these transplants.

2) We are concerned that mobilization with G-CSF may cause disease exacerbation and will mobilize with the combination of cyclophosphamide and G-CSF in our future phase II study.

3) TBI can be safely employed in the immuno-ablative regimen without observable CNS toxicities specific for MS.

4) Engraftment has occurred rapidly in these patients and no unexpected infections were encountered.

5) Use of this treatment regimen has resulted in no MS-specific toxicities and appears at this point to be a well tolerated regimen.

6) The use of an expert Outside Panel to certify the eligibility of patients resulted in no inordinate delays and proved reassuring to patients and the investigators.

7) Although the Phase I study was primarily to determine toxicities and feasibility, disease has stabilized in all patients treated to date, although follow-up is short.

CLINICAL RESULTS OF OUR PHASE I AUTOLOGOUS HEMATOPOIETIC STEM CELL TRANSPLANT STUDY IN SYSTEMIC LUPUS ERYTHEMATOSUS

Beginning in 1995, we started developing a phase I study to perform lymphocyte depleted autologous hematopoietic stem cell transplantation in patients with poor prognosis systemic lupus erythematosus. The trial received Northwestern University IRB approval on 7-26-96 and opened on 1-31-97 following U.S. FDA approval. Seven patients have been enrolled on the protocol and five have undergone transplant. Two were not taken to transplant due to opportunistic infections diagnosed prior to treatment. We recently reported the first patient as a letter to the New England Journal of Medicine (4). The reasoning that went into the development of that protocol is recounted here.

Selection of Immunosuppressive (Transplant) Regimen
Cyclophosphamide was chosen because of its established effectiveness at conventional dosage in the treatment of lupus. Since all transplant candidates would have failed monthly pulse cyclophosphamide at 500-1000 mg/m^2, there was concern that the patient's lymphocytes may have become cyclophosphamide resistant. However, patients who fail low dose daily oral cyclophosphamide (150 mg/day), often respond to higher dose monthly pulse cyclophosphamide (PCy) (500-1000 mg/m^2) (63). We, therefore, speculated that patients resistant to monthly PCy would respond by escalating cyclophosphamide to transplant doses (TDCy) (200 mg/kg). This, in fact, was the case.

We recognized that the dose limiting toxicity of cyclophosphamide, unlike most alkylating agents, is not hematopoietic. Even without reinfusion of stem cells, cyclophosphamide induced cytopenias will resolve. In recognition of this fact some investigators have performed immunosuppressive trials in autoimmune diseases using TDCy without stem cell reinfusion. We chose to reinfuse hematopoietic stem cells in order to minimize the duration of cyclophosphamide induced neutropenia. We reasoned that the patients who met our eligibility criteria, having been heavily pretreated with immunosuppressive medications, would be at high risk of opportunistic infection. This proved true. Two patients who met our eligibility criteria could not be taken to transplant because of opportunistic infections (cytomegalovirus viremia and mucormycosis). Both were diagnosed prior to transplantation and after a transient period of neutropenia (ANC < 500/ul for 2-3 days) associated with stem cell mobilization.

Type of transplant
As we mentioned earlier, animal models of lupus-like illnesses appear to be genetically determined. In animals, allogeneic transplant from an unaffected strain, by transferring stem cells with normal wild type alleles, is capable of both preventing and curing established disease. These experiments could be interpreted to indicate that an allogeneic transplant will be needed in order to cure lupus. However, in humans the relative contributions of genes and environment to the development of SLE is probably somewhat different. Approximately two-thirds of identical twins are discordant for the disease, indicating that penetrance of a genetic predisposition to disease is not complete and that environmental selection may play a role (64). SLE disease activity also fluctuates, characterized by flares and long term remissions. Investigators have suggested the existence of regulatory cells (65).

Autologous transplantation performed for malignant disease is associated with a prolonged, post transplant "immunosuppressive" phenotype, which has recently been reported by our group to exist after autologous transplantation of autoimmune diseases as well (6). This generalized "suppressor" phenotype is manifest by a low CD4 count, elevated CD8 percentage, an inverted CD4/CD8 ratio, and an early predominance of CD45RO memory cells followed after 3-6 months by recurrence of CD45RA naive cells. We and others have speculated that high dose immunosuppression, by inducing apoptosis of disease causing lymphocytes and imposing a post transplant suppressor phenotype, may be beneficial in inducing a sustained remission of lupus. We, therefore, chose the safer autologous stem cells over an allogeneic source of stem cells.

METHOD OF HARVESTING STEM CELLS

Hematopoetic stem cells were mobilized with cyclophosphamide (2 g/m^2) and G-CSF. Engraftment kinetics are faster with G-CSF mobilized peripheral blood stem cells compared to marrow. Due to the anticipated high risk of infection in patients with SLE, we felt that the rapid engraftment of peripheral blood stem cells would be superior to that of marrow. In fact, most autologous transplants for malignancies now use peripheral blood mobilized stem cells rather than marrow due to more rapid engraftment, less infections, and more rapid hospital discharge. We were concerned that attempts to mobilize peripheral blood stem cells with G-CSF (an inflammatory cytokine) would be dangerous in patients with active SLE. For this reason cyclophosphamide (2.0 mg/m^2) was given first with G-CSF started 4-5 days later. This dose of cyclophosphamide, caused neutropenia of 1-3 days duration. Leukapheresis was initiated when the post nadir white blood cell count reached more than 1,000/ul (1.0 x 10^9/liter). Apheresis was continued daily until the number of harvested progenitor cells reached a minimum of 1.4 x 10^6 CD34$^+$ cells/kg body weight after selection. The mobilized peripheral blood stem cells were lymphocyte depleted via selection for CD34 positive cells using the CEPRATE SC Stem Cell Concentrator (CellPro, Bothell, Washington).

Patient selection
Mortality from lupus improved significantly due to the introduction of better anti-hypertensive medications and PCy (500-1000 mg/m^2 monthly for 6 months). Still, as a rule of thumb, mortality remains 1% per year for all patients with SLE (66-69). In order to select for patients at high risk for early mortality, we chose patients with active visceral disease despite corticosteroids and PCy. Cyclophosphamide must have been given for at least 6 months in patients with nephritis (WHO class III or class IV glomerulonephritis). With other visceral organ involvement, failure to prevent life-threatening manifestations (e.g. cerebritis, transverse myelitis, pulmonary hemorrhage, restrictive lung disease or cardiac failure) between pulses of cyclophosphamide was also an indication. Seven patients were enrolled; two were not taken to transplant because of opportunistic infections; four patients have undergone transplantation, a seventh patient is currently undergoing transplant.

RESULTS

Patients mobilized but not transplanted
Of the two patients who were not treated, one patient, despite being asymptomatic with a normal chest radiograph, had a resting O$_2$ saturation of 78%. Bronchoscopy revealed CMV. She was treated with ganciclovir and discharged home after being denied a transplant. Three months later, she died from active lupus cerebritis. The second patient developed seizures that were thought to be lupus-related prior to starting conditioning. The patient progressed rapidly with uncal herniation. Autopsy revealed hematogenously disseminated mucormycosis.

Patients transplanted
A total of four patients, ages 15-26 years, with SLE have undergone transplant. All were corticosteroid dependent with daily prednisone dose ranging from 60 to 100 mg per day. All had been treated with and failed between 8 to 18 monthly cycles of Pcy.

Table 3 -Pre Tx profile of first 2 patients who underwent transplant

Patient	1	2
Age (years)	24	15
Disease duration (years)	13	<1
Corticosteroids (years)	13	<1
Prior Immune suppressive medications	Prednisone, Plaquenil PCy	Prednisone , Plaquenil PCy
SLEDAI	37	35
Anti-ds DNA titer	1:1280	1:1280
Creatinine clearance	14 cc/min	56 cc/min
Proteinuria/ 24 hours.	23,000 mg/24 hrs.	5,400 mg
Renal pathology	WHO Class III, IV	Class IIIC
Left ventricle shortening fraction	24% (30-45%)	27%
CNS history	CVA, headache	Fatigue
Hepatic involvement	none	Transaminase, 2xNL.
Hematologic cytopenias	Hemoglobin 8.0 G/dl	Hemoglobin 7.8 G/dl

Post transplant follow-up ranges from 6 to 24 months with a median of 11
months. All patients are currently without evidence of active disease and all
have experienced marked improvements. All patients have been off
cyclophosphamide since transplant. Two patients have been off corticosteroid
for 6 and 12 consecutive months, respectively. Two other patients have been
tapered to less than 10 mg of prednisone a day. Two patients are off anti-
hypertensive medications, and two have been reduced from four to one anti-
hypertensive agent. Anti-depressants have also been discontinued in two
patients.

Figure 1 - Renal function of 1st patient with SLE who underwent autologous transplantation.

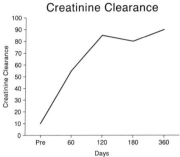

How do our results compare to other published data? Recently, investigators at Johns Hopkins have used TDCy (200 mg/kg) without stem cell support (70). In their publication of 8 patients, most had hematologic autoimmune diseases, however, two had systemic lupus. Their early response also appeared promising, however, they selected a much healthier subset of patients by using the usual transplant exclusion criteria for end organ dysfunction. For example, patients with a creatinine > 2.0 mg/dl were excluded. Neither patient reported by the Hopkins group had received and subsequently failed prior cyclophosphamide therapy. Therefore, given the more advanced and refractory nature of our patients, there are no comparable outcomes for this subset of patients with severe and refractory lupus.

Our preliminary conclusions from this ongoing Phase I lupus study are:
1) Mobilization using cyclophosphamide and G-CSF has been well tolerated.
2) Despite renal, cardiac, pulmonary, and other end-organ lupus-related toxicities, use of this treatment regimen has resulted in no lupus-specific flares and appears at this point to be a well tolerated regimen.
3) Engraftment occurred rapidly.
4) Patients with lupus, due to prior long term immunosuppressive medications as well as possibly the disease itself, are at a high risk of opportunistic infection and the transplant associated neutropenic period must be kept as short as possible.
5) Although this Phase I study is primarily to determine toxicities and feasibility, disease has remitted in all previously refractory patients with gradual and continuing improvement in organ function for up to 20 months.

CLINICAL RESULTS OF OUR PHASE I AUTOLOGOUS HEMATOPOIETIC STEM CELL TRANSPLANT STUDY IN RHEUMATOID ARTHRITIS

In 1995, we began planning a trial of hematopoietic stem cell transplantation in patients with refractory rheumatoid arthritis. We reasoned that despite currently available therapy, some patients with rheumatoid arthritis (RA) fail to respond and although most RA patients have a normal life expectancy, subsets of patients can be identified who have a 5-year survival of between 40% to 70%. Our trial received IRB approval on July 19, 1996 and U.S. FDA approval (IDE number BB-IDE 6778) in October 1996. To date four patients have been enrolled and all have undergone transplantation. We have previously published our results on the first two patients with RA who were treated by autologous hematopoietic stem cell transplantation (6).

Immunosuppressive conditioning (transplant regimen)
We initially chose the same immunosuppressive regimen for RA as we used for Lupus. This regimen of cyclophosphamide (200 mg/kg) and ATG (90 mg/kg) was based on our own and others successful experience using this regimen in aplastic anemia, which, in many cases represents an autoimmune suppression of hematopoiesis. We wanted to avoid total body irradiation due to concerns about pulmonary toxicity in patients with possible rheumatoid-related interstital lung disease. However, one patient also received low dose TBI given in a single fraction of 400cGy. These regimens were easily tolerated with no unexpected non-hematopoietic toxicity. Hematopoietic stem cells were reinfused to shorten the duration of neutropenia.

Type of transplant
Using the same philosophy employed for lupus and multiple sclerosis, we chose to initiate this process with the safer and less toxic stem cell source, i.e. autologous stem cells. If relapses occurred, then we could determine changes in the patient's immune system before transplant, while in remission, and upon relapse. If a high relapse rate occurred, we could also consider altering the immunosuppressive regimen by advancing to a more aggressive myeloablative regimen or using an allogeneic source of stem cells from a healthy sibling. In fact, before considering transplant for RA, we evaluated the literature for cases of patients with a malignancy or hematologic disease and coincidental RA who had received a transplant. We could find no reports of autologous hematopoietic transplants in patients with RA. However, nine allogeneic transplants have been reported in patients who had coincidental RA (71-76). In 7 out of the 9 reported patients with coexistent RA that have undergone allogeneic HSCT for the treatment of aplastic anemia, three died within 3 months, but the other 4 patients remained free of symptoms at 2, 11, 13, and 20 years, respectively (71-73).

Another patient had a flare at 2 years, but subsequently the disease followed an attenuated course, with treatment free remission for 11 years (73). The other patient developed a relapse at 3 years.

Method of Harvesting Stem Cells

We chose the same method to harvest stem cells as employed for mobilizing progenitor cells from patients with lupus. We reasoned that cyclophosphamide ($2g/m^2$) would prevent a possible G-CSF-induced flare of disease while at the same time provide a partial in vivo purge of lymphocytes prior to stem cell collection. All patients experienced a transient improvement of their symptoms after cyclophosphamide mobilization of stem cells. In all but one patient, baseline symptoms returned prior to administration of the conditioning regimen. After receiving cyclophosphamide, G-CSF did not cause a flare in disease activity. Similar to our MS and SLE protocols, the mobilized peripheral blood stem cells were lymphocyte depleted in vitro via selection for CD34 positive cells using the CEPRATE SC Stem Cell Concentrator.

Patient selection

In RA, prognostic factors for a poor survival rate include the presence of many involved joints, and the functional disability as assessed by the Health Assessment Questionnaire (HAQ) (77-79). We felt that the risk of autologous hematopoietic stem cell transplantation would be justified in these patients provided that they had failed corticosteroids and at least two disease modifying antirheumatic drugs (DMARD). We defined failure as more than six swollen joints and either 30 involved joints (swelling, tenderness, deformity, pain on motion, or decreased motion), or answering less than 75% of 20 Health Assessment Questionnaire (HAQ) questions "without any difficulty".

Results

Four patients (3 females, 1 male) with RA, according to the 1987 ARA criteria for the classification of RA, were treated (80). All had severe seropositive RA, with functional disability and characteristic radiographic findings. Two patients had rheumatoid nodules, and one patient had pulmonary involvement (interstitial lung infiltrates on CT scan, and reduced DLCO). Their disease was resistant to nonsteroidal antiinflammatory drugs and oral corticosteroids, and each patient had failed at least 5 DMARDs (Table 2). All patients were markedly limited in their daily activities, answering 0 to 3 of 20 questions "without any difficulty".

Table 4 Characteristics of first 2 RA patients prior to transplant

	patient 1	patient 2
Age/sex	46/F	42/F
RA duration (years)	7	7
Prior Tx	Hcq, Ssz, gold, MTX, CSA, Dpsn, Mncin	Hcq, Ssz, gold, MTX, CSA,
Swollen/ tender joints	27/41	18/21
HAQ-ADL "without difficulty"	0	1

Hcq=hydroxychloroquine, Ssz=sulfasalazine, MTX=methotrexate, CSA=cyclosporine, Dpsn=dapsone, Mincin=minocyclin, Aza=azathioprine, CYC=cyclophosphamide, leuk=chlorambucil

All patients had an initial marked improvement (Figure 4). At 8 months and 20 months after Tx, two patients meet the ACR 70 criteria for improvement (81,82).

Figure 2. Swollen joint count of 1st patient with RA who underwent autologous transplantation.

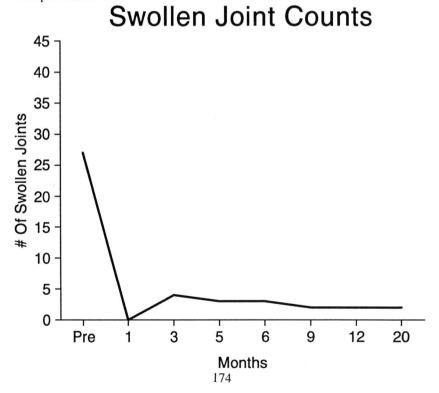

Swollen Joint Counts

How do our results compare to other published data? Brooks et. al. found that in patients undergoing autologous transplant for RA, all relapsed after an initial improvement with 100 mg/kg of cyclophosphamide, while in those receiving 200mg/kg, 3 out of 4 patients have maintained remission although follow up does not exceed 6 months (83). These findings could be interpreted to suggest a conditioning regimen-related dose response curve. In a non-transplant but relatively new therapy for RA, soluble TNF receptor given twice weekly for three months at three doses (0.25, 2, or 16 mg/m^2) was compared to placebo (84). In this 3 month trial for patients who had failed one to four disease modifying agents, a dose response curve was seen with 75% of patients in the highest dose group having at least a 20% or more improvement in symptoms. In our trial of refractory RA, in which every patient failed at least 5 disease modifying agents, one patient has maintained an ACR 70 response for 20 months while another has maintained an ACR 70 response for 8 months and two had early relapses. Although our patient experience is limited, the results suggest that further investigation with a myeloablative regimen is justified.

Our preliminary conclusions from this ongoing Phase I study in RA are:
1) Intense immunosuppression with autologous hematopoietic stem cell support is very well tolerated and safe in these four patients with refractory RA.
2) All the patients experienced an initial improvement and 2 of 4 patients have maintained the ACR criteria for 70% improvement for more than 20 months.
3) The reason(s) for failure to obtain sustained improvement in 2 of 4 patients is unclear.

Relapse may be due to: 1) inability of the conditioning regimen to ablate disease-causing immune cells, 2) reinfusion with the autologous hematopoietic stem cells of disease-causing immune effector cells, 3) regeneration of disease-mediating immune cells from the autologous hematopoietic stem cell compartment, or 4) failure of the hypothesis that RA is an autoimmune disease that can be cured by immune ablation and regeneration of immunity from an autologous stem cell compartment. Therefore, considerations in designing a new trial include: 1) Although the conditioning regimen was dose-intense compared to standard therapies for RA, it is a relatively mild transplant regimen and is non-myeloablative. An easily tolerated but myeloablative regimen should be considered. 2) Lowering the target or acceptable T cell dose reinfused with the autograft may be beneficial. With aggressive T cell depletion ($< 5 \times 10^4$ T cells/kg), even without immunosuppression, major HLA barriers such as haploidentical allogeneic transplantation may be crossed without GVHD (85). Since an allograft containing less than 5×10^4 T cells/kg can develop tolerance to foreign MHC mismatched tissue, it remains possible that an autologous graft containing a similar reduction of T cells could regenerate tolerance to self epitopes. 3) It may be that RA is an autoimmune disease that arises from an inherited $CD34^+$ progenitor stem cell disorder. Alternatively, RA may not be autoimmune in etiology, but rather immune mediated and due, for example, to an infectious agent, although no adverse infectious event occurred as a result of transplant or neutropenia. In either case, an allogeneic graft containing a new stem cell compartment may be curative by overcoming the previous stem cell predisposition for autoimmunity or immune-mediated clearance of infectious complications.

It has long been known that allogeneic transplantation prevents relapse of hematologic malignancies by means of a graft versus malignancy effect (86-88). Allogeneic allular transplantation may also provide a graft versus autoimmune (GVA) effect. Two observations support the possibility that immunologic mismatch between donor and recipient may be important in maintaining long term remission in RA. First, maternal-fetal HLA-DR and HLA-DQ disparity was associated with remission of RA during pregnancy (89). Second, immunization with allogeneic mononuclear cells resulted in remission in patients with rheumatoid arthritis (90).

GENERAL CONCLUSIONS IN TRANSPLANT STUDIES FOR ALL THREE AUTOIMMUNE DISEASES: MULTIPLE SCLEROSIS, RHEUMATOID ARTHRITIS, SYSTEMIC LUPUS ERYTHEMATOSUS

We selected these three diseases because: 1) they are common diseases, 2) they may be associated with significant morbidity or even mortality, and 3) they affect a wide variety of ages, with SLE predominately affecting children and young adults and MS middle aged individuals, while the incidence of RA increases with age but can be disabling in middle-aged individuals. We have learned that not all autoimmune diseases will respond the same or require the same type of conditioning regimen. Durable remissions (>two years) have occurred in patients with previously refractory SLE using a non-myeloablative regimen of cyclophosphamide (200 mg/kg) and ATG (90 mg/kg). However, SLE patients are unusually susceptible to opportunistic infections due to both chronic corticosteroid dependence and disease-related impaired immunity to intracelluar, viral, and fungal organisms. Therefore, it is imperative to keep the duration of treatment related neutropenia as short as possible in patients with SLE, necessitating the reinfusion of mobilized stem cells. SLE patients who have aggressive disease and are candidates for hematopoietic stem cell transplantation often have multi-organ dysfunction which, at least in our patients, has been readily reversible, but has also complicated the transplant procedure. Our experience has, therefore, taught us that most patients with active SLE (that has failed pulse cyclophosphamide) cannot have the transplant performed safely as an outpatient.

For patients with RA, we have learned that the transplants are remarkably uncomplicated. In fact, during the transplant procedure, the patients performance status and sense of well being normalize often for the first time in years. They claim to be pain free and can button shirts, coomb hair, and function normally, again often for the first time in years. Their general lack of other organ involvement (unlike SLE) also makes for an uncomplicated transplant procedure. For rheumatoid arthritis, transplant can be easily performed in an outpatient setting, markedly decreasing the cost of the procedure. We have also learned that despite the early marked improvement, relapses following transplant have occurred using non-myeloablative regimens such as cyclophosphamide (200 mg/kg) and ATG (90 mg/kg). We, therefore, anticipate that a truely myeloablative regimen is necessary to attempt curative therapy in RA. For MS, our myeloablative regimen has been well tolerated, and transplants could be easily performed as an outpatient. However, we have learned that G-CSF by itself for stem cell mobilization may cause disease exacerbation and have consequently modified the method of stem cell mobilization to include both cyclophosphamide and G-CSF.

REFERENCES:

1. Fassas A, Anagnostopoulos A, Kazis A, Kapinas K, Sakellari I, Kimiskidis V, Tsompanakou A. Peripheral blood stem cell transplantation in the treatment of progressive multiple sclerosis: first results of a pilot study. Bone Marrow Transplantation 1997; 20: 631-638.
2. Burt RK, Traynor AE, Cohen B, Karlin KH, Davis FA, Stefoski D, Terry C, Lobeck L, Russell EJ, Goolsby C, Rosen S, Gordon LI, Keever-Taylor C, Burns WH. T cell depleted autologous hematopoietic stem cell transplantation for multiple sclerosis: report on the first three patients. Bone Marrow Transplantation1998; 21: 537-541.
3. Joske DJ. Autologous bone-marrow transplantation for rheumatoid arthritis. (letter) Lancet 1997;350: 337-338.
4. Burt RK, Traynor AE, Ramsey-Goldman R. Hematopoietic stem-cell transplantation for systemic lupus erythematosus. (letter) New England Journal of Medicine 1997; 337 (24): 1777-1778.
5. Tyndall A, Black C, Finke J, Winkler J, Mertlesmann R, Peter H H, Gratwohl A. Treatment of systemic sclerosis with autologous hematopoietic stem cell transplantation. (letter) Lancet 1997; 349(9047): 254.

6. Burt RK, Traynor AE, Pope R, Schroeder J, Cohen B, Karlin KH, Lobeck L, Goolsby C, Rowlings P, Davis FA, Stefoski D, Terry C, Keever-Taylor C, Rosen S, Vesole D, Fishman M, Brush M , Mujias S, Villa M, Burns WH. Treatment of autoimmune disease by intense immunosuppressive conditioning and autologous hematopoietic stem cell transplantation. Blood 1998; 92 (10); 3505-3514.
7. McSweeney PA, Furst DE, Storek J, Nash RA, Nelson JL, Wener M, Sullivan KM. High dose immunosuppressive therapy (HDIT) using total body irradiation (TBI), cyclophosphamide (CY) and ATG with autologous CD34 selected peripheral blood stem cell (PSC) rescue as treatment for severe systemic sclerosis. Blood 1998; (abst 1208) 92 (10) Suppl 1: 295a.
8. Wulffraat NM, Vlieger A, Brinkman D, Vossen JP, Kuis W. Autologous stem cell transplantation (ASCT) in refractory polyarticular and systemic JCA. Arth Rheum 1998 (abst 581); 41 (9) Suppl: S131.
9. Brooks PM, Snowden J, Biggs J, Millikin S. A pilot dose escalation of high dose cyclophosphamide (CY) and autologous stem cell therapy (ASCT) in active rheumatoid arthritis (RA). Arth Rheum 1998 (abst 598); 41 (9) Suppl: S132.
10. Burt RK, Pope R, Schroeder J, Rosa RM, Rosen S, Traynor AE. Hematopoietic stem cell transplantation of autoimmune disease. Arth Rheum 1998; (abst 1253), 41 (9) Suppl: S241.
11. Burt RK, Burns WH, Cohen B, Karlin KH, Lobeck L, Schroeder J, , Pope R, , , Goolsby C, Schuening F, Graziano F, Rosa R, Keever-Taylor C, Rosen S, Traynor AE. T cell depleted autologous hematopoietic stem cell transplantation in patients with severe autoimmune diseases. Blood 1998; (abst 1327) 92 (10) Suppl 1: 324a.
12. Huhn RD, Read EJ, Rick M, Leitman SF, Kimball J, Gratwahl A, Young NS, Barrett AJ, Dunbar CE. Intensive immunosuppression with high dose cyclophosphamide and autologous CD34+ selected hematopoietic stem cell support for chronic refractory autoimmune thrombocytopenia. Blood 1998; (abst #719) 92 (10) Suppl 1: 178a.
13. Lui Yin JA, Jowitt SN. Resolution of immune-mediated diseases following bone marrow transplantation for leukemia. Bone Marrow Transplant 1992; 9: 31-33.
14. Lowenthal RM, Cohen ML, Atkinson K, Biggs JC. Apparent cure of rheumatoid arthritis by bone marrow transplantation. J Rheumatol 1993; 20: 137-140.
15. Meloni G, Capria SD, Vignetti M, Mandelli F. Blast crisis of chronic myelogenous leukemia in long-lasting systemic lupus erythematosus: regression of both diseases after autologous bone marrow transplantation. (letter) Blood 1997; 12: 4659.

16. McKendry RJR, Huebsch L, Leclair B. Progression of rheumatoid arthritis following bone marrow transplantation. A case report with 13 year follow-up. Arthritis and Rheumatism 1996; 39 (7): 1246-1253.
17. McAllister LD, Beatty, PG, Rose J Allogeneic bone marrow transplantation for chronic myelogenous leukemia in a patient with multiple sclerosis: case study. Bone Marrow Transplantation 1997; 19(4): 395-397.
18. Salzman P, Tami J, Jackson C, et al. Clinical remission of myasthenia gravis after high dose chemotherapy and autologous transplantation with CD34$^+$ stem cells. Blood 1994; 84(10) Suppl I: 206a, (abstract 808).
19. Fastenrath S, Dreger P, Schmitz N. Autologous unpurged bone marrow transplantation in a patient with lymphoma and SLE: short term recurrence of antinuclear antibodies. Arthritis and Rheumatology 1995; 38(9): 53Q3.
20. Euler HH, Marmont AM, Bacigalupo A, et al. Early recurrence or persistence of autoimmune diseases after unmanipulated autologous stem cell transplantation. Blood 1996; 88(9): 3621-3625.
21. Lopez-Cubero S, Sullivan K, McDonald G.B. Course of Crohn's disease after allogeneic marrow transplantation. Gastroenterology 1998; 114, 433-440.
22. Ikehara S, Yasumizu R, Inaba M, Izui S, Hayakawa K, Sekita K, Toki J, Sugiura K, Iwai H, Nakamura T, Muso E, Hamashima Y, Good RA. Long-term observations of autoimmune-prone mice treated for autoimmune disease by allogeneic bone marrow transplantation. Proc Natl Acad Sci USA 1989, 86: 3306-3310.
23. Himeno K, Good RA. Marrow transplantation from tolerant donors to treat and prevent autoimmune diseases in BXSB mice. Proc Natl Acad Sci USA 1988; 85: 2235-2239.
24. Ikehara S, Good RA, Nakamura T, Sekita K, Inque S, OO MM, Muso E, Ogawa K, Hamashima Y. Rationale for bone marrow transplantation in the treatment of autoimmune diseases. Proc Natl Acad Sci USA 1985; 82: 2483-2487.
25. Laface DM, Peck AB. Reciprocal allogeneic bone marrow transplantation between NOD mice and diabetes non-susceptible mice associated with transfer and prevention of autoimmune diabetes. Diabetes 1989; 38: 894-901.
26. Knaan-Shanzer S, Houben P, Kinwewl-Bohre EPM, van Bekkum DW. Remission induction of adjuvant arthritis in rats by total body irradiation and autologous bone marrow transplantation. Bone Marrow Transplantation 1991; 8: 333-338.
27. van Bekkum DW, Bohre EPM, Houben PFJ, Knaan-Shanzer S. Regression of adjuvant-induced arthritis in rats following bone marrow transplantation. Proc Natl Acad Sci USA 86, 10090-10094, 1989.

28. van Gelder M, Kinwel-Bohre EPM, van Bekkum DW. Treatment of experimental allergic encephalomyelitis in rats with total body irradiation and syngeneic BMT. Bone Marrow Transplantation 1993; 11: 233-241.
29. Burt RK, Hess A, Burns W, et al. Syngeneic bone marrow transplantation eliminates v_b8.2T lymphocytes from the spinal cord of Lewis rats with experimental allergic encephalomyelitis. Journal of Neuroscience Research 1995; 41: 526-531.
30. van Gelder M, van Bekkum DW. Treatment of relapsing experimental autoimmune encephalomyelitis in rats with allogewneic bone marrow transplantation from a resistant strain. Bone Marrow Transplantation 1995; 16: 343-351.
31. van Gelder M, Mulder AH, van Bekkum DW. Treatment of relapsing experimental autoimmune encephalomyelitis with largely MHC-matched allogeneic bone marrow transplantation. Bone Marrow Transplant 1996; 62: 810-818.
32. van Gelder M, van Bekkum DW. Effective treatment of relapsing experimental autoimmune encephalomyelitis with pseudoautologous Bone Marrow Transplantation 1996; 18(6): 1029-1034.
33. Karussis DM, Vourka-Karussis U, Lehmann D, et al: Prevention and reversal of adoptively transferred, chronic relapsing experimental autoimmune encephalomyelitis with a single high dose cytoreductive treatment followed by syngeneic bone marrow transplantation. J Clin Invest 1993; 765-772.
34. Burt RK, Padilla J, Begolka WS, Dal Conto C, Miller SD. Effect of disease stage on clinical outcome after syngeneic bone marrow transplantation for relapsing experimental autoimmune encephalomyelitis. Blood 1998; 91(7): 2609-2616.
35. Heyler BJ, Howie JB. Renal disease associated with positive lupus erythematosus tests in a cross bred strain of mice. Nature 197, 197, 1963.
36. Putterman C, Naparstek Y. Murine models of spontaneous systemic lupus erythematosus. Autoimmune Disease Models: A guidebook, 1994; 217-243.
37. Akizuki M, Reeves JP, Steinberk AD. Expression of autoimmunity by NZB/NZW Marrow. Clinical Immunology and Immunopathology 1978; 10: 247-250.
38. Jimenez SD, Christner P. 1994. Animal models of systemic sclerosis. Clinics in Dermatology. 12:425-436.
39. Kasturi KN, Shibata S, Muryoi T et al. Tight-skin mouse: an experimental model for scleroderma. Intern. Rev. Immunol 1994; 11: 253-271.
40. van de Water J, Boyd R, Wick G et al. The immunologic and genetic basis of avian scleroderma, an inherited fibrotic disease of line 200 chickens. Inter Rev Immunol 1994; 11: 273-282.

41. Rose NR. Avian models of autoimmune disease: lessons from the birds. Poultry Science 1994; 73: 984-990.
42. Warren BF, Watkins PE. Animal models of inflammatory bowel disease. Journal of Pathology 1994;172: 313-316.
43. Mendez JD, Ramos HG. Animal models in diabetes research. Archives of Medical Research 1994; 25(4): 367-375.
44. Hanfusa T, Miyagawa J, Nakajima H, et al. The NOD Mouse. Diabetes Res. Clin. Pract 1994; 24 Supppl: S307-S311.
45. Cohen PL, Eisenberg RA. The lpr and gld genes in systemic autoimmunity: life and death in the Fas lane. Immunol Today 1992; 13 (11): 427-428.
46. Drappa J, Brot N, Elkon KB. The Fas protein is expressed at high levels on double positive thymocytes and activated mature T cells in normal but not MRL/lpr mice. Proc Natl Acad Sci USA 1993; 90: 10340-10344.
47. Hayashida K, Ochi T, Fujimoto M, et. al. Bone marrow changes in adjuvant-induced and collagen-induced arthritis. Arthritis and Rheumatism 1992;35(2): 241-245.
48. Durie FH, Fava RA, Noelle RJ. Collagen-induced arthritis as a model of rheumatoid arthritis. Clinical Immunology and Immunopathology 1994; 73(1): 11-18.
49. Patrick J, Lindstrom J. Autoimmune response to acetylcholine receptor. Science 1973; 180: 871-872.
50. Vincent A. Experimental autoimmune myasthenia gravis. in <u>Autoimmune Disease Models: A Guidebook</u>, San Diego, Academic Press, Inc 1994; 83-106.
51. Brocke S, Gijbels K, Steinman L: 1994. Experimental autoimmune encephalomyelitis in the mouse. in <u>Autoimmune Disease Models: A Guidebook</u>, San Diego, Academic Press, Inc 1994; 1-14.
52. Steinman L, Schwartz G, Waldor M, et al. in <u>EAE: A Good Model for MS</u>, San Diego, Academic Press, Inc 1984; 393-397.
53. Rosenberg N. Experimental models of inflammatory myopathies. Bailliere's Clinical Neurology 1993; 2(3): 693-703.
54. Kamiya M, Sohen S, Yamane T, et al. Effective treatment of mice with type II collagen induced arthritis with lethal radiation and bone marrow transplantation. The Journal of Rheumatology 1993; 20: 225-230.
55. Knaan-Schanzer S, Houben P, Kinwel-Bohre EP, et al. Remission induction of adjuvant arthritis in rats by total body irradiation and autologous bone marrow transplantation. Bone Marrow Transplantation 1991; 8: 333-338.
56. Pestronk A, Drachman DB, Teoh R, et al. Combined short-term immunotherapy cures experimental autoimmune myasthenia gravis. Ann Neurol 1983; 14: 235-241.
57. Noseworthy JH, Ebers GC, Vandervoot MK, Farquhar RE, Yetisir E, Roberts R. The impact of blinding on the results of a randomized, placebo-controlled multiple sclerosis trial. Neurology 1994; 44: 16-20.

58. Ebstein WV. Expectation bias in rheumatoid arthritis clinical trials. The anti-CD4 monoclonal antibody experience. Arth Rheum 1996; 39 (11): 1773-1780.
59. Pocock SJ. Clinical Trials: A Practical Approach. New York, John Wiley and Sons, 1983.
60. Burt RK, Burns W, Hess A. Bone marrow transplantation for multiple sclerosis. Bone Marrow Transplantation 1995; 16: 1-6.
61. Cook SD, Devereux C, Trioano R, et. al. Effect of total lymphoid irradiation in chronic multiple sclerosis. Lancet 1986; 1: 1405-1409.
62. European Study Group on interferon beta-1b in Secondary Progressive MS. Placebo controlled multicentre randomized trial of interferon beta-1b in treatment of disability in secondary progressive multiple sclerosis. Lancet 1998; 352: 1491-1497.
63. Boumpas DT, Austin HA, Vaughn EM, Klippel JH, Steinberg AD, Yarboro CH, Balow JE. Controlled trial of pulse methylprednisolone versus two regimens of pulse cyclophosphamide in severe lupus nephritis. Lancet 1992; 340: 741-745.
64. Deapen D, Escalate A, Weinrib L, Horwitz D, Bachman B, Roy-Burman P, Walker A, Mack TM. A revised estimate of twin concordance in systemic lupus erythematosus. Arthritis Rheum 1992; 35: 311-318.
65. Horowitz DA. Impaired delayed hypersensitivity in systemic lupus erythematosus. Arthritis Rheum 1972; 353-9.
66. Seleznick MJ, Fries JF. Variables associated with decreased survival in Systemic lupus erythematosus. Seminars in Arthritis and Rheumatism 1991; 21(2): 73-80.
67. Gladman DD. Prognosis of systemic lupus erythematosus and factors that affect it. Rheumatology 1992; 4: 681-687.
68. Cohen MG, Li EK. Mortality in systemic lupus erythematosus: active disease is the most important factor. NZ J Med 1992; 22: 5-8.
69. Austin HA III, Muenz LR, Joyce KM, et al. Prognostic factors in lupus nephritis. Contribution of renal histology data. Am J Med 1983; 75: 382-391.
70. Brodsky RA, Petri M, Smith BD, Steifter J, Spivak JL, Styler M, Dang CV, Bridsky I, Jones R. Immunablative high dose cyclophosphamide without stem cell rescue for refractory severe autoimmune disease. Ann Intern Med 1998; 129: 1031-1035.
71. Baldwin JL, Storb R, Thomas ED, et al. Bone marrow transplantation in patients with gold-induced marrow aplasia. Arthritis Rheum 1977; 20: 1043-8.
72. Nelson JL, Torrez R, Louie FM, et al. Pre-existing autoimmune disease with long term survival after allogeneic bone marrow transplantation. J Rheumatol 1997; 24(suppl 48): 23-9.

73. Snowden JA, Kearney P, Kearney A, et al. Long term outcome of autoimmune disease following allogeneic bone marrow transplantation. Arthritis Rheum 1998; 41(3): 453-9.
74. Jacobs P, Vincent MD, Martell RW. Prolonged remission of severe refractory rheumatoid arthritis following allogeneic bone marrow transplantation for drug-induced aplastic anaemia. Bone Marrow Transplant 1986; 1(2): 237-9.
75. McKendry RJ, Huebsch L, Leclair B. Progression of rheumatoid arthritis following bone marrow transplantation. A case report with a 13-year follow up. Arthritis Rheum 1996; 39(7): 1246-53.
76. Snowden JA, Atkinson K, Kearney P, et al. Allogeneic bone marrow transplantation from a donor with severe active rheumatoid arthritis not resulting in adoptive transfer of disease to recipient. Bone Marrow Transplant 1997; 20(1): 71-3.
77. Pincus T, Brooks RH, Callahan LF. Prediction of long-term mortality in patients with rheumatoid arthritis according to simple questionnaire and joint count measures. Ann Intern Med 1994; 120: 26-34.
78. Callahan LF, Pincus T, Huston JW, et al. Measures of activity and damage in Rheumatoid Arthritis: depiction of changes and prediction of mortality over five years. Arthritis Care Res 1997; 10(6): 381-394.
79. Pincus T, Callahan LF. Rheumatology function tests: grip strength, walking time, button test and questionnaires document and predict longterm morbidity and mortality in rheumatiod arthritis. The Journal of Rheumatology 1992; 19(7): 1051-1057.
80 Amett F, Edworthy S, Bloch D, et al. The American Rheumatism Association 1987 revised criteria for the classification of rheumatoid arthritis. Arthritis Rheum 1988; 31: 315-24.
81. Feldson DT, Anderson JJ, Boers M, et al. American College of Rheumatology preliminary definition of improvement in rheumatoid arthritis. Arthritis Rheum 1995; 38: 727-35.
82. Guidance for industry: clinical development programs for drugs, devices, and biological products for the treatment of rheumatoid arthritis (RA): draft guidance. Washington, D.C.: Food and Drug Administration, 1998 March. Available from: http://www.fda.gov/cder/guidance/index.htm.
83. Brooks PM, Snowden J, Biggs J et al. A pilot dose escalation of high dose cyclophosphamide and autologous stem cell therapy in active rheumatoid arthritis. Arthritis Rheum 1998; 41, No 9 (Suppl): 598.

84. Moreland LW. Baumgartner SW, Schiff MH, Tindall EA, Fleischmann RM, Weaver AL, Ettlinger RE, Cohen S, Foopman WJ, Mohler K, Widman MB, Blosch CM. Treatyment of rheumatoid arthritis with a recombinant human tumor necrosis factor receptor (p75)-Fc fusion protein. N Engl J Med 1997; 337 (3), 141-147.

85. Aversa F, Tabilio A, Velardi A, Cunnigham I, Terenzi A, Falzetti F, Ruggeri L, Barbabietola G, Aristei C, Latini P, Reisner Y, Martelli MF. Treatment of high risk acute leukemia with T cell depleted stem cells from related donors with one fully mismatched HLA haplotype. N Engl J Med 1998; 339 (17): 1186-1192.

86. Horowitz MM, Gale RP, Sondel PM, Goldman JM, Kersey J, Kolb HJ, Rimm AA, Ringden O, Rozman C, Speck B. et.el. Graft versus leukemia reactions after bone marrow transplantation. Blood 1990; 75(3): 555-562.

87. Sullivan KM, Weiden PL, Storb R, Witherspoon RP, Fefer A, Fisher L, Buckner CD, Anasetti C, Appelbaum FR, Badger C. et al. Influence of acute and chronic graft-versus-host disease on relapse and survival after bone marrow transplantation from HLA-identical siblings as treatment of acute and chronic leukemia (published erratum appears in Blood Aug 15, 74(3), 1180, 1989.) Blood 1989; 73: 1720-8.

88. Kolb HJ, Schattenberg A, Goldman JM, Hertenstein B, Jacobsen N, Arcese W, Ljungman P, Ferrant A, Verdonck L, Niederwieser D, van Rhee F, Mittermueller J, de Witte T, Holler E, Ansari H: Graft-versus-leukemia effect of donor lymphocyte transfusions in marrow grafted patients. Blood 1995; 86: 2041-2050.

89. Nelson JL, Hughes KA, Smith AG, Nisperos BB, Branchard AM, Hansen JA. Remission of rheumatoid arthritis during pregrancy and maternal-fetal class II alloantigen disparity. Am J Reprod Immunol. 1992; 28 (3-4): 226-7.

90. Smith JB, Fort JG. Treatment of rheumatoid arthritis by immunization with mononuclear white blood cells: results of a preliminary trial. J Rheumatology 1996; 23(2): 220-5.

9

ADVANCES IN THE CONTROL OF CYTOMEGALOVIRUS DISEASE IN BONE MARROW TRANSPLANT PATIENTS

William H. Burns, M.D.
Medical College of Wisconsin, Milwaukee, WI 53226

Human cytomegalovirus (CMV) was first noted as inclusion bodies in the salivary glands of children and initially was thought to be protozoa. The high prevalence of this infection was evident when in 1932 Farber and Wolbach reported the occurrence of these lesions in the salivary glands of 12% of 183 children dying for various reasons (1). Isolation of the virus was subsequently reported independently by three groups led by Smith, Rowe and Weller (2-4). In 1971 Weller published a seminal two part article with the apt title, "The cytomegaloviruses: ubiquitous agents with protean clinical manifestations" (5,6). CMV has continued to reveal itself in many clinical settings from the brain of newborns to the retina of AIDS patients.

Until the introduction of effective antiviral agents such as ganciclovir (GCV) and foscarnet, CMV infections represented the most serious infectious complication of allogeneic BMT patients. In some centers it accounted for the deaths of 20% of allogeneic patients and today it remains an important complication. It was last reviewed in this series in 1990 (7). At that time partially effective treatment of CMV pneumonia with GCV and immunoglobulin had recently been reported (8-10). Since then new methods to monitor patients after BMT and strategies to prevent CMV disease have emerged and are now in widespread clinical use. This review assesses these advances and speculates on future developments.

BIOLOGY OF CMV

The virus is a double-stranded DNA virus with a genome of about 240 kb. This value is approximate because the commonly used laboratory strains, including the strain AD169 which was sequenced, are lacking about 15 kb present in most clinical isolates (11). It is unclear why approximately the same genetic segment is lost during multiple passages of human CMV through fibroblasts, nor are the functions of these lost genes known. In addition, there is considerable heterogeneity among clinical strains which allows for easy characterization of isolates from individuals using restriction patterns.

Cytomegaloviruses are highly species-specific, restricting investigations of human CMV to clinical and in vitro studies and the use of imperfect animal models (e.g., murine CMV). Like all herpesviruses, CMV can cause acute, productive infections in which the infected cells are lysed, and also poorly understood quiescent states of persistence or latency from which the virus can be reactivated to productive infections. BMT patients seropositive prior to transplant typically reactivate endogenous virus. This was demonstrated in four patients from whom pre-BMT isolates of CMV with unique restriction patterns were found to be identical to those of isolates obtained post transplant (12). However, analysis of restriction patterns of isolates obtained from multiple sites of individual patients revealed that 6 of 11 such BMT patients were infected with more than a single strain of virus (Burns, unpublished observations). Similar observations have been made for AIDS patients (13,14). Thus, patients may acquire additional strains of the virus from the stem cell source or from blood products. Patients seronegative for CMV pre-transplant may similarly acquire the virus from the marrow graft or from transfused blood products. Transmission of CMV in this manner, particularly to seropositive persons, occurs in the presence of antibody to the virus and probably occurs by cell-to-cell spread from leukocytes. Details of this process are not known. Can the viral genome pass from latently infected cells directly to uninfected cells or must it first be reactivated? If the latter, what factors are involved in reactivation (e.g., immune stimulation of the cell or cytokine milieu). Most studies in animal models of CMV infection and of human CMV in tissue culture use large inoculums of extracellular virus, usually laboratory strains, and are thus difficult to interpret in the context of the typical human patient.

Although the molecular basis of the latent state is unknown, the immediate early region of the viral genome is implicated because the CpG dinucleotide frequency of this region is markedly lower than that of the remaining genome (15). It is likely that immediate early genes are exposed to host methylating enzymes during the latent state as there is no evidence for methylation of the viral genome during lytic infection. Low levels of immediate early 1 (IE1) transcripts with novel start sites as well as antisense transcripts in the same region were detected during the latent state in hematopoietic cells and may be important in the establishment or maintenance of the latent state (16-18). Virus has been detected in hematopoietic precursors and particularly in monocytes, from which it can be induced to the productive state with cytokines (19,20).

186

Infection can involve many organs including liver, kidney, salivary glands, esophagus, intestines, brain, retina, heart, and lungs as well as many pervasive cell types such as endothelial cells and progenitor cells of the hematopoietic system. Plachter et al have recently reviewed the evidence for the widespread infection of various cell types by CMV in humans (21). This contrasts with the limited repertoire of cell types, mainly fibroblasts, in which human CMV can be efficiently propagated in tissue culture.

MONITORING ASSAYS

In contrast to shedding of CMV in urine or the throat, viremia and presence of the virus in bronchoalveloar (BAL) fluid correlate with the development of CMV pneumonia (22,23). These observations form the basis for current methods to monitor for clinically significant infection. The following methods performed on blood or BAL fluid are commonly used: 1) Rapid culture using the shell vial technique in which leukocytes are centrifuged onto fibroblast monolayers and these are fixed and examined with antibody specific for CMV 24 to 72 hours later for signs of infection. 2) Antigenemia assay in which leukocytes are centrifuged onto slides, fixed and examined with antibody for the virion matrix protein pp65 (UL83). 3) A hybrid capture assay (HCA) – a method to quantitate viral nucleic acid in leukocytes (e.g., the MUREX assay or the Digene Hybrid Capture System assay). 4) PCR of plasma for viral DNA. 5) PCR of whole blood extract for viral DNA. Each assay has strengths and weaknesses. For example, the antigenemia assay must be performed immediately for reliable quantitation of viremia (24) .

Many reports have compared these assays for their sensitivity, specificity and clinical usefulness to detect viremia, predict CMV disease or assess antiviral therapy. Table 1 lists representative comparative studies reported since this subject was last reviewed in this series. Because of their greater sensitivity and ability to predict CMV disease earlier than other assays, the PCR-based assays should prove most helpful in the initiation of pre-emptive therapy. Their chief drawback is their considerable variability from center to center which makes comparisons of data across centers difficult. However, they should become more standardized as the services of commercial vendors or their kits become more widely used. An improved hybrid capture assay is currently being tested and may have sensitivity approaching that of PCR-based assays and be more easily standardized than the latter.

Table 1. Comparative studies of assays to monitor for CMV viremia

Reference	Assays compared
Einsele et al 1991 (25,26)	PCR, culture
Vlieger et al 1992 (27)	PCR, antigenemia
Einsele et al 1995 (28)	PCR, culture
Mazzulli et al 1996 (29)	HCA, antigenemia, culture
Veal et al 1996 (30)	HCA, antigenemia, culture
Boeckh et al 1997 (31)	PCR. Antigenemia, culture
Hiyoshi et al 1997 (32)	PCR, antigenemia
Barrett-Muir et al 1998 (33)	PCR, HCA, culture
Hebart et al 1998 (34)	PCR, HCA, culture
Kanda et al 1998 (35)	PCR, antigenemia

STRATEGIES TO PREVENT CMV DISEASE AFTER AUTOLOGOUS BMT

Although the incidence of CMV infection is similar in autologous and allogeneic patients following transplant, the incidence of CMV disease is much lower in autologous transplants. Wingard et al reported a 2% incidence of CMV disease in 143 patients at Johns Hopkins (36) while Reusser et al reported from Seattle an incidence of 7.7% in 88 seronegative (pre-BMT) patients and 11.3% in 71 seropositive patients (37). This high incidence may reflect the use of TBI in Seattle regimens since CMV disease occurred only in those autologous patients receiving TBI. More recently Ljungman reported an incidence of 0.8% with a variation among centers of 0 to 8.6% based on 2252 patients reported in the European Group for BMT (38). In these reports, the mortality associated with CMV pneumonia was similar to that for allogeneic recipients and is therefore a serious complication when it occurs. Since the incidence varies so much among centers and the costs for monitoring patients is considerable, a center's experience with this complication should guide the decision of whether or not to monitor autologous patients for viremia.

STRATEGIES TO PREVENT CMV DISEASE AFTER ALLOGENEIC BMT

Seronegative patients
There are several strategies to prevent CMV disease in BMT patients. The first strategy is to prevent seronegative patients from exposure to the virus. In early

reports the use of seronegative blood products for seronegative recipients of stem cells from seronegative donors resulted in CMV infection of 13% of such patients (39). An alternative to blood products from seronegative donors are blood products filtered to remove leukocytes (40,41). In a large study of over 500 seronegative marrow transplant patients, the infection rate among those receiving seronegative blood products was 1.3% compared to 2.4% for those receiving filtered blood products (42). Both approaches can be successfully employed and the choice depends on local factors such as seronegative donor availability and the costs of filters. Should a seronegative patient have a seropositive stem cell donor, provision of screened or filtered blood products is still useful since about 30% of such patients so treated will remain uninfected. Newer methods to sterilize blood products of all nucleic acid pathogens using psoralen derivatives and light exposure are being investigated and may obviate the need to screen or filter blood products.

Seropositive patients
There are three strategies to prevent CMV disease (mainly pneumonia) in seropositive patients. The first is pre-emptive treatment of patients found to be viremic or to have virus detected in BAL fluid (22,23,43). This approach depends on monitoring patients with one of the above methods and usually commences at engraftment when enough cells are present for the assay (with the exception of plasma PCR which can begin at any time). Usually one of the following will trigger treatment with GCV: 1) two consecutive positive PCR-based assays, 2) a positive shell vial assay, 3) a positive antigenemia assay based on the number of cells positive for pp65 protein and the concurrent presence of GVHD, 4) a nucleic acid capture assay positive above a certain threshold. The usual treatment is 5 mg/kg twice daily for 2 to 3 weeks, followed by half that dose 5 to 7 times per week until 100 days post-BMT or until a monitoring assay for viremia is negative. The main side effect of GCV is marrow suppression which occurs in about 30% of patients and often requires growth factor administration or a switch to foscarnet. Although foscarnet is sometimes used if neutropenia is a problem, it and cidofovir are not used in initial therapy because most BMT patients in the peri-transplant period are on nephrotoxic drugs such as cyclosporine or amphotericin.

A second strategy is GCV prophylaxis beginning after engraftment and continuing usually until 100 days post-BMT or discontinuation due to drug toxicity. The first truly prophylaxis report using GCV was by Atkinson et al (44), recently updated to include 88 patients (45). This group showed that GCV prophylaxis was more effective in reducing CMV disease in recipients of related (10%) than unrelated (33%) transplants. There was an increase in CMV disease after the prophylaxis period which ended 84 days after transplant. This study had no control or pre-emptive arm for comparison. The post-transplant dose of

GCV (5 mg/kg 3 times per week) was less than that used in later studies and may account for a higher incidence of CMV disease. Also, 4 of 14 patients receiving marrow from unrelated donors concurrently received foscarnet.

Two GCV prophylaxis studies were reported that compared the pre-emptive approach to true prophylaxis(46,47). Prophylaxis results in a lower incidence of CMV disease than the pre-emptive approach, but due to GCV-related neutropenia there is no survival advantage because of a higher mortality from bacterial and fungal infections. In a large study of 226 patients randomized to GCV prophylaxis versus the pre-emptive approach (monitoring pp65 antigenemia), during the first 100 days after transplant more patients developed CMV disease in the pre-emptive group (14%) compared to the prophylaxis group (2.7%) (48). However, after 180 days following transplant and thereafter there was no difference in the incidence of CMV disease between the two groups as there was more late disease in the prophylaxis group. The latter group experienced an increase in invasive fungal disease and overall there were no differences in CMV-related deaths or transplant survival.

A prophylaxis study using oral GCV (1 gram three times per day) or placebo beginning when neutrophils were > 750/ μL and continuing until 100 days post BMT prevented CMV infection in 11 of 12 patients receiving GCV compared to 4 of 15 patients on placebo (49). In no patients did the neutrophils drop below 500/ μL. However, there was an increase in opportunistic infections during the six month study period in the GCV prophylaxis group. Thus, in this small study, there was effective antiviral prophylaxis without the severe neutropenia usually observed in GCV prophylaxis studies. Long-term follow-up has not been reported but one patient who received GCV prophylaxis died from CMV pneumonia following the prophylaxis period. These results are encouraging for preventing disease in the peri-transplant period but one would predict that after the prophylaxis period patients would be less likely to have developed adequate immune responses to the virus and might be more susceptible to late CMV disease.

A third strategy, adoptive cellular immunotherapy, was developed at Seattle and is practiced there and at only a few other institutions (including the Medical College of Wisconsin) because of the expense and resources needed. However, it offers clear advantages to the other approaches and in time may become cost effective. In this approach clones of T cells with specificity for CMV are derived from donor lymphocytes and expanded ex vivo to 10^8 to 10^9 and infused into the patient commencing within 6 weeks of transplant. Theoretically, there is little chance of causing GVHD with these infusions since clones of T cells are employed.

The basis for this approach includes animal studies of the murine CMV (MCMV) and earlier observations of CMV disease in humans following BMT. Extensive studies in mice by Koszinowski and his colleagues demonstrated a need for CD8$^+$ cells to control virus from most organs (50,51). Interestingly, clearance of virus from salivary glands required CD4$^+$ cells. Repeated observations that seropositive BMT recipients have less CMV disease if transplanted from seropositive rather than from seronegative donors might be interpreted as resulting from adoptive immune cell transfer (52,53).

In humans Quinnan et al demonstrated the presence of CMV-specific cytotoxic lymphocytes (CTL) in assays of the peripheral blood mononuclear cells (PBMC) of patients beginning several weeks following BMT. The presence or absence of CMV-specific CTL activity correlated with survival from CMV infection (54,55). The Seattle group has used a re-stimulation assay in which PBMC are stimulated for 12 to 14 days with CMV-infected fibroblasts before measuring CTL activity (56) . Their studies have demonstrated the requirement for CD8$^+$ CTL for prevention of CMV disease following BMT (57). CD4$^+$ lymphocytes were always present whenever CD8$^+$ CTLs were detected but could not alone prevent CMV disease (58,59). These investigators noted that the main targets of the CTLs were present on cells infected in the presence of transcription inhibitors and further showed that they are derived from virion matrix proteins introduced into the cells during viral entry (56). Immune responses directed towards the peptides derived from these proteins may be effective prior to the expression of viral proteins capable of down regulating MHC and evading the immune system. Detailed studies of a small number of patients revealed that CTL responses to viral glycoproteins localized to the cell membrane (e.g., gB and gH) and to viral proteins primarily retained in the nucleus (i.e., IE1) are relatively minor, suggesting that these proteins may not be as readily available to the proteasome/TAP system as the cytoplasmic virion matrix proteins (56,59-61). In fact one of these matrix proteins (pp65) can phosphorylate an immediate early protein (IE1) of CMV and prevent it from effective processing and presentation as antigen (62).

Riddell, Greenberg and their colleagues have developed a method of cloning CD8$^+$ T cells from seropositive bone marrow donors and expanding them to the billions ex vivo (59,63,64). The details of these procedures that produce clinically useful numbers of CD8$^+$ cells which retain antigen specificity and cytolytic potential are a major contribution to antigen specific immunotherapy. Fibroblasts derived from donor skin biopsies are infected with human CMV (the AD169 strain) and used as a source of antigen for lymphocyte stimulation. Monocytes/macrophages/dendritic cells in the PBMC used as a source of lymphocytes presumably are the antigen processing and presenting cells for the lymphocytes. After multiple stimulations over two weeks, CTL activity can be demonstrated in these bulk cultures. These cultures are the source of lymphocytes cloned by limiting dilution cultures in 96-well plates with feeder cells and CMV-infected fibroblasts. Wells with proliferating cells are then identified and the cells examined for CMV-specificity using infected fibroblasts as targets. These are then further expanded by the addition of IL-2 and either antibody to CD3 or repeated antigen stimulation using infected fibroblasts, always in the critical presence of feeder cells. Riddell has reported that with the above procedure 2% to 10% of T cells plated from the bulk cultures produce clones, 30% to 80% of which are CMV-specific (59). Our cloning efficiency has been lower at about 0.1% of T cells plated from bulk cultures. The CTL assays of CD8[+] clones specific for CMV derived from one of our donors using infected (or mock infected control) HLA-matched fibroblasts as targets are shown in Figure 1.

Figure 1. Lysis of CMV-infected and mock-infected fibroblast targets by CD8[+] T cell clones after expansion.

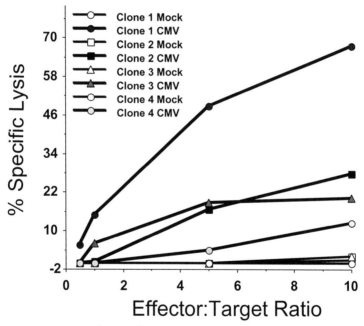

Clones of T cells (10^8 to 10^9 cells) are then infused weekly for 4 weeks beginning 5 to 6 weeks after transplant. After infusion, CD8[+] cytotoxic activity can be measured for at least three months and reach levels similar to those of the donors, particularly if CMV-specific CD4[+] cells concurrently (endogenously)

develop (64). The infused clones were also monitored by detection of the variable genes (V_α and V_β) of the T-cell receptor (TCR) of the infused clones and clones isolated later from the patient. Clones of CD4$^+$ T cells can be derived by stimulating lymphocytes with supernatants prepared from CMV-infected fibroblasts followed by limiting dilution cultures. Infusion of these clones with CD8$^+$ clones theoretically would lead to the sustained presence of the latter through helper effects. Administration of low dose IL-2 might also perpetuate the CD8$^+$ cells but the use of the CD4$^+$ cells obviates the toxicity and cost of IL-2 administration and may provide for a longer term stimulation of the CTL clones.

Persistence of infused clones will also be influenced by concurrent immunosuppressive therapy. Presumably all 14 patients in the report from Seattle were receiving cyclosporine or tacrolimus during and after the T cell infusions, yet the clones were active weeks later. Furthermore, cytotoxic T cell clones persisted even after the administration of high doses of steroids (1-3 mg/kg) for GVHD treatment (64).

The timing of infusion of the T cell clones is important since CMV pneumonia peaks during the second month after BMT. Another concern is that CMV pneumonia may have an immunological component to its pathogenesis and restoring the immune capacity of the patient after the lungs have been seeded with the virus may potentially result in the clinical pneumonia syndrome or exacerbate it. One approach might be to treat patients prophylactically with GCV after engraftment and discontinue it after T cell clones are infused. This would allow more time for preparation of the clones and a later deadline for their safe infusion. Suppression of viral replication by prophylaxis is effective and marrow suppression should not be a problem if the lymphocytes are not infused too late .

A requirement of the Seattle approach to cloning T cells specific for CMV is the availability of donor fibroblasts. Cells not autologous to the T cell donor might elicit reactions to minor histocompatibility antigens. Although theoretically clones of T cells against CMV peptides in the context of genetically identical MHC proteins should not elicit graft-versus-host (GVH) reactions unless there is cross reactivity of the viral peptide with host peptides, the use of the patient's fibroblasts to stimulate donor T cells is undesirable. It generally takes a month to obtain sufficient fibroblasts from skin biopsies to begin the bulk stimulation cultures. This logistical problem precludes using this approach for patients undergoing unrelated donor transplants since skin biopsies must be obtained a month before the stem cell donation if cytotoxic clones are to be available within 6 weeks after transplant. Also, many unrelated donors may refuse skin biopsies. This situation is unfortunate as recipients of stem cells from unrelated donors have more severe and long term CMV disease than related donor recipients.

Dermal fibroblasts have the advantage over other cell types known to be infected by CMV in that they are readily available from normal persons. Dendritic cells (DC) may be an excellent alternative to fibroblasts since they can be obtained from the blood of normal donors and should provide superb stimulation of both CD4$^+$ and CD8$^+$ lymphocytes. We have not been able to infect them with laboratory strains of human CMV; however, it may be possible to infect them by exposing them to infected fibroblasts (unpublished observations). The desire not to expose lymphocytes to genetically non-identical cells in the stimulatory process would nevertheless still require donor fibroblasts, although possibly fewer. The finding that virion matrix proteins provide the immunodominant peptides of CMV allows one to restrict the cloning to T cells that recognize these peptides. Riddell et al used peptides derived from pp65 and by pulsing cultures of PBMC were able to derive T cell clones cytotoxic for CMV-infected cells (65). This approach depends on the prior determination of the relevant peptides for different HLA types and unknown factors might influence antigen presentation in certain HLA contexts. Indeed, in two donors studied in detail MHC preferences were noted for CMV-specific polyclonal CTLs (59). There is also concern that antigen stimulation by peptide pulsing may produce clones with low avidity TCR that might be less active and more prone to cross-reactivities with self. Our approach is to use DC expressing pp65 and/or pp150 as stimulators. DC can be readily prepared from PBMC in a few days, greatly simplifying procurement of stimulator cells from unrelated or other donors and decreasing the time to initiate bulk stimulation. The CMV matrix gene could be introduced into the DC by a retrovirus, adenovirus or other means. CTL assays could use EBV-transformed cells infected with a vaccinia recombinant expressing pp65 or pp150 and obviate any need for fibroblasts. These approaches are currently being explored at the Medical College of Wisconsin.

There are many advantages of an adoptive immunity approach to preventing CMV disease in BMT patients. With this approach one is restoring control of the virus infection in a more natural and lasting manner than the transient pharmacological approach. Indeed, there is evidence that suppression of viral growth with GCV results in a delay in development of CTL against the virus (46,58). In this investigation advantage was taken of a study in which GCV or placebo was administered prophylactically beginning with engraftment. Some patients receiving GCV developed CTLs against CMV shortly after engraftment (day 30 post BMT), but those that did not were unlikely to develop CTL to CMV by day 90. In contrast, patients receiving placebo were likely to develop CTL to CMV from day 30 to day 90.

It is likely that patients failing to develop a T cell immune capacity for CMV will develop late CMV disease. An increase in late CMV disease has been noted in most of the pre-emptive and prophylaxis reports cited previously. A CMV-specific T cell proliferation assay has been used to screen patients around day 120 post-transplant to predict for late CMV disease (66). No patient with a positive proliferative response by that time later developed CMV disease compared to 31% of those with negative tests. These results support the need to acquire a T cell immune capacity for long-term prevention of CMV disease.

The toxicities and costs of GCV and foscarnet treatment would also be reduced. These costs include growth factor for marrow suppression associated with GCV, multiple laboratory tests to monitor electrolytes for patients on foscarnet, and repeat hospitalizations for late CMV disease. An added benefit more difficult to quantify would be the prevention of fevers, immunosuppression and other morbidities associated with recurring or chronic CMV infections.

CONCLUSIONS

CMV disease is no longer the lethal complication of allogeneic BMT it once was. The development of surveillance methodologies to identify patients at great risk of CMV disease, the availability of effective antiviral drugs and an appreciation of their toxicities have clearly altered the outlook during the first few months following BMT. The overall survival is comparable whether one employs the pre-emptive approach based on surveillance for viremia or the truly prophylactic approach which commences GCV after engraftment for all patients at risk. The former has increased occurrence of CMV disease in some patients while the latter suffers from GCV toxicity (mainly neutropenia and increased severe bacterial and especially fungal infections). Unfortunately, both suppress the development of effective immune responses to CMV in many patients. The price to be paid later is recurring manifestations of CMV infection and occasionally death from CMV. The financial cost of the drug therapy, viral surveillance and other laboratory assays, the cost of growth factor administration for GCV-related neutropenia, and the re-hospitalizations related to recurring CMV infection are substantial. A direct financial comparison of adoptive immunotherapy versus prophylaxis or pre-emptive GCV treatment would be of great interest.

The development of adoptive CMV specific immunotherapy by investigators at Seattle is thus a very attractive alternative both for financial reasons as well as the logic involved in restoring a faulty immune system to eliminate the problem more definitively and, with the administration of $CD4^+$ as well as $CD8^+$ T cell clones, for the long term. The ability of these clones to persist with activity and specificity despite concurrent immunosuppressive therapy for GVHD is encouraging. Improvement in the methods of stimulation (DC cells) and cloning for a limited number of specificities (pp65, pp150) should result in economies of cost and time of preparation. It is probable that this approach will supplant others in the future.

REFERENCES

1. Farber S, Wolbach S: Intranuclear and cytoplasmic inclusions ("protozoan-like bodies") in the salivary glands of infants. Am J Pathol Children 1932;8:123-126.
2. Smith M: Propagation in tissue cultures of a cytopathogenic virus from human salivary gland virus disease. Proc Soc Exptl Biol Med 1956;92:424-430.
3. Rowe W, Hartley J, Waterman S, et al: Cytopathogenic agents resembling human salivary gland virus recovered from tissue cultures of human adenoids. Proc Soc Exptl Biol Med 1956;92:418-424.
4. Weller TH, Macaulay JC, Craig JM, et al: Isolation of intranuclear inclusion producing agents from infants with illnesses resembling cytomegalic inclusion disease. Proc Soc Exptl Biol Med 1957;94:4-12.
5. Weller TH: The cytomegaloviruses: ubiquitous agents with protean clinical manifestations. I. N Engl J Med 1971;285:203-214.
6. Weller TH: The cytomegaloviruses: ubiquitous agents with protean clinical manifestations. II. N Engl J Med 1971;285:267-274.
7. Winston DJ, Ho WG, Champlin RE: Cytomegalovirus infection and interstitial pneumonia after bone marrow transplantation. Cancer Treat Res 1990;50:113-128.
8. Emanuel D, Cunningham I, Jules-Elysee K, et al: Cytomegalovirus pneumonia after bone marrow transplantation successfully treated with the combination of ganciclovir and high-dose intravenous immune globulin. Ann Intern Med 1988;109:777-782.
9. Reed EC, Bowden RA, Dandliker PS, et al: Treatment of cytomegalovirus pneumonia with ganciclovir and intravenous cytomegalovirus immunoglobulin in patients with bone marrow transplants. Ann Intern Med 1988;109:783-788.
10. Schmidt GM, Kovacs A, Zaia JA, et al: Ganciclovir/immunoglobulin combination therapy for the treatment of human cytomegalovirus-associated interstitial pneumonia in bone marrow allograft recipients. Transplantation 1988;46:905-907.
11. Cha TA, Tom E, Kemble GW, et al: Human cytomegalovirus clinical isolates carry at least 19 genes not found in laboratory strains. J Virol 1996;70:78-83.

12. Winston DJ, Huang ES, Miller MJ, et al: Molecular epidemiology of cytomegalovirus infections associated with bone marrow transplantation. Ann Intern Med 1985;102:16-20.

13. Drew WL, Sweet ES, Miner RC, et al: Multiple infections by cytomegalovirus in patients with acquired immunodeficiency syndrome: documentation by Southern blot hybridization. J Inf Dis 1984;150:952-953.

14. Spector SA, Hirata KK, Newman TR: Identification of multiple cytomegalovirus strains in homosexual men with acquired immunodeficiency syndrome. J Inf Dis 1984;150:953-956.

15. Honess RW, Gompels UA, Barrell BG, et al: Deviations from expected frequencies of CpG dinucleotides in herpesvirus DNAs may be diagnostic of differences in the states of their latent genomes. J Gen Virol 1989;70:837-855.

16. Kondo K, Kaneshima H, Mocarski ES: Human cytomegalovirus latent infection of granulocyte-macrophage progenitors. Proc Natl Acad Sci USA 1994;91:11879-11883.

17. Kondo K, Mocarski ES: Cytomegalovirus latency and latency-specific transcription in hematopoietic progenitors. Scandinavian Journal of Infectious Diseases 1995;99:63-67.

18. Sarisky RT, Gao Z, Lieberman PM, et al: A replication function associated with the activation domain of the Epstein-Barr virus Zta transactivator. J Virol 1996;70:8340-8347.

19. Taylor-Wiedeman J, Sissons JG, Borysiewicz LK, et al: Monocytes are a major site of persistence of human cytomegalovirus in peripheral blood mononuclear cells. J Gen Virol 1991;72:2059-2064.

20. Taylor-Wiedeman J, Sissons JG, Sinclair J: Induction of endogenous human cytomegalovirus gene expression after differentiation monocytes from healthy carriers. J Virol 1994;68:1597-1604.

21. Plachter B, Sinzger C, Jahn G: Cell types involved in replication and distribution of human cytomegalovirus. Adv Virus Res 1996;46:195-261.

22. Goodrich JM, Mori M, Gleaves CA, et al: Early treatment with ganciclovir to prevent cytomegalovirus disease after allogeneic bone marrow transplantation. N Engl J Med 1991;325:1601-1607.

23. Schmidt GM, Horak DA, Niland JC, et al: A randomized, controlled trial of prophylactic ganciclovir for cytomegalovirus pulmonary infection in recipients of allogeneic bone marrow transplants; The City of Hope-Stanford-Syntex CMV Study Group. N Engl J Med 1991;324:1005-1011.

24. Boeckh M, Woogerd PM, Stevens-Ayers T, et al: Factors influencing detection of quantitative cytomegalovirus antigenemia. J Clin Microbiol 1994;32:832-834.

25. Einsele H, Ehninger G, Steidle M, et al: Polymerase chain reaction to evaluate antiviral therapy for cytomegalovirus disease. Lancet 1991;338:1170-1172.
26. Einsele H, Steidle M, Vallbracht A, et al: Early occurrence of human cytomegalovirus infection after bone marrow transplantation as demonstrated by the polymerase chain reaction technique. Blood 1991;77:1104-1110.
27. Vlieger AM, Boland GJ, Jiwa NM, et al: Cytomegalovirus antigenemia assay or PCR can be used to monitor ganciclovir treatment in bone marrow transplant recipients. Bone Marrow Transplant 1992;9:247-253.
28. Einsele H, Ehninger G, Hebart H, et al: Polymerase chain reaction monitoring reduces the incidence of cytomegalovirus disease and the duration and side effects of antiviral therapy after bone marrow transplantation. Blood 1995;86:2815-2820.
29. Mazzulli T, Wood S, Chua R, et al: Evaluation of the Digene Hybrid Capture System for detection and quantitation of human cytomegalovirus viremia in human immunodeficiency virus-infected patients. J Clin Microbiol 1996;34:2959-2962.
30. Veal N, Payan C, Fray D, et al: Novel DNA assay for cytomegalovirus detection: comparison with conventional culture and pp65 antigenemia assay. J Clin Microbiol 1996;34:3097-3100.
31. Boeckh M, Gallez-Hawkins GM, Myerson D, et al: Plasma polymerase chain reaction for cytomegalovirus DNA after allogeneic marrow transplantation: comparison with polymerase chain reaction using peripheral blood leukocytes, pp65 antigenemia, and viral culture. Transplantation 1997;64:108-113.
32. Hiyoshi M, Tagawa S, Takubo T, et al: Evaluation of the AMPLICOR CMV test for direct detection of cytomegalovirus in plasma specimens. J Clin Microbiol 1997;35:2692-2694.
33. Barrett-Muir WY, Aitken C, Templeton K, et al: Evaluation of the murex hybrid capture cytomegalovirus DNA assay versus plasma PCR and shell vial assay for diagnosis of human cytomegalovirus viremia in immunocompromised patients. J Clin Microbiol 1998;36:2554-2556.
34. Hebart H, Gamer D, Loeffler J, et al: Evaluation of Murex CMV DNA hybrid capture assay for detection and quantitation of cytomegalovirus infection in patients following allogeneic stem cell transplantation. J Clin Microbiol 1998;36:1333-1337.
35. Kanda Y, Chiba S, Suzuki T, et al: Time course analysis of semi-quantitative PCR and antigenaemia assay for prevention of cytomegalovirus disease after bone marrow transplantation. Brit J Hematol 1998;100:222-225.

36. Wingard JR, Chen DY, Burns WH, et al: Cytomegalovirus infection after autologous bone marrow transplantation with comparison to infection after allogeneic bone marrow transplantation. Blood 1988;71:1432-1437.
37. Reusser P, Fisher LD, Buckner CD, et al: Cytomegalovirus infection after autologous bone marrow transplantation: occurrence of cytomegalovirus disease and effect on engraftment. Blood 1990;75:1888-1894.
38. Ljungman P, Biron P, Bosi A, et al: Cytomegalovirus interstitial pneumonia in autologous bone marrow transplant recipients. Bone Marrow Transplant 1994;13:209-212.
39. Bowden RA, Sayers M, Flournoy N, et al: Cytomegalovirus immune globulin and seronegative blood products to prevent primary cytomegalovirus infection after marrow transplantation. N Engl J Med 1986;314:1006-1010.
40. Bowden RA, Slichter SJ, Sayers MH, et al: Use of leukocyte-depleted platelets and cytomegalovirus-seronegative red blood cells for prevention of primary cytomegalovirus infection after marrow transplant. Blood 1991;78:246-250.
41. Bowden RA: Transfusion-transmitted cytomegalovirus infection. Hematol Oncol Clinics N Am 1995;9:155-166.
42. Bowden RA, Slichter SJ, Sayers M, et al: A comparison of filtered leukocyte-reduced and cytomegalovirus (CMV) seronegative blood products for the prevention of transfusion-associated CMV infection after marrow transplant. Blood 1995;86:3598-3603.
43. Goodrich JM, Boeckh M, Bowden R: Strategies for the prevention of cytomegalovirus disease after marrow transplantation. Clin Infect Dis 1994;19:287-298.
44. Atkinson K, Downs K, Golenia M, et al: Prophylactic use of ganciclovir in allogeneic bone marrow transplantation: absence of clinical cytomegalovirus infection. Brit J Hematol 1991;79:57-62.
45. Atkinson K, Arthur C, Bradstock K, et al: Prophylactic ganciclovir is more effective in HLA-identical family member marrow transplant recipients than in more heavily immune-suppressed HLA-identical unrelated donor marrow transplant recipients. Australasian Bone Marrow Transplant Study Group. Bone Marrow Transplant 1995;16:401-405.
46. Goodrich JM, Bowden RA, Fisher L, et al: Ganciclovir prophylaxis to prevent cytomegalovirus disease after allogeneic marrow transplant. Ann Intern Med 1993;118:173-178.
47. Winston DJ, Ho WG, Bartoni K, et al: Ganciclovir prophylaxis of cytomegalovirus infection and disease in allogeneic bone marrow transplant recipients. Results of a placebo-controlled, double-blind trial. Ann Intern Med 1993;118:179-184.

48. Boeckh M, Gooley TA, Myerson D, et al: Cytomegalovirus pp65 antigenemia-guided early treatment with ganciclovir versus ganciclovir at engraftment after allogeneic marrow transplantation: a randomized double-blind study. Blood 1996;88:4063-4071.

49. Pineiro LA, Skettino S, Tan J, et al: A study of the safety and efficacy of oral ganciclovir for the prevention of cytomegalovirus disease in bone marrow transplant recipients. Blood 1997;90 (supplement):544a

50. Koszinowski UH, del Val M, Reddehase MJ: Cellular and molecular basis of the protective immune response to cytomegalovirus infection. Curr Top Microbiol Immunol 1990;154:189-220.

51. Koszinowski UH, Reddehase MJ, Jonjic S: The role of CD4 and CD8 T cells in viral infections. Curr Opinion Immunol 1991;3:471-475.

52. Grob JP, Grundy JE, Prentice HG, et al: Immune donors can protect marrow-transplant recipients from severe cytomegalovirus infections. Lancet 1987;1:774-776.

53. Humar A, Wood S, Lipton J, et al: Effect of cytomegalovirus infection on 1-year mortality rates among recipients of allogeneic bone marrow transplants. Clin Infect Dis 1998;26:606-610.

54. Quinnan GV, Jr., Kirmani N, Rook AH, et al: Cytotoxic t cells in cytomegalovirus infection: HLA-restricted T- lymphocyte and non-T-lymphocyte cytotoxic responses correlate with recovery from cytomegalovirus infection in bone-marrow- transplant recipients. N Engl J Med 1982;307:7-13.

55. Quinnan GV, Jr., Burns WH, Kirmani N, et al: HLA-restricted cytotoxic T lymphocytes are an early immune response and important defense mechanism in cytomegalovirus infections. Rev Infect Dis 1984;6:156-163.

56. Riddell SR, Rabin M, Geballe AP, et al: Class I MHC-restricted cytotoxic T lymphocyte recognition of cells infected with human cytomegalovirus does not require endogenous viral gene expression. J Immunol 1991;146:2795-2804.

57. Reusser P, Riddell SR, Meyers JD, et al: Cytotoxic T-lymphocyte response to cytomegalovirus after human allogeneic bone marrow transplantation: pattern of recovery and correlation with cytomegalovirus infection and disease. Blood 1991;78:1373-1380.

58. Li CR, Greenberg PD, Gilbert MJ, et al: Recovery of HLA-restricted cytomegalovirus (CMV)-specific T-cell responses after allogeneic bone marrow transplant: correlation with CMV disease and effect of ganciclovir prophylaxis. Blood 1994;83:1971-1979.

59. Riddell SR, Greenberg PD: Therapeutic reconstitution of human viral immunity by adoptive transfer of cytotoxic T lymphocyte clones. Curr Top Microbiol Immunol 1994;189:9-34.

60. Borysiewicz LK, Hickling JK, Graham S, et al: Human cytomegalovirus-specific cytotoxic T cells. Relative frequency of stage-specific CTL recognizing the 72-kD immediate early protein and glycoprotein B expressed by recombinant vaccinia viruses. J Exp Med 1988;168:919-931.
61. Borysiewicz LK, Sissons JG: Cytotoxic T cells and human herpes virus infections. Curr Top Microbiol Immunol 1994;189:123-150.
62. Gilbert MJ, Riddell SR, Plachter B, et al: Cytomegalovirus selectively blocks antigen processing and presentation of its immediate-early gene product. Nature 1996;383:720-722.
63. Riddell SR, Watanabe KS, Goodrich JM, et al: Restoration of viral immunity in immunodeficient humans by the adoptive transfer of T cell clones. Science 1992;257:238-241.
64. Walter EA, Greenberg PD, Gilbert MJ, et al: Reconstitution of cellular immunity against cytomegalovirus in recipients of allogeneic bone marrow by transfer of T-cell clones from the donor. N Engl J Med 1995;333:1038-1044.
65. McLaughlin-Taylor E, Pande H, Forman SJ, et al: Identification of the major late human cytomegalovirus matrix protein pp65 as a target antigen for CD8+ virus-specific cytotoxic T lymphocytes. J Med Virol 1994;43:103-110.
66. Krause H, Hebart H, Jahn G, et al: Screening for CMV-specific T cell proliferation to identify patients at risk of developing late onset CMV disease. Bone Marrow Transplant 1997;19:1111-1116.

10

ADOPTIVE IMMUNOTHERAPY FOR EBV-ASSOCIATED MALIGNANCIES

Kenneth G. Lucas, M.D. and J. Christian Barrett, M.D.
University of Alabama-Birmingham, Birmingham, AL

The recognition of an increased risk of certain malignancies in immunocompromised individuals has led to a growing understanding of the role of the immune system in the surveillance for and prevention of neoplasms. This fact, combined with the limitations and toxicities associated with currently available cytotoxic agents, has provided the impetus to investigate alternative therapeutic approaches. Over the past decade there has been an increased interest in biologic approaches to augment the immune system in its anti-neoplastic efforts including the use of biologic agents (ie. interferons and interleukins), vaccines, and adoptive immunotherapy. This chapter will discuss aspects of the Epstein-Barr virus and the human immune response against EBV. The clinical role of adoptive immunotherapy in the treatment of EBV-induced malignancies will be presented, as well as the areas of current investigation.

EPSTEIN-BARR VIRUS

The Epstein-Barr virus (EBV) is a ubiquitous agent with 90% of adults worldwide having serologic evidence of EBV infection (1). The virus primarily infects B-cells. While the number of infected B-cells decreases rapidly as the immune response against EBV develops, a small population of resting B-cells escapes the immune response, establishing a population of latently infected cells which persists throughout the life of the infected individual (2,3,4). These latently infected cells are transformed into immortalized lymphoblasts both *in vitro* and *in vivo* (5,6). Viral shedding occurs intermittently from the oropharyngeal epithelium over the lifetime of the infected individual and is increased in immunocompromised patients (7,8). Following allogeneic bone marrow transplantation, virus being shed can be traced to donor origin suggesting that latently infected B-cells can serve as a source of infection and, as discussed later in this chapter, lymphomagenesis (9).

EBV and the Human Immune Response
Following primary infection by EBV, the virus is rapidly internalized within the B-cell where the viral DNA circularizes as an episome. Lytic genes are

expressed to affect the replication, packaging, and release of new virions from the host cell. Conversely, resting B-cells infected by EBV express a group of latent genes which act in concert to affect the transformation of the cell into immortalized lymphoblastoid cells (10). A humoral immune response develops against antigens on the viral capsule and envelope. However, it is the subsequent cellular immune response which is required for clearance of infected cells harboring intracellular virus.

It has long been recognized that the major component of viral-induced cellular immune response involves HLA-restricted CD8$^+$ T-cells (11). Viral antigens presented in complex with MHC class I molecules on the infected cell surface serve as the target of this cytotoxic response (12,13). Similar mechanisms appear to be in operation in the immune response against EBV. Carriers of latent EBV infection maintain a population of cytotoxic T-lymphocytes (CTL) which can be reactivated when exposed to autologous EBV-infected B-cells in an HLA-restricted manner (14). Murray *et al* transfected human fibroblasts using recombinant vaccinia virus genetically manipulated to express one of eight EBV latent proteins (15). They then tested CTL preparations from sixteen donors with EBV-induced immunity and known HLA typing to determine the specific antigen(s) recognized by EBV-specific CTLs and to determine the specific HLA class I type associated with the recognition of these target antigen(s). This work demonstrates that the cytoxic T-cell response of an individual against EBV consistently recognizes a specific panel of latent EBV proteins and that this panel of recognized latency proteins varies among individuals. Moreover, each HLA class I molecule presents a restricted array of latency proteins. Therefore, the viral proteins targeted by an individual are determined by their specific HLA type, and the variation of recognized targets among individuals reflects differing HLA expression. Among the sixteen donors tested, EBNA-3a, EBNA-3b, and EBNA-3c represented the predominant antigenic targets with responses also seen against EBNA-2 and LMP-2. No response against LMP-1 and EBNA-1 were elicited. Though there has been an occasional CTL response to LMP-1 reported, there have been no reported responses to EBNA-1, suggesting these proteins are less antigenic (16). Selective expression of these viral proteins may serve as the basis of immune evasion by latently infected cells.

Differences in expression of the EBV proteins by various EBV-associated tumors have lead to the following classification scheme. Latency Type I (LAT I) infected cells express only EBNA-1 as seen in most Burkitt's lymphomas. LAT II cells express both EBNA-1 and LMP-1 as frequently seen in nasopharyngeal carcinoma and Hodgkin's disease. LAT III cells express a full range of the known EBV proteins as seen in the post-transplant lymphomas of stem cell and solid organ transplant patients (17).

LYMPHOPROLIFERATIVE DISORDERS AND THE IMMUNOCOMPROMISED PATIENT

An increased incidence of lymphoproliferative diseases (LPD) has been reported among immunocompromised individuals following solid organ transplantation, bone marrow transplantation (BMT), and infection with the human immunodeficiency virus (HIV)(Table 1). Among organ transplant recipients, the risk of a lymphoproliferative disorder is particularly increased among those patients undergoing a heart or heart/lung transplant and among those treated with OKT3 or cyclosporin A (18,19) Crawford *et al* examined the CTL responses against autologous EBV-infected B-cell cultures from cadaveric renal transplant patients with serologic evidence of prior EBV infection and compared these responses to seropositive and seronegative controls (20). This work demonstrated a functional impairment of CTLs among patients receiving cyclosporin A with no such impairment noted among those patients receiving azathioprine and prednisone.

Table 1. Clinical Factors Associated with Impaired Cellular Immunity and EBV Lymphoproliferative Disorders

Quantitative Defects in T-Lymphocytes
> Congenital Deficiencies (ie Wiscott-Aldrich; Severe
> > Combined Immunodeficiency Syndrome)
> HIV Infection
> Marrow –Ablative Chemotherapy
> T-Cell Depletion of Stem Cell Transplantation Products
> Anti-T-Cell Antibodies (ie ATG; OKT3)

Qualitative Defects in T-Lymphocytes
> Immunosuppressive Agents (ie Cyclosporin A)

Impaired EBV-Antigen Recognition
HLA-Mismatching

A variety of lymphoproliferative disorders have been described following solid organ transplantation, ranging from plasmacytic hyperplasia to immunoblastic lymphoma, accounting for the varied clinical course and therapeutic responses reported in the literature. EBV DNA has been detected in 85-100% of specimens tested (21,22) though cases of B-cell LPD without genetic evidence of EBV have been reported (21,23,24). Immunohistochemical staining of the EBV[+]

lymphoproliferative lesions in organ transplant patients demonstrates that these tissues express a variety of latent EBV proteins without expression of lytic proteins. Specifically, all specimens studied expressed EBNA-1 and EBNA-2, and most expressed EBNA-3 and/or LMP, indicating a LAT-III phenotype (25). Classification of these disorders is best accomplished by combining morphology and assessment of clonality based on immunoglobulin gene rearrangement studies. Plasmacytic hyperplasia is characterized by normal nodal architecture with expansion of the interfollicular area predominately by plasmacytoid lymphocytes. These tumors exhibit a lack of clonality and a benign clinical course typically confined to the tonsillar and nodal tissues with regression following withdrawal of immunosuppressive medications (21,26). Polymorphic B-cell hyperplasia and polymorphic B-cell lymphomas are characterized by increasing cellular atypia and necrosis with architectural distortion. These tumors exhibit monoclonal gene rearrangements and increased extranodal tissue involvement (21). The clinical behavior of this group is variable, with some regressing following withdrawal of immunosuppression while others progress despite the change. Moreover, the presence of monoclonal gene rearrangements does not necessarily correlate with benign or malignant clinical behavior although it has been suggested that increased intensity of the clonal band may correlate to more malignant behavior (21,22). Finally, immunoblastic B-cell lymphomas (IBL) exhibit monoclonal gene rearrangements, additional genetic aberrations involving tumor suppressor or protooncogenes, and a widely disseminated, malignant disease course not responsive to withdrawal of immunosuppressive agents (21) One model of pathogenesis would involve the polyclonal expansion of latently-infected, EBV-immortalized B-cells resulting from a suppressed EBV-specific immunosurveillance. This expansion would allow additional mutations to occur within this proliferating population, culminating in the malignant transformation of subset of clonal cells (Figure 1).

Figure 1. Model of Progression for EBV$^+$ Lymphoproliferative Disorders

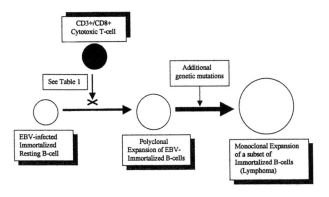

Using cytogenetics or HLA-typing to determine the origin of the malignant lymphocytes, most of the tumors reported in the literature have been of host origin following solid organ transplantation (25,27-29) Other investigators have reported tumors of donor origin; however, neither case had detectable molecular evidence of EBV (23,24) As the EBV⁺ LPDs express a LAT III phenotype in the context of host HLA-molecules, evasion of immunosurveillance is not attributable to failure of target recognition. Rather, it results from the quantitative and qualitative defects in the CTL resulting from the immunosuppressive agents necessary to insure organ engraftment.

Similarly, bone marrow transplant recipients develop lymphoproliferative disorders of B-cell origin with 75-100% having molecular evidence of EBV (30,31) The risk of developing an LPD is particularly increased among those undergoing partially-matched related allogeneic transplants (32-34), those manipulated by T-cell depletion (TCD) techniques during the processing of donor stem cells (32-35), and those treated with anti-T-cell immunoglobulins such as anti-thymocyte globulin (ATG) (36) or T-cell specific monoclonal antibodies. (30,37) Histologically, the spectrum of LPDs seen following bone marrow transplantation is similar to that reported following solid organ transplantation. The University of Minnesota reviewed their institution's experience following 506 patients having undergone allogeneic transplantation (34) They found only one case of a post-transplant LPD among 424 matched sibling allogeneic transplants without T-cell depletion and no case of a LPD among 47 matched sibling transplants with TCD. On the other hand, their experience found one case among only ten matched-unrelated (MUD) transplants without TCD and a surprising six cases of an LPD among the 25 mismatched sibling transplants utilizing TCD. In addition, they reported a median time from transplant to onset of the LPD of 72 days with only two of the eight tumors occurring later than ninety days after the transplant (at days 484 and 1488). Studies to determine the origin of the tumors were performed on seven of the eight specimens and revealed that five specimens were of donor origin while only two specimens were of host origin. Notably, the two patients developing a LPD beyond the immediate post-transplant period had the two tumors of host origin, and both had congenital immunodeficiencies--severe combined immunodeficiency disease (SCID) and Wiscott-Aldrich Syndrome-- which are themselves associated with an increased risk of LPD, raising the possibility that these cases were not related to the transplant but to the underlying diseases. Other retrospective studies have reported similar experiences with incidence ranges as follows: 0-0.45% following matched sibling allogeneic BMT, 0-0.45% following MUD BMT, 0-6.7% following matched sibling allogeneic BMT with TCD, 6.16-18.3% following MUD BMT with TCD and 13-24% following mismatched BMT with TCD (30,34,35,38)

The reported experiences raise many questions regarding the pathogenesis of these tumors. Unlike in solid organ transplantation, the host lymphocytes in BMT patients are nearly ablated during the preparative chemotherapy and are replaced by the donor's cells. Thus, the LPDs arising following BMT are typically of donor origin though rare cases of host origin tumors have been observed (30,31,34,36,39,40) The numbers of LPDs noted among recipients of a MUD transplant without TCD are too small to make meaningful assessment of the relative contribution to the risk for developing a LPD by this technique. Nevertheless, following an unmanipulated MUD and matched sibling BMT where surveillance by donor T-cells remains relatively intact, the risk of developing LPD appears to be small. While no statistical comparisons have been drawn, T-cell depletion appears to increase the risk of developing a LPD following all types of transplants, suggesting that the removal from the donor T-cells in itself is sufficient to allow an increased proliferation of EBV-transformed B-cells. Most patients are reported to have received ATG alone or in combination with other agents for engraftment and the prophylaxis of graft-versus-host disease (GVHD), suggesting that depletion of host and donor T-cell by immunoglobulins by itself may not be sufficient to increase lymphoproliferation. However, the patients reported to have developed a LPD often received higher doses of ATG such that there may be a dose-response relationship. HLA mismatching, perhaps even at the molecular level in the case of MUD BMT, may play a pivitol role in the development of a LPD following bone marrow transplantation by allowing infected cells expressing antigens in a HLA-restricted fashion not recognized by any residual T-cells to escape host recognition. This evasion of immunosurveillance would be compounded by T-cell depletion techniques and ATG which would result in the further removal of donor EBV-specific CTL, therefore, allowing the proliferation of EBV-transformed B-lymphocytes to proceed unchecked.

Following bone marrow transplantation, the immune function of the host remains compromised by both the preparative regimens and the graft-versus-host disease prophylaxis. The nature and duration of the immunosuppression have been subjects of investigation. An early study evaluated the recovery of EBV-specific immunity following HLA-matched allogeneic BMT using total body irradiation and cyclophosphamide as the preparative regimen and cyclosporin A as GVHD prophylaxis (41) Using [51]chromium release assays to detect CTL function, all patients studied recovered EBV-specific CTL function by 6 months post-transplantation. Following HLA-matched-related transplantation combined with T-cell depletion, no difference in the time to engraftment, in the absolute number of T-cells, or in the CD4:CD8 ratio is seen when compared with HLA-matched-related transplantation without T-cell depletion (42) EBV-specific CTLs have also been studied following T-cell depletion and appear quantitatively similar at 3 and 6 months to unmanipulated allogeneic transplants though the small number of patients studied, particularly at the later time points, limits the ability to detect subtle differences. However, [51]chromium release assays evaluating lysis of donor-derived, EBV-transformed B-lymphoblastoid cell lines (BLCL) suggest the possibility of a delay in development of EBV-specific CTL response to donor infected cells among T-cell depleted marrow recipients (Figure 2) (38) Differences may result from qualitative or quantitative differences in donor-specific CTLs following the use of ATG or the removal of donor-specific T-cells. No study of EBV-specific CTL recovery following allogeneic, HLA-mismatched transplantation with or without T-cell depletion has been reported. Nevertheless, the limited available data confirms that the most severe deficiency in CTL immunity--including that specific for EBV--is within the first six months post-transplant coinciding with the period of highest risk for development of lymphoproliferative disorders.

Figure 2. The log of EBV CTLp frequency is represented over time for recipients of unmodified BMT, related TCD BMT, and unrelated TCD BMT. The time at which past cases (28) of EBV-LPD have occurred in BMT patients at MSKCC is depicted below. The majority of past cases of EBV-LPD have occurred in the same time interval in which our study patients have been found to have deficient cytotoxicity against the donor BLCL.

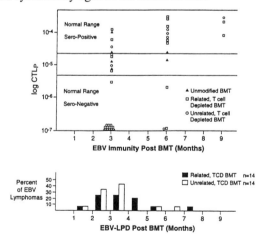

Infection with Human Immunodeficiency Virus-I (HIV) leads to the gradual destruction of $CD4^+$ T-lymphocytes and the acquired immunodeficiency syndrome (AIDS) which is defined by the degree of immunodeficiency and the resultant infectious and malignant manifestations of the compromised T-cell mediated immunity. AIDS-related Non-Hodgkin's lymphoma represents the second most common malignancy affecting the HIV infected individual with an incidence estimated between 4-10% (43,44) Protease inhibitors and combinations of anti-retroviral agents have been shown to decrease the incidence of AIDS-associated opportunistic infections and Kaposi's sarcoma; however, the impact of such therapy on NHL incidence remains uncertain with no clear decrease observed (45-47). Histologically, the majority are aggressive B-cell lymphomas (Burkitt's-type--BL, immunoblastic--IBL, and diffuse large cell lymphoma--DLCL). In systemic AIDS-associated NHL, evidence suggests an association with EBV in 42% of these malignancies though the association varies significantly depending upon the histologic type (25% of DLCL, 31% of BL, and 100% of IBL) (48). Immunohistochemical staining for LMP-1 and EBNA-2 among AIDS-associated NHL with DNA and/or RNA evidence of EBV infection demonstrates that among Burkitt's-like tumors 73% express a LAT I phenotype and 27% a LAT II phenotype while among immunoblastic/large cell NHL phenotypic expression is as follows: 27% LAT I; 32% LAT II; and 41% LAT III (49).

Primary Central Nervous System Lymphoma (PCNSL)--a rare malignancy among individuals not infected by HIV--is estimated to occur in 2-13% of HIV infected individuals over the life-time of their infection.(50) Histologically, these malignancies are of B-lymphocyte origin in 95% of cases—with >90% being either large cell lymphoma (LCL) or immunoblastic lymphoma (IBL).(51-53) Nearly 100% of B-cell, HIV-associated PCNSL have evidence of EBV mRNA.(51,54) In addition, immunohistochemical staining of AIDS-associated PCNSL reveals that 100% express EBV-associated antigens with 54-91% expressing a LAT III phenotype.(54,55) None of the reported studies evaluated these tumors for the more immunogenic antigens—EBNA-3a, 3b, and 3c.

Figure 3.

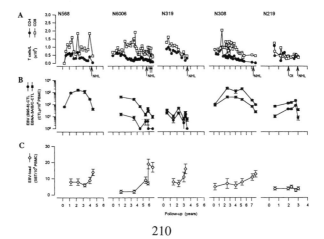

210

Using serial measures in HIV infected patients, CTL responses to HIV-1 and to EBV have been shown not to be parallel in their deterioration over the course of the HIV infection (56). Of note, in all five patients studied with progression to NHL, EBV-specific CTLs were noted to decrease--corresponding in four of the five with an increase in the EBV load as measured by a spontaneous B-cell transformation assay—during the months preceding the development of the NHL (Figure 3). Interestingly, one of the five patients experienced a brief spontaneous remission of a high grade B-cell lymphoma temporally associated with a transient increase in EBV-specific CTLs which subsequently became undetectable prior to recurrence of disease months later.

CELLULAR ADOPTIVE IMMUNOTHERAPY: RATIONALE AND BACKGROUND

Whether congenital, drug-induced, immunologically-induced, or viral-mediated and whether qualitative or quantitative, deficiency in T-lymphocyte cell-mediated immunity plays a critical role in the development of lymphoproliferative disorders in post-transplant and HIV-infected patients. Restoration of immunosurveillance, therefore, provides an attractive theoretical approach to the treatment and prevention of the infectious or neoplastic sequelae of immunodeficiency with the potential to avoid potentially toxic and/or ineffective therapies.

The feasibility of the transfer of lymphocytes was first demonstrated in animal models. Reddehase *et al* investigated the transfer of lymphocytes from immunocompetent mice to syngeneic, immunosuppressed mice (57,58). They demonstrated that the transfer of cytotoxic ($CD8^+$) T-lymphocytes was able to protect the recipient against both a cytomegalovirus (CMV) challenge and established CMV infection. Moreover, helper ($CD4^+$) T-cells provided no such benefit. Transfer of cellular immunity among humans was initially investigated in patients having relapsed after allogeneic transplantation for chronic myelogenous leukemia (CML) (59,60). Infusion of donor mononuclear cells into the patients with relapsed CML induced a graft-versus-leukemic reaction with cytogeneic remissions obviating the need for additional cytotoxic therapies; however, acute and/or chronic GVHD of varying degrees occurred in nine of the eleven patients (60). Subsequently, to reduce the acute and chronic toxicity of GVHD associated with the use of mononuclear cells, investigators isolated and cultured CMV-specific $CD8^+$ T-lymphocytes from the peripheral blood of CMV^+ allogeneic donors (61). They infused the cells into allogeneic bone marrow transplantation patients starting one month after the transplant. None of the patients developed CMV viremia or CMV disease, and, impressively, no major toxicity was observed in any of the fourteen patients.

Table 2. Summary of the Clinical Experience in Cellular Immunotherapy for Post-BMT EBV+ LPD

Author	# Pts	Patient Type	Effector Cells	Dose	Response	Notes
Papadopoulos[62]	5	Allogeneic TCD Matched	PBMC	0.8-2 x 10^6/kg	5/5 CR	2 died ARF 2 Grade II AGVHD 2 Chronic GVHD
Heslop[63]	1	Allogeneic TCD Mismatched	PBMC	1 x 10^6/kg	1/1 CR	Grade IV GVHD
Lucas[64]	5	Allogeneic TCD MUD/Mismatched	PBMC	0.7-1.2 x 10^6/kg	1/5 CR	2 died GVHD 1 died ARF 2 died LPD
Rooney[65]	1	Allogeneic TCD MUD	EBV-CTL	12 x 10^7/m^2 (over 4 doses)	1/1 CR	No Toxicity
Lucas[64]	1	Allogeneic TCD MUD	EBV-CTL	2 x 10^5/kg	1/1 CR	No Toxicity

TCD=T-cell depletion; MUD=matched, unrelated donor; PBMC=peripheral blood mononuclear cells; EBV-CTL=Epstein-Barr virus specific cytotoxic T-lymphocytes; CR=complete response; ARF=acute respiratory failure; AGVHD=acute graft versus host disease; GVHD=graft versus host disease

CELLULAR ADOPTIVE IMMUNOTHERAPY FOR POST-BONE MARROW TRANSPLANTATION LYMPHOPROLIFERATIVE DISORDERS

Progress in the development of adoptive cellular immunotherapy for EBV-related lymphoproliferative disorders in the post-transplant patient has followed closely the work in CML and CMV (Table 2). In 1990, Papadopoulos *et al* reported their clinical experience using donor leukocytes in five patients for established EBV-related large cell NHL following allogeneic BMT for leukemia (62). All five patients had received HLA-matched, T-cell depleted transplants (four related and one unrelated). with four of the five receiving ATG and methylprednisolone for the prevention of graft rejection. The patients received infusions of unirradiated donor peripheral-blood mononuclear cells at a total dose range of 0.8-2.0 x 10^6 CD3$^+$ cells/kg patient weight. Clinical remissions were achieved 14-30 days after the first infusion. However, two of the patients died of respiratory failure 7-17 days after the first infusion of donor cells though both had already developed respiratory distress before the treatments. Neither had evidence of active lymphoma at autopsy. The other three patients had a complete response without evidence of recurrence 7-11 months after the first infusion of PBMC. Whether the infusions contributed to the respiratory failure of the two patients who died is uncertain. While alloreactive cytotoxicity could result from leukocyte infusions with subsequent inflammation and capillary leak and while infectious agents could potentially be transmitted, both patients were experiencing respiratory deterioration before receiving the PBMC infusions. Of the remaining three patients, two developed grade II cutaneous GVHD, and all developed mucocutaneous chronic GVHD. However, these were easily managed with corticosteroids. A second group reported similar clinical benefit following the infusion of 1×10^6 donor $CD3^+$ cells/kg in a three year old boy developing an immunoblastic lymphoma eight months following a HLA-mismatched, T-cell depleted transplant (63). Though the patient remained clinically free of recurrence 16 months after the infusion, the therapy precipitated Grade IV GVHD of the skin, gastrointestinal tract, and liver resulting in much therapy-related morbidity.

More recent data raises some caution against over-optimism regarding the efficacy of cellular immunotherapy for the posttransplant EBV LPD. Lucas *et al* reported eight cases of EBV-associated lymphomas developing after TCD BMT (64). Five cases were treated with donor PBMCs at total doses of 0.7-1.2×10^6 cells/kg. Of these patients only one had a disease response corresponding to a rise in EBV-CTLs and decline in detectable EBV-DNA (Figure 4). This patient and one other, however, died of complications related to GVHD; two additional patients died of acute respiratory failure. More sobering is the fact that two patients died with persistence of disease and that two died from progression of their LPD despite therapy and an increase in EBV-specific cytotoxic activity (Figure 5).

To minimize the risk of non-specific alloreactivity and the resulting GVHD, the use of EBV-specific CTL instead of nonspecific PBMC infusions—as previously studied using CMV-specific CTL (61)--provides a theoretical advantage in specificity of the targeted tissue. The use of donor-derived EBV-specific CTL has been evaluated in patients receiving T-cell depleted, partially-matched related or MUD bone marrow transplants in which both the patient and the donor had pre-transplantation evidence of EBV-DNA (65). Using EBV-transformed B-lymphoblastoid cell lines (BLCL) prepared from donor peripheral blood, EBV-specific donor CTL have been generated and subsequently infused into ten such transplant patients at total dose levels of 4-12 $\times 10^7$ EBV-CTL/m^2 divided in four weekly infusions. Seven patients were infused for prophylaxis against EBV disease; none of whom developed disease nor increased EBV-DNA concentrations. Two patients were infused following elevations in EBV-DNA concentrations consistent with reactivation of disease; both patients experienced normalization of the EBV-DNA concentrations within three weeks of the first infusion. Finally, one patient was infused following a rise in EBV-DNA associated with the development of an immunoblastic lymphoma with LAT III EBV-antigen expression. Clinical improvement was observed within one week following the first infusion, and complete resolution of adenopathy was noted by four weeks. The patient remained free of disease eight months following the therapy. Importantly, none of the patients experienced GVHD or any serious toxicity as a result of the infusions. Similar success has been reported in a patient treated with a smaller total dose of only 2 x 10^5 donor EBV-CTL/kg with complete resolution of the lymphoma (64). EBV-specific T-cells, therefore, appear to be an effective and safe approach to the management of EBV-associated disease occurring following bone marrow transplantation and warrants further investigation.

Figure 4.

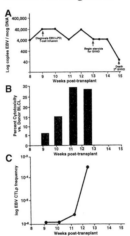

The number of patients studied is too small to determine whether the prophylactic use of such infusions would be efficacious and cost-effective in selected transplant patients at high risk of developing EBV-related post-transplant complications. Using a *scid* mouse model, Buchsbaum *et al* demonstrated that human-derived EBV-specific CTL given with interleukin-2 prevented the development of autologous human EBV-associated lymphomas following concomitant intraperitoneal injection of EBV-transformed B-cells (66). Conversely, nearly 100% of mice not injected with EBV-specific CTL died of these tumors 10-26 weeks following inoculation with EBV-infected cells. While this study is limited by the fact that it is an animal model and transformed cells were directly inoculated concurrent with the administration of the protective CTL (albeit at separate sites), these preclinical observations combined with the apparent safety provide the rationale supporting studies to examine the use of EBV-specific CTL as prophylaxis against EBV-associated LPD in humans undergoing allogeneic T-cell depleted bone marrow transplantation. Furthermore, serial measures of EBV DNA by semiquantitative

214

PCR may help identify patients at high risk for developing an EBV LPD and target populations for the study of prophylactic cellular immunotherapy (64).

Figure 5.

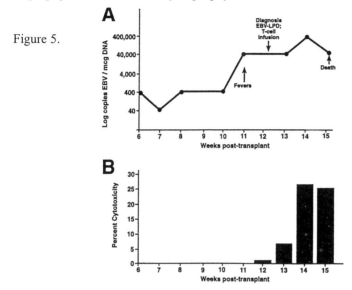

Rooney *et al* used the G1Na retroviral vector containing the neomycin resistance gene (*neo*[R]) to genetically mark EBV-specific CTLs and estimated that following an infusion of EBV-specific donor CTL at doses of 2-12 x 10^7 CTL/m^2, donor EBV-CTL comprise 1/100-1/1000 of circulating lymphocytes (65,67). Given the small number of infused cells relative to the total *in vivo* lymphocyte population, it is believed that this represents a 2-3 log expansion *in vivo* of the marked CTL following the infusion (67). The duration of detectable *neo*[R] marked CTL ranged from 3-16 weeks (median 10 weeks)(Figure 6) (65,67). However, following an EBV-antigenic challenge the cytotoxic response remained intact with appropriate expansion of CTL resulting in detection of *neo*[R] marked CTL as long as 18 months after the CTL infusions both *in vitro* and *in vivo* (65,67). Therefore, following adoptive transfer of EBV-specific donor CTL into BMT patients, the donor CTL are capable of sustained expansion and cytotoxic function.

CELLULAR ADOPTIVE IMMUNOTHERAPY FOR POST-SOLID ORGAN TRANSPLANTATION LYMPHOPROLIFERATIVE DISORDERS

Clinical experience in the use of cellular adoptive immunotherapy in EBV-associated LPD following solid organ transplantation has been more limited (Table 3). While these tumors exhibit a LAT III phenotype and histology

215

comparable to the LPDs following bone marrow transplantation and should, therefore, be amenable to cellular immunotherapy, issues regarding the source of the CTLs deserve special consideration. With the exception of living related donors of kidneys, solid organ donors are typically deceased and, thus, not available following the initial organ harvest. As the tumors are typically of host origin and express EBV antigens in the context of host MHC-molecules, autologous CTLs would be a logical choice and do not require any delay in further HLA-typing. Problems with using autologous CTLs include potential difficulty expanding functional cytotoxic cells from the immunocompromised patient particularly while immunosuppressive therapies are ongoing, failure to recognize the EBV antigen epitopes presented by the tumor especially in the donor-origin tumors, and precipitation of graft rejection particularly with the use of nonspecific PBMCs. Camoli *et al* demonstrated that EBV-specific CTLs can be expanded from the peripheral blood of organ transplant patients, and these cells exhibit functional, HLA-restricted lysis of autologous, EBV-transformed BLCL (68). Three heart transplant patients have been infused with autologous EBV-CTLs and have demonstrated that the infusions can result in decreased detection of EBV DNA without evidence of graft rejection by serial myocardial biopsies (68)

Figure 6

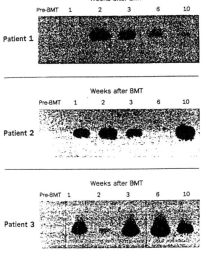

Allogeneic cells procured from a second donor provide the third potential source of CTLs. In addition to the considerations described above for autologous CTLs, use of a second donor entails the time necessary to find a suitable HLA-match and a potential risk for both GVHD and graft rejection. Nevertheless, one patient with a host-origin, monoclonal B-cell lymphoma of the brain following cadaveric lung transplantation for cystic fibrosis has been infused with 1×10^6 CD3$^+$ PBMC/kg from an EBV-seropositive HLA-identical sibling resulting in a marked decrease in the size of his tumor (69). Following an increase in his immunosuppressive therapy, the patient experienced a local recurrence of disease which was treated by two additional infusions of CD3$^+$ PBMC from his sibling resulting in a complete remission with no evidence of disease confirmed by brain biopsy. Thus, adoptive immunotherapy using autologous or allogeneic CTLs appears to be feasible and safe, warranting further clinical investigation in the use of this modality in the organ transplant recipients developing EBV-associated LPDs. Additional issues requiring study include the duration of CTL survival and efficacy following infusion and the optimal use of immunosuppressive therapies during and following the infusions.

POTENTIAL ROLE IN AIDS-ASSOCIATED NHL

There has been little experience with the use of adoptive immunotherapy for HIV-associated EBV-induced lymphoproliferative disorders; however, in light of the limited efficacy of currently available therapies for most of these patients, the modality has obvious potential benefits (Table 3). With many of the AIDS-NHL cases—particularly the immunoblastic subtype—exhibiting evidence of EBV DNA and/or RNA and with many of these exhibiting a LAT III phenotype, these tumors are potentially amenable to targeting by CTL (48,49)

Table 3. Summary of the Experience in Cellular Immunotherapy in Organ Transplant and HIV Patients

Author	# Pts	Patient Type	Effector Cells	Dose	Response	Notes
Camoli[68]	3	Heart TX	EBV-CTL	NS	3/3 EBV-DNA decreased	No graft rejection
Emanuel[69]	1	Lung TX	PBMC	3 x 10^6/kg	1/1 CR	
Wheatley[72]	1	HIV-NHL	EBV-CTL		1/1 CR	

TX=transplant; HIV-NHL=human immunodeficiency virus-associated non-Hodgkin's lymphoma; PBMC=peripheral blood mononuclear cells; EBV-CTL=Epstein-Barr virus specific cytotoxic T-lymphocytes;NS=not specified; CR=complete response

One issue in the use of cellular immunotherapy in the AIDS patient is the source of the cytotoxic cells. As the lymphomas seen in this population are of host origin and, therefore, express the viral antigens in the context of the patients own MHC class I proteins, the use of autologous CTL would appear to be a potential option. Advantages to the use of autologous PBMC or EBV-CTL include the following: (1) a readily available donor from whom to obtain the necessary blood samples, (2) viral antigens presented in the appropriate MHC-restricted context for cellular recognition, and (3) minimal risk of toxicity related to GVHD. However, while EBV-specific CTLs have been demonstrated in HIV-infected individuals, these cells markedly decrease prior to the development of EBV-associated NHL in these patients (56). This decline is part of the cellular immune deterioration resulting directly from the underlying HIV infection, and for most patients, no subsequent rise in EBV-CTL with the development of the EBV-associated LPD—an antigenic challenge—has been observed. The possibility that immunosurveillance may be recovered has been raised by anecdotal cases of spontaneous regression of established lymphomas following the initiation of protease inhibitor therapy for the HIV infection resulting in a rise in the $CD4^+$ T-cells (70,71). More exciting is the case report of an HIV infected individual with a AIDS-associated EBV^+ B-cell NHL refractory to conventional chemotherapy treated with autologous EBV-specific CTL expanded *in vitro* without apparent toxicity and with a complete response (72). Therefore, the use of autologous cellular immunotherapy appears to be potentially feasible. Whether sufficient numbers of EBV-specific CTL could be isolated from most patients with AIDS-associated NHL remains uncertain, and clinical investigation into the possibility continues.

The use of allogeneic PBMC or EBV-CTL provides a second potential option. This approach would eliminate the potential difficulties of expanding sufficient numbers of EBV-CTL from the HIV infected patient; however, disadvantages include the following: (1) need for tissue typing and the associated time delays to identify a potential donor, (2) potential differences in HLA-restricted antigen presentation allowing for lack of cellular recognition—particularly in partially-matched donor candidates, and (3) potential toxicity related to GVHD—particularly if PBMC infusions are employed. While HLA-identical CTL would have the greater likelihood of inducing a cytotoxic response, haplo-identical CTL may also induce a response against lymphoma cells if the CTL are capable of recognizing EBV peptides in the context of the shared HLA antigens (44,72). Indeed, haploidentical related EBV-CTL and partially-matched, unrelated EBV-specific CTL sharing at least 1 or 2 HLA class I antigens have demonstrated strong EBV-specific lysis of patient BLCL *in vitro* without nonspecific alloreactivity (73). As such, the possibility of using partially-matched EBV-specific CTL with effective recognition and lysis of patient EBV-infected cells greatly increases the likelihood of identifying an appropriate donor and makes the use of allogeneic CTL a widely available therapeutic consideration. One problem of infusing allogeneic CTL would be the risk of inducing graft versus host disease (GVHD)—particularly if using a partially-matched donor. The risk of this complication would be minimized by the infusion of EBV-specific CTL as discussed previously, especially if similarly small doses of EBV-specific CTL are required in the HIV-associated NHL patient as suggested in the bone marrow transplant population (65). The use of matched or partially-matched, allogeneic T-cells in EBV[+] AIDS-NHL is currently under investigation in an ongoing clinical trial.

Various studies have shown that CTL penetrate the blood-brain barrier and may play a protective and/or pathologic role in various viral-mediated diseases of the CNS (74-76). As nearly 100% of AIDS-PCNSL demonstrate EBV DNA and/or RNA and as many exhibit a LAT III phenotype, these tumors also are potentially amenable to targeting by CTL (48,49). The amenability of PCNSL to immunomodulation is highlighted in the case report of an HIV[+] patient with a large cell CNS lymphoma who refused radiation and chemotherapy (71). He was, therefore, managed with dexamethasone, and anti-retrovirals including a protease inhibitor were initiated. Anti-retroviral therapy sustained a CD4[+] increase $>100/mm^3$, and the patient remained asymptomatic with a complete clinical and radiographic response 22 months after the initial presentation. As discussed previously, the infusion of PBMC from an EBV-seropositive HLA-identical sibling into a non-HIV infected patient with a host-origin, monoclonal B-cell lymphoma of the brain following cadaveric lung transplantation resulted in a complete remission with no evidence of disease confirmed by brain biopsy (69). Thus, the use of adoptive cellular immunotherapy for the treatment of EBV-associated PCNSL appears to be both feasible and potentially effective, providing an alternative to the current standard where median survival has been a disappointing 3 months. Investigation into the use of matched or partially-matched, allogeneic T-cells in EBV[+] AIDS-PCNSL is ongoing.

CD4[+] T-helper cells are necessary to sustain host CD8[+] CTL responses during chronic viral infections (77). CD4[+] T-helper cells are also pivotal in the maintenance of CD8[+] CTL responses following adoptive transfer (61). In bone marrow transplant patients infused with CMV-specific CTL, recovery of CD4[+] T-helper cell responses following the infusion is associated with a sustained or increased CD8[+] CTL response while patients in whom T-helper function does not recover following CTL infusions experience a gradual decline in CTL responses. Therefore, the fate of adoptively transferred CTL in the AIDS patient is unknown. Whether the sustained CTL responses observed as long as 18 months after infusion in bone marrow transplant patients will be seen in a patient population where the HIV results in progressive deterioration of the

CD4$^+$ lymphocytes remains to be seen. Though some EBV-specific CD4$^+$ T-cells are expanded and transferred along with the EBV-specific CD8$^+$ T-cells, sustained responses following the infusions may be best achieved in those patients in whom effective anti-retroviral therapy can lead to some degree of viral control and immune "reconstitution". The kinetics of adoptively transferred CTL in AIDS patients needs to be formally investigated with additional attention to the influence of highly active anti-retroviral therapy (HAART).

POTENTIAL ROLE IN BURKITT'S LYMPHOMA

While nearly all cases of endemic (African) Burkitt's lymphoma are associated with EBV,(78,79) the association in the sporadic form seen elsewhere is less frequently observed. Among cases of AIDS-associated Burkitt's lymphoma, only half of the tumors exhibit DNA and/or RNA evidence of EBV (49). The potential role of adoptive cellular immunity in Burkitt's lymphoma is tempered by the limited expression of EBV antigens with most cases exhibiting a latency type I phenotype in which antigen expression is limited to EBNA-1 and the remainder exhibiting a latency type II phenotype (17,49). The limited expression of less immunogenic antigens provides a means for escaping immunosurveillance. In maintained cultures of Burkitt's cell lines, tumor cells phenotypically shift gradually toward a lymphoblastoid (BLCL)-type phenotype with a LAT-III expression of the full array of EBV latency antigens (80,81). Along with the changing EBV antigen expression, the expression of cellular adhesion molecules (LFA-1, LFA-3, and ICAM-1) increases dramatically (81). Using allogeneic, HLA-matched, EBV-specific T-lymphocytes exhibiting lysis of autologous BLCL derived from patients with Burkitt's, the Burkitt's lymphoma cells from the same patients are able to evade cytolysis by the viral-specific T-cells (80,81). Even after Burkitt's cell lines exhibit a shift in EBV antigen expression, EBV-specific cytotoxic T-cells are able to effectively lyse tumor cells only if upregulation of the cellular adhesion molecules has also been achieved (81). Burkitt's lymphoma cells *in vivo* evade cellular immunosurveillance by downregulation of both EBV-latency antigens and cellular adhesion molecules, and both need to be overcome for effective immune recognition.

Unless upregulation of EBV-latency antigens and cellular adhesion molecules can be achieved *in vivo*, the clinical role of adoptive cellular immunotherapy in the management of EBV$^+$ Burkitt's lymphoma appears to be unlikely. Two promoters (Wp and Cp) have been identified which appear to be involved in the generation of the transcript from which the full compliment of EBNAs are derived (82). Alternatively, the promoter located in the F-Q region generates a shorter transcript encoding only for EBNA-1 (83). In contrast to cells with a LAT-III phenotype, Burkitt's lymphoma and other cell-types with a limited

EBV latency antigen expression have inactivated Wp and Cp promoters and use the F-Q promoter instead (83). The Burkitt's cells switch to the Wp and Cp promoters *in vitro* during the observed phenotypic drift and with exposure to 5-azacytadine (17). Thus, if activation of the Wp and Cp promoters could be induced *in vivo* resulting in upregulation of EBV antigens, and if upregulation of the cellular adhesion molecules could be similarly induced, enhanced immune-recognition by cytotoxic T-cells may make investigation of adoptive cellular immunotherapy more reasonable and feasible.

POTENTIAL ROLE IN HODGKIN'S DISEASE

The role of EBV in the pathogenesis of Hodgkin's disease (HD) remains unclear. However, using in situ hybridization techniques, the EBV genome has been identified as clonal within the Reed-Sternberg cells (RS cells) in half of patients seropositive for EBV, particularly among the mixed cellularity and nodular sclerosis histologic subtypes (84-91). Expression of EBV antigens by the RS cells in EBV$^+$ tumors follows a LAT II phenotype limited to EBNA-1, LMP-1 and LMP-2 (17,87,92,93). The limited expression of the non-immunogenic EBNA-1 and the less immunogenic LMPs provides the RS cell with the potential for a weakened immunosurveillance by CTLs though not complete evasion. HLA class I molecule expression by RS cells has been demonstrated in approximately half of studied specimens, but expression has not been universal and may, therefore, limit the appropriate presentation of viral antigens to the cytotoxic T-cells in some patients (94). Moreover, Frisan *et al* noted that EBV-specific CTLs could not be expanded *in vitro* from EBV$^+$ HD specimens despite the ability to stimulate the expansion of functional EBV-specific CTLs from the peripheral blood of the same patients and from EBV- HD specimens (95). This work suggests that local inhibition of EBV-specific CTLs may contribute to the ability of EBV antigen expressing RS cells to evade a cytoxic immune response.

The use of adoptive cellular immunotherapy in Hodgkin's disease may, therefore, be limited to the subset of patients with EBV$^+$ tumors and with HLA class I expression. It may also have to overcome unknown local inhibitors of EBV-specific CTLs. Nevertheless, it has been demonstrated *in vitro* that functional EBV-specific CTLs targeting LMP-2 could be generated and expanded from the peripheral blood mononuclear cells of patients with HD (96). Despite nondetectable responses against LMP-2 from polyclonal EBV-CTLs in which EBNA-2 and EBNA-3a were the dominant antigenic targets, autologous BLCLs could be used to further expand a clone of CTLs with cytolytic activity against transfected cells with EBV-antigen expression restricted to LMP-2. Additionally, expansion of EBV-LMP-2-specific CTLs could be accomplished more efficiently using autologous fibroblasts transfected with a recombinant vaccinia virus encoding EBV LMP-2 as the stimulator cell in cultures. These LMP-2 specific CTLs demonstrate effective lysis of both transfected target cells expressing LMP-2 and autologous BLCL. Allogeneic CTL have been expanded *in vitro* with demonstrated cytotoxic activity against HD cell lines in culture in an HLA-restricted fashion (96). While the use of EBV-directed immunotherapy may be applicable to only a subset of Hodgkin's disease patients, it appears the approach may be feasible and warrants further clinical investigation.

Alternatively, a novel approach to cellular immunotherapy may include the use of targeted immunoglobulins. Bispecific monoclonal antibodies directed against the Hodgkin's disease-associated CD30 and either the T-cell-associated CD3 or CD28 have been generated (97). In the murine model, these antibodies result in tumor clearance even when innoculated in mice with advanced, established xenografted HD tumors. The anti-tumor action required the presence of both human $CD8^+$ and $CD4^+$ lymphocytes; T-cells from both healthy human controls and Hodgkin's disease patients were effective. Moreover, the cytotoxic effects are antigen-specific ($CD30^+$ cells) but are not MHC-restricted. Though these antibodies have not been evaluated in human clinical trials, they suggest an alternative means of augmenting the cellular immunity against Hodgkin's disease, potentially without the need for *in vitro* expansion of autologous or allogeneic CTLs and without the limitations posed by the issues of the restricted LAT II phenotype and MHC-restricted presentation. In patient's with compromised cellular immunity such as in patient's with AIDS, the potential of a combined cellular and humoral immunotherapy approach could be investigated.

POTENTIAL IN NASOPHARYNGEAL CARCINOMA

Nasopharyngeal carcinoma is an EBV-associated malignancy most prevalent in China and Southeast Asia. Like Hodgkin's disease, EBV antigen expression is of the LAT II phenotype. Therefore, the issues discussed for HD also apply in the case of nasopharyngeal carcinoma—(1) limited immunogenicity of the expressed EBV-antigens, (2) need for MHC- class I molecule expression on the tumor surface, and (3) CTL-recognized presentation of the EBV antigens by the MHC class I molecules. As discussed above, the ability to generate a sufficient quantity of functional CTLs specific for EBV LMP-2 raises the possibility that the lesser immunogenicity of LMP-2 can be overcome (96) The presentation of LMP-2 by HLA alleles commonly found within the Chinese population has been demonstrated to produce a functional CTL response (98). Moreover, the LMP-2 epitopes expressed by nasopharyngeal carcinoma specimens appear to be the same as those presented and recognized on peripheral blood cells (98). Therefore, while it remains possible that functional CTL responses could be directed against nasopharyngeal carcinoma, no clinical experience exists in the use of cellular immunotherapy for these tumors.

FUTURE DIRECTIONS

Despite the considerable work achieved over the last decade in the use of adoptive cellular immunotherapy, much work remains to be done to explore the potential of this novel therapeutic approach. Clinical issues pertinent to each of the EBV-related malignancies have been raised in each of the corresponding sections. The use of EBV-specific CTLs has provided a safer alternative to PBMCs with a reduction in the risk of GVHD and, potentially, graft rejection. However, the considerable time required to generate EBV-specific CTLs hinders the broad application of the modality particularly for those patients whose clinical condition and the potentially rapid disease course of their LPD does not allow for the 6-8 weeks delay. If dendritic cells are substituted for BLCLs as the antigen-presenting cells used to stimulate CTL generation, the necessary time delay can be reduced by nearly 3-4 weeks (99). This may substantially improve the availability of the modality to many such patients. Applicability may also be increased using methods capable of improving the generation of CTLs directed against specific EBV antigens particularly for those tumors with restricted antigen expression. This can be achieved using dendritic cells or cells transfected with a restricted portion of the EBV genome (96,100). Conversely, tumor cells may be able to be manipulated to express a broader array of antigens to allow greater immunorecognition, ie. with 5-azacytadine (17)

In murine studies, IL-2 and IL-7 have been shown *in vivo* to increase the antiviral activity of transferred T-cells against the herpes simplex virus corresponding with a seven-fold and twenty-fold decrease in viral load, respectively (101). The concomitant use of biologic agents may enhance the effectiveness of CTLs though these agents may additionally enhance CTL-related toxicities such as GVHD and/or graft rejection. An alternative approach to augmenting the antitumor effects of natural and/or transferred CTLs may include the use of bispecific antibodies engineered both to target tumor-specific antigens and to recruit and stimulate cytotoxic lymphocytes (97,102). Such antibodies might provide enhanced activity directed specifically against the tumor while minimizing non-specific toxicities to non-tumor tissues.

Toxicities associated with transfer of cellular immunity may be minimized by molecularly altering the transferred CTLs to provide a means of terminating them. Transfecting CTLs with a retroviral vector containing the thymidine kinase gene provides one such possibility. The transfected cells could be eliminated using the thymidine kinase dependent antiviral, ganciclovir (103,104). A significant problem with the clinical application of this approach has been the *in vivo* development of immunity against the transfected cells thereby eliminating the cells even in the absence of ganciclovir (105)

CONCLUSIONS

EBV-associated malignancies remain a significant problem both for the immunocompromised and the immunocompetent host. Cellular immunotherapy provides a novel modality in our armamentarium though requires further investigation to define its clinical role. Early clinical studies indicate that PBMCs confer protection against EBV-related lymphoproliferative disorders in the post-transplant patient although toxicities may be considerable. The use of EBV-specific CTLs have demonstrated similar potential in post-transplant and HIV-infected patients with minimal toxicity although the substantial amount of time required to generate such cells may limit their applicablity. Investigation into the application of this modality to more prevalent diseases worldwide such as Burkitt's lymphoma, Hodgkin's disease, and nasopharyngeal carcinoma is needed and provides hope for future generations of cancer victims.

REFERENCES

1. Henle G et al. Antibodies to epstein-barr virus in burkitt's lymphoma and control groups. Journal of the National Cancer Institute 1969; 43(5):1147-1157.
2. Diehl V, et al. Demonstration of a herpes group virus in cultures of peripheral leukocytes from a patient with infectious mononucleosis. Journal of Virology 1968; 2(7):663-669.
3. Svedmyr E et al. Virologic, immunologic, and clinical observations on a patient during the incubation, acute, and convalescent phases of infectious mononucleosis. Clinical Immunology and Immunopathology 1984; 30(3):437-450.
4. Lewin N et al. Characterization of ebv-carrying b-cell populations in healthy seropositive individuals with regard to density, release of transforming virus, and spontaneous outgrowth. International Journal of Cancer 1987; 39(4):472-476.
5. Henle G, Henle W, and Diehl V. Relation of burkitt's tumor-associated herpes-type virus to infectious mononucleosis. Proceedings of the National Academy of Sciences of the United States of America 1968; 59(1):94-101.
6. Klein G et al. EBV-determined nuclear antigen (ebna)-positive cells in the peripheral blood of infectious mononucleosis patients. International Journal of Cancer 1976; 17(1):21-26.
7. Miller G et al. Prolonged oropharyngeal excretion of epstein-barr virus after infectious mononucleosis. New England Journal of Medicine 1973; 288(5):229-232.

8. Strauch B et al. Oropharyngeal excretion of epstein-barr virus by renal transplant recipients and other patients treated with immunosuppressive drugs. Lancet 1974; 1(7851):234-237.

9. Gerber P et al. Association of eb-virus infection with the post-perfusion syndrome. Lancet 1969; 1 (7595):593-595.

10. Kaye KM and Kieff E. Epstein-Barr virus. Infectious Diseases, 2nd Edition, SL Gorbach, JG Bartlett, and NR Blacklow, editors. WB Sanders Company, Philadelphia, 1998; 2067-2073.

11. Zinkernagel RM et al. MHC-Restricted cytotoxic T-Cell: studies on the biological role of polymorphic major transplantation antigens determining t-cell restriction specificity, function, and responsiveness. Advances in Immunology 1979; 27:51-177.

12. Townsend A et al. The epitopes of influenza nucleoprotein recognized by cytotoxic t-lymphocytes can be defined with short synthetic peptides. Cell 1986; 44(6):959-968.

13. Townsend A et al. Antigen recognition by class i restricted t-lymphocytes. Annual Reviews in Immunology 1989; 7:601-624.

14. Rickinson AB et al. Cellular immunologic responses to infection by the virus. In the epstein barr virus: recent advances, MA Epstein and BG Achong, editors. William Heinemann Medical Books Ltd., London, 1986; 75-125.

15. Murray RJ et al. Identification of target antigens for the human cytotoxic t cell response to epstein-barr virus (ebv): implications for the immune control of ebv-positive malignancies. Journal of Experimental Medicine 1992; 176(1):157-168.

16. Khanna R et al. Localization of epstein-barr virus cytotoxic t cell epitopes using recombinant vaccinia: implications for vaccine development. Journal of Experimental Medicine 1992; 176(1):169-176.

17. Klein G and Klein E. Epstein-barr virus and human lymphomas. In Canellos et al (editors) The Lymphomas, Philadelphia, Saunders Company 1998; 63-73.

18. Swinnen LJ et al. Increased incidence of lymphoproliferative disorder after immunosuppression with the monoclonal antibody okt3 in cardiac-transplant recipients. New England Journal of Medicine 1990; 323(25):1723-1728.

19. Wilkinson AH et al. Increased frequency of posttransplant lymphomas in patients treated with cyclosporine, azothioprine, and prednisone. Transplantation 1989; 47(2):293-296.

20. Crawford DH et al. Studies on the long-term t cell mediated immunity to epstein-barr virus in immunosuppressed renal allograft recipients. International Journal of Cancer 1981; 28(6):705-709.

21. Knowles DM et al. Correlative morphologic and molecular genetic analysis demonstrates three distinct categories of posttransplantation lymphoproliferative disorders. Blood 1995; 85(2);552-565.
22. Locker J and Nalesnik M. Molecular genetic analysis of lymphoid tumors arising after organ transplantation. American Journal of Pathology 1989; 135(6);977-987.
23. Hjelle B et al. A poorly differentiated lymphoma of donor origin in a renal allograft recipient. Transplantation 1989; 47(6):945-948.
24. Gambacorta M et al. Malignant lymphoma in the recipient of a heart transplant from a donor with malignant lymphoma. Lymphoma Transplantation or De Novo Disease? Transplantation 1991; 151(4):920-922.
25. Thomas JA et al. Immunohistology of epstein-barr virus-associated antigens in B cell disorders from immunocompromised individuals. Transplantation 1990; 49(5);944-953.
26. Nalesnik MA et al. The pathology of posttransplant lymphoproliferative disorders occuring in the setting of cyclosporine a-prednisone immunosuppression. American Journal of Pathology 1988; 133(1):173-192.
27. Penn I. Host origin of lymphomas in organ transplant recipients. Transplantation 1979; 27(3):214.
28. Randhawa PS et al. Epstein-barr virus-associated lymphoproliferative disease in a heart-lung allograft. Demonstration of host origin by restriction fragment-length polymorphism analysis. Transplantation 1990; 49(1):126-130.
29. Thomas JA et al. Immunohistology of epstein-barr virus-associated antigens in b-cell disorders from immunocompromised individuals. Transplantation 1990; 49(5):944-953.
30. Zutter MM et al. Epstein-barr virus lymphoproliferation after bone marrow transplantation. Blood 1988; 72(2),520-529.
31. List AF et al. Lymphoproliferative diseases in immunocompromised hosts: the role of epstein-barr virus. Journal of Clinical Oncology 1987; 5(10):1673-1689.
32. McGlave P et al. Unrelated donor bone marrow transplantation therapy for chronic myelogenous leukemia. Blood 1987; 70(3):877-81.
33. Miller WJ et al. Molecular genetic rearrangements distinguish pre- and post-bone marrow transplantation lymphoproliferative processes. Blood 1987; 70(3):882-885.
34. Shapiro RS et al. Epstein-barr virus associated b cell lymphoproliferative disorders following bone marrow transplantation. Blood 1988; 71(5):1234-1243.

35. Antin JH et al. Selective depletion of bone marrow t lymphocytes with anti-cd5 monoclonal antibodies: effective prophylaxis for graft-versus-host disease in patients with hematologic malignancies. Blood 1991; 78(8):2139-2149.
36. Schubach WH et al. A monoclonal immunoblastic sarcoma in donor cells bearing epstein-barr virus genomes following allogeneic marrow grafting for acute lymphoblastic leukemia. Blood 1982; 60(1):180-187.
37. Martin PJ et al. Fatal epstein-barr virus-associated proliferation of donor b-cells after treatment of acute graft-versus-host disease with a murine anti-t-cell antibody. Annals of Internal Medicine 1984; 101(3):310-315.
38. Lucas KG et al. The development of cellular immunity to epstein-barr virus after allogeneic bone marrow transplantation. Blood 1996; 87(6):2594-2603.
39. Gossett TC et al. Immunoblastic sarcoma in donor cells after bone marrow transplantation. New England Journal of Medicine 1979; 300(16):904-907.
40. Bloom et al. Lymphoma of host origin in a marrow transplant recipient in remission of acute myeloid leukemia and receiving cyclosporin a. American Journal of Haematology 1985; 18(1):73-83.
41. Crawford DH et al. Epstein-barr virus infection and immunity in bone marrow transplant recipients. Transplantation 1986; 42(1):50-54.
42. Keever CA et al. Immune reconstitution following bone marrow transplantation: comparison of recipients of t-cell depleted marrow with recipients of conventional marrow grafts. Blood 1989; 73(5):1340-1350.
43. Biggar RJ et al. Cancer trends among young single men in the seer registries of the united states. Presented at the International Conference on AIDS, Paris, June 1986.
44. Levine AM. Acquired immunodeficiency-related lymphoma. Blood 1992; 80(1):8-20.
45. Hammer SM et al. A controlled trial of two nucleoside analogues plus indinavir in persons with human immunodeficiency virus infection and cd4 cell counts of 22 per cubic millimeter or less. New England Journal of Medicine 1997; 337(11):725-733.
46. Buchbinder SP et al. Declines in aids incidence associated with highly active anti-retroviral therapy (Haart) are not reflected in ks and lymphoma incidence. Presented at the Second National AIDS Malignancy Conference, Bethesda, April 1998.
47. Jacobson LP. Impact of highly active anti-retroviral therapy on the incidence of malignancies among hiv-infected individuals. Presented at the Second National AIDS Malignancy Conference, Bethesda, April 1998.
48. Knowles DM and R Dalla-Favera. Aids-associated malignant lymphoma. In Broder et al (editors) Textbook of AIDS Medicine, Baltimore, Williams & Wilkins 1994; 431-463.

49. Hamilton-Dutoit SJ et al. Epstein-barr virus latent gene expression and tumor cell phenotype in acquired immunodeficiency syndrome-related non-hodgkin's lymphoma. American Journal of Pathology 1993; 143(4):1072-1085.
50. Forsyth PA et al. Biology and management of aids-associated primary central nervous system lymphomas. Hematology-Oncology Clinics of North America 1996; 10(5):1125-1134.
51. MacMahon EM et al. Epstein-Barr virus in AIDS-Related primary central nervous System Lymphomas. Lancet 1991; 338(8773):969-973.
52. Nakhleh RE et al. Central nervous system lymphomas. Immunohistochemical and Clinicopathologic Study of 26 Autopsy Cases. Archives of Pathology and Laboratory Medicine 1989; 113(9):1050-1056.
53. Camilleri-Broet S et al. AIDS-Related primary brain lymphomas: histopathologic and immunohistochemical study of 51 cases. Human Pathology 1997; 28(3):367-374.
54. Camilleri-Broet S et al. High expression of latent membrane protein 1 of epstein-barr virus and bcl-2 oncoprotein in acquired immunodeficiency syndrome-related primary brain lymphomas. Blood 1995; 86(2):432-435.
55. Auperin I et al. Primary central nervous system malignant non-hodgkin's lymphomas from hiv-infected and non-infected patients: expression of cellular surface proteins and epstein-barr viral markers. Neuropathology and Applied Neurobiology 1994; 20(3):243-252.
56. Kersten MJ et al. Epstein-barr virus-specific cytotoxic t cell responses in hiv-1 infection. Journal of Clinical Investigation 1997; 99(7):1525-1533.
57. Reddehase MJ et al. Interstitial murine cytomegalovirus pneumonia after irradiation: characterization of cells that limit viral replication during established infection of the lungs. Journal of Virology 1985; 55(2):264-273.
58. Reddehase MJ et al. Cd8-positve t-lymphocytes specific for murine cytomegalovirus immediate-early antigens mediate protective immunity. Journal of Virology 1987; 61(10):3102-3108.
59. Kolb HJ et al. Donor leukocyte transfusions for treatment of recurrent chronic myelogenous leukemia in marrow transplant patients. Blood 1990; 76(12):2462-2465.
60. Porter DL et al. Induction of graft-versus-host disease as immunotherapy for relapsed chronic myeloid leukemia. New England Journal of Medicine 1994; 330(2):100-106.
61. Walter EA et al. Reconstitution of cellular immunity against cytomegalovirus in recipients of allogeneic bone marrow by transfer of t-cell clones from the donor. New England Journal of Medicine 1995; 333(16):1038-1044.

62. Papadopoulos EB et al. Infusions of donor leukocytes to treat epstein-barr virus-associated lymphoproliferative disorders after allogeneic bone marrow transplantation. New England Journal of Medicine 1994; 330(17):1185-1191.

63. Heslop HE et al. Donor t-cells to treat EBV-associated lymphoma. (letter) New England Journal of Medicine 1994; 331(10):679-680.

64. Lucas KG et al. Semiquantitative epstein-barr virus (EBV) polymerase chain reaction for the determination of patients at risk for EBV-induced lymphoproliferative disease after stem cell transplantation. Blood 1998; 91(10):3654-3661.

65. Rooney CM et al. Use of gene-modified virus specific t lymphocytes to control epstein-barr-virus-related lymphoproliferation. Lancet 1995; 345(8941):9-13.

66. Buchsbaum RJ et al. EBV-specific cytotoxic t lymphocytes protect against human EBV-associated lymphoma in scid mice. Immunology Letters 1996; 52(2,3):145-152.

67. Heslop HE et al. Long-term restoration of immunity against epstein-barr virus infection by adoptive transfer of gene-modified virus-specific t lymphocytes. Nature Medicine 1996; 2(5):551-555.

68. Camoli P et al. Autologous ebv-specific cytotoxic t cells to treat EBV-associated post-transplant lymphoproliferative disease (PTLD). Blood 1997; 90(10)suppl 1(part1):249a,abstract 1097.

69. Emanuel DJ et al. Treatment of posttransplant lymphoproliferative disease in the central nervous system of a lung transplant recipient using allogeneic leukocytes. Transplantation 1997; 63(11):1691-1694.

70. Lemas MV et al. EBV-specific cd4$^+$ t cell responses in immune compromised HIV$^+$ Individuals with Lymphoma. Blood 1997; 90(10)suppl 1(part 1):134a, abstract 589.

71. McGowan JP et al. Long-term remission of AIDS-related primary central nervous system lymphoma (PCNSL) with the use of highly active antiretroviral therapy (HAART). 2nd National AIDS Malignancy Conference, Bethesda, Maryland. Journal of Acquired Immune Deficiency Syndromes and Human Retrovirology 1998; 17(4):A30, abstract 74.

72. Wheatley GH et al. Adoptive immunotherapy using autologous EBV-specific cytotoxic t-lymphocytes in an HIV-infected patient with refractory epstein-barr virus expressing b-cell lymphoma. 1st National AIDS Malignancy Conference, Bethesda, Maryland. Journal of Acquired Immune Deficiency Syndromes and Human Retrovirology 1997; 14(4):A53, abstract 147.

73. Lemas MV et al. Large-scale expansions of ebv-specific cytotoxic t lymphocyte (ctl) lines lyse EBV-infected haploidentical target cells but not uninfected autologous or hapoloidentical cells. Blood 1997; 90(10)suppl 1(part 1):134a-135a, abstract 590.

74. Lavi E and Way Q. The protective role of cytotoxic t cells and interferon against coronavirus invasion of the brain. Talbot and Levy (editors). Corona and Related Viruses 1995.

75. Stohlman S et al. JHM virus-specific cytotoxic t-cells derived from the central nervous system. Laude and Vautherot (editors). Coronaviruses 1994.

76. Hudson SL and Streilein JW. Functional cytotoxic T cells are associated with focal lesions in the brains of SJL mice with experimental herpes simplex encephalitis. Journal of Immunology 1994; 152(11):5540-5547.

77. Matloubian M et al. CD4$^+$ T cells are required to sustain CD8$^+$ cytotoxic T cell responses during chronic viral infection. Journal of Virology 1994; 68(12):8056-8063.

78. Niedobitek G et al. Heterogeneous expression of epstein-barr virus latent proteins in endemic burkitt's lymphoma. Blood 1995; 86(2):659-665.

79. Shiramizu B et al. Patterns of chromosomal breakpoint locations in burkitt's lymphoma: relevance to geography and epstein-barr virus association. Blood 1991; 77(7):1516-1526.

80. Rooney CM et al. Epstein-barr virus-positive burkitt's lymphoma cells not recognized by virus-specific t-cell surveillance. Nature 1985; 317(6038):629-631.

81. Gregory CD et al. Downregulation of cell adhesion molecules LFA-3 and ICAM-1 in epstein-barr virus-positive burkitt's lymphoma underlies tumor cell escape from virus-specific T cell surveillance. Journal of Experimental Medicine 1988; 167(6):1811-1824.

82. Woisetschlaeger M et al. Mutually exclusive use of viral promoters in epstein-barr virus latently infected lymphocytes. Proceedings of the National Academy of Sciences of the United States of America 1989; 86(17):6489-6502.

83. Sample J et al. The epstein-barr virus nuclear protein 1 promoter active in type 1 latency is autoregulated. Journal of Virology 1992; 66(80:4654-4661.

84. Weiss LM et al. Epstein-barr viral DNA in tissues of hodgkin's disease. American Journal of Pathology 1987; 129(1):86-91.

85. Weiss LM et al. Detection of epstein-barr viral genomes in reed-sternberg cells of hodgkin's disease. New England Journal of Medicine 1989; 320(8):502-506.

86. Anagnostopoulos I et al. Demonstration of monoclonal EBV genomes in hodgkin's disease and KI-1-positive anaplastic large cell lymphoma by combined southern blot and in situ hybridization. Blood 1989; 74(2):810-816.

87. Wu TC et al. Detection of EBV gene expression in reed-sternberg cells of hodgkin's disease. International Journal of Cancer 1990; 46(5):801-804.

88. Weiss LM et al. Epstein-Barr virus and hodgkin's disease. A correlative in situ hybridization and polymerase chain reaction study. American Journal of Pathology 1991; 139(6):1259-1265.

89. Herbst H et al. High incidence of epstein-barr virus genomes in hodgkin's disease. American Journal of Pathology 1990; 137(1):13-18.

90. Herbst H et al. Distribution and phenotype of epstein-barr virus-harboring cells in hodgkin's disease. Blood 1992; 80(2):484-491.

91. Boiocchi M et al. Association of epstein-barr virus genome with mixed cellularity and cellular phase nodular sclerosis hodgkin's disease subtypes. Annals of Oncology 1992; 3(4):307-310.

92. Herbst H et al. Epstein-barr virus latent membrane protein expression in hodgkin and Reed-Sternberg cells. Proceedings of the National Academy of Sciences of the United States of America 1991; 88(11):4766-4770.

93. Pallesen G et al. Expression of epstein-barr virus latent gene products in tumour cells of hodgkin's disease. Lancet 1991; 337(8737):320-322.

94. Poppema S and Visser L. Absence of hla class i expression by reed-sternberg cells. American Journal of Pathology 1994; 145(1):37-41.

95. Frisan T et al. Local suppression of epstein-barr virus (EBV)-specific cytotoxicity in biopsies of EBV-Positive hodgkin's disease. Blood 1995; 86(4):1493-1501.

96. Sing AP et al. Isolation of epstein-barr virus (EBV)-specific cytotoxic t lymphocytes that Lyse Reed-Sternberg cells: implications for immune-mediated therapy of EBV$^+$ hodgkin's disease. Blood 1997; 89(6):1978-1986.

97. Renner CR et al. Cure of disseminated xenografted human hodgkin's tumors by bispecific monoclonal antibodies and human T cells: the role of human t-cell subsets in a preclinical model. Blood 1996; 87(7):2930-2937.

98. Lee SP et al. Conserved epitopes within ebv latent membrane protein 2: a potential target for ctl-based tumor therapy. Journal of Immunology 1997; 158(7):3325-3334.

99. Romani N et al. Proliferating dendritic cell progenitors in human blood. Journal of Experimental Medicine 1994; 180(1):83-93.

100. Roskrow MA et al. Genetically modified dendritic cells generate primary and memory tumor antigen-specific cytotoxic t lymphocytes. Blood 1996; 88(10)suppl 1(part1):87a,abstract 337.

101. Wiryana P et al. Augmentation of cell-mediated immunotherapy against herpes simplex virus by interleukins: comparison of in vivo effects of IL-2 and IL-7 on adoptively transferred T cells. Vaccine 1997; 15(5):561-563.
102. Hombach A et al. Specific activation of resting t cells against ca 19-9[+] tumor cells by an anti-CD3/CA19-9 bispecific antibody in combination with a costimulatory anti-CD28 antibody. Journal of Immunotherapy 1997; 20(5):325-333.
103. Mavilo F et al. Peripheral blood lymphocytes as target cells of retroviral vector-mediated gene transfer. Blood 1994; 83(7):1988-1997.
104. Tiberghien P et al. Ganciclovir treatment of herpes simplex thymidine kinase transduced primary t lymphocytes: an approach for specific in vivo donor t-cell depletion after bone marrow transplantation? Blood 1994; 84(4):1333-1341.
105. Riddell SR et al. T-cell mediated rejection of gene-modified HIV-specific cytotoxic T lymphocytes in HIV-infected patients. Nature Medicine 1996; 29(2):216-223.

11

ADOPTIVE IMMUNOTHERAPY USING DONOR LEUKOCYTE INFUSIONS TO TREAT RELAPSED HEMATOLOGIC MALIGNANCIES AFTER ALLOGENEIC BONE MARROW TRANSPLANTATION

William R. Drobyski

Department of Medicine and the Bone Marrow Transplant Program, Medical College of Wisconsin, Milwaukee, WI 53226

Allogeneic bone marrow transplantation (BMT) is the only curative therapy for a number of patients with hematologic malignancies. The therapeutic efficacy of allogeneic marrow transplantation derives from the conditioning regimen which is myeloablative and the allogeneic marrow graft itself which is able to exert an antileukemic effect against residual malignant cell populations. This phenomenon which has been termed the graft-versus-leukemia (GVL) effect is mediated by immunocompetent cells resident in the donor marrow graft (1). Support for the existence of the GVL effect has come from both animal models (2,3) and epidemiological studies in man (4) which have provided strong evidence that allogeneic marrow transplantation is a potent demonstration of effective adoptive immunotherapy.

Unfortunately, GVL reactivity in man has typically been coexpressed with graft-versus-host disease (GVHD) which is the major complication of allogeneic BMT (4,5). This has hindered the effective application and expansion of this therapy into broader clinical settings since morbidity and mortality from GVHD have been inversely proportional to the degree of donor/recipient histocompatibility. Consequently, patients who lack HLA-identical sibling donors are either not offered allogeneic BMT or for those patients who are transplanted with marrow grafts from HLA-disparate donors, there is a high likelihood that they may ultimately succumb from GVHD-related complications. Any potential salutory GVL effect in this setting is therefore efficacy while minimizing GVHD-associated complications has emerged as one of the major goals of clinical and experimental BMT research.

BACKGROUND

Clinical studies have indicated that patients who develop GVHD after allogeneic marrow transplantation have a lower risk of subsequent disease relapse (4,5). In an effort to augment GVL reactivity, this observation led to studies designed to enhance GVHD in the hope that relapse rates would be decreased. The largest clinical study to test this hypothesis was conducted by Sullivan and colleagues (6) who sought to increase the severity of GVHD in allogeneic BMT patients at high-risk for relapse by either shortening the duration of posttransplant immunosuppression or by infusing donor buffy coat cells early posttransplant. Patients transplanted with unmodified marrow grafts from HLA-identical siblings were randomly assigned to a standard GVHD prophylaxis regimen consisting of long term methotrexate or one of the above experimental arms. In both experimental groups, the incidence of grade II-IV acute GVHD was increased two-three fold. While this goal of increasing acute GVHD severity was achieved, there was no salutory corresponding decrease in relapse or improvement in survival. Rather transplant-related mortality was increased in these groups due to a higher rate of infectious deaths occurring in the setting of concurrent GVHD.

An alternative approach to this problem has been to temporally dissociate GVH and GVL reactivity by delaying the administration of donor immunocompetent effector cells posttransplant in the hope that this will mitigate GVHD yet not compromise GVL reactivity. Studies as far back as 1962 (7) had shown that the delayed infusion of donor spleen cells to irradiated mice which had been transplanted with allogeneic bone marrow could abrogate lethal GVHD. This was in direct contrast to mice administered donor spleen cells at the time of transplant which were not protected from this complication. Subsequent studies in murine and canine models confirmed these results (8,9), but this strategy was not applied clinically until many years later. Reports from Kolb (10) and Slavin (11) in the 1980s were the first in which donor leukocyte infusions (DLI) were employed as a form of adoptive immunotherapy in the posttransplant period. Notably, however, the goal of these studies was not the abrogation of GVHD but rather the eradication of recurrent disease after allogeneic BMT. What was observed though was that the administration of donor T cells far in excess of the number given at the time of BMT not only eliminated recurrent leukemia, but did not result in the degree of GVHD which one would have predicted had the same number of T cells been given at initial BMT. In the study by Kolb and colleagues, three patients who had relapsed with overt chronic myelogenous leukemia (CML) after undergoing HLA-identical sibling marrow transplants were each administered a series of leukocyte infusions from their original marrow donors (10). While patients did develop GVHD, unlike the experience in animal models, all patients subsequently went into both clinical and cytogenetic remissions which appeared to be durable. This observation was particularly noteworthy in that the antileukemic effect was accomplished in the absence of any chemotherapy or radiation treatment providing conclusive evidence for an immunologically-mediated donor-derived antileukemic response. Several other important observations were derived from this clinical experience. First of all, all patients in this small series were in hematologic relapse indicative of a substantial leukemic cell burden. The elimination of these cells after infusion of donor leukocytes therefore indicated that this therapy was capable of eradicating multiple logs of leukemia cells. This was further evidence that the GVL effect was not merely relevant or restricted to patients with minimal residual disease posttransplant. Secondly, there was a period of several months before the elimination of leukemia cells could be demonstrated by cytogenetic analysis. These data suggested that the GVL effect required prolonged interaction between donor effector cells and leukemic target populations and was not an immediate event. These early reports provided proof of principle for the potency of this form of adoptive immunotherapy and opened the door for future application of this strategy in preclinical animal models and clinical studies in man.

PRE-CLINICAL ANIMAL MODELS OF DLI

Since the early work of Vos (7), Thompson (8), and Weiden (9), there have been been more recent studies aimed directly at further elucidating mechanistic aspects related to the use of DLI as adoptive immunotherapy in animal models. These studies which have been conducted primarily in mice have either sought to define why GVHD is abrogated in these murine models or how GVL reactivity can be further augmented in this setting. Johnson and colleagues (12) demonstrated that the transplantation of a specific dose of allogeneic spleen cells which caused lethal GVHD if given to recipients at the time of transplant failed to cause GVHD if given three weeks post BMT, confirming the earlier studies of Thompson. Similar results have also been recently observed by van Bekkum and colleagues (13). Experiments by Johnson and coworkers were performed in donor/recipient strain combinations that were either major histocompatibility complex (MHC) matched but differed at multiple minor histocompatibility antigens (B10.BR→AKR/J) or MHC- haplotype mismatched (SJL→ SJL/AKRF1). Three weeks appeared to be a critical time point in these studies as the administration of spleen cells at earlier time points was capable of eliciting GVHD, although the intensity of the reaction diminished the longer from transplant cells were transfused (Figure 1). Animals treated with delayed splenocyte infusions three weeks posttransplant were also capable of resisting a supralethal challenge of leukemia cells, indicating that an antileukemic response could be preserved in the absence of clinically evident GVHD (Figure 2). Subsequent studies demonstrated that T helper cell frequencies as determined by limiting dilution analysis were no different from bone marrow control (non-GVHD) mice (14). Conversely, cytolytic T cell precursor frequencies were 4 to 9 fold higher than control mice indicating that IL-2 secreting $CD4^+$ T cells were preferentially inhibited as opposed to cytolytic $CD8^+$ T cells. These data provided a potential mechanism for the lack of GVHD, since $CD4^+$ T cells are critical for the induction of GVHD in the examined strain combination (B10.BR→AKR/J). The reason $CD4^+$ T cells failed to make IL-2 was postulated to be due to the presence of suppressor cells which downregulated the helper T cell population early after BMT. Additional studies have since provided evidence for a donor-derived (Thy 1.2^+) cell population which plays an important role in suppressing GVH reactivity after DLI (B. Johnson, personal communication).

Figure 1: GVH-associated mortality in AKR chimeras infused with donor cells at various time points after BMT. Survival curves are shown for AKR hosts conditioned with 900 rads total body irradiation before intravenous injection with 1 x 10^7 B10.BR bone marrow cells admixed with 3 x 10^7 B10.BR spleen cells ($\square$; n = 12), or 1 x 10^7 bone marrow cells alone followed by the infusion of 3 x 10^7 donor spleen cells on day 3 ($\blacksquare$; n = 12), 7 (O; n = 27), 10 ($\bullet$; n = 20), 14 ($\wedge$; n = 21), 17 ($\blacktriangle$; n = 21) or 21 (X; n = 21) after transplant.

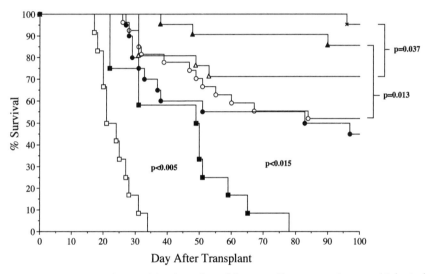

The data represent the combined results of three replicate experiments. (Adapted from reference 14).

Studies focusing on the antileukemic effect of DLI have been performed by Blazar and colleagues (15) who examined variables which influenced the magnitude of the GVL effect after DLI in mice with either acute lymphoblastic leukemia (ALL) or acute myeloid leukemia (AML). Both AML and ALL respond much less well to DLI in man (see below). These studies therefore sought to examine whether the GVL effect after DLI could be enhanced using an MHC-disparate strain combination as a preclinical model. Both ALL and AML leukemia cell lines were transfected with the costimulatory molecules B7-1 or B7-2 in order to augment anti-tumor immunity after DLI. The results of these studies demonstrated that B7-1 transfection of either ALL or AML cell lines reduced relapse rates after DLI. This was the result of an enhanced donor-derived antileukemic effect which was due to either CD8[+] or a combination of CD8[+] and CD4[+] T cells depending upon the specific leukemia examined. These data suggested that the low response rate seen in relapsed acute leukemic patients after DLI may be in part attributable to the lack of effective T cell costimulatory signals and suggested a potential mechanism whereby the GVL effect in man might be augmented.

Figure 2: GVL reactivity in leukemic B10.BR/AKR chimeras given multiple infusions of donor cells after BMT and long term persistence of the antileukemic affect of the infused cells. (A) Primary leukemia challenge: AKR hosts, preconditioned with 900 rads total body irradiation were transplanted by intravenous injection with 1 x 10[7] B10.BR bone marrow cells. On day 18 after transplant, all mice were intravenously injected with a lethal dose of 100 AKR leukemia cells and randomized into two groups: one group received no additional treatment (O; n =24); the other group was given 3 x 10[7] B10.BR spleen cells intravenously on days 21, 28, and 35 after transplant (●; n = 24). Normal, nontransplanted AKR mice (∧; n = 5) were also challenged with 100 leukemia cells. (B) Secondary leukemia challenge: the surviving animals from A (●, n = 13; O, n = 8) were rechallenged with 100 AKR leukemia cells between 99 and 111 days post-BMT.

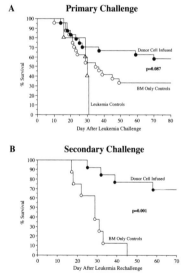

The survival curves represent the combined results of two experiments. (Adapted from reference 14).

THERAPEUTIC EFFICACY

A variety of hematologic malignancies have been evaluated for response to donor leukocyte infusions. The efficacy of this treatment in each of the primary disease states for which data on DLI therapy is currently available is detailed below. Epstein Barr virus (EBV)-associated lymphoproliferative disorders which are one of the major disease entities for which DLI have been used (16) are reviewed in another chapter in this book and will therefore not be further discussed here.

Chronic myelogenous leukemia

CML has been the prototypical disease for which DLI has been the most effective at inducing disease remission. In two large retrospective reviews totalling approximately 140 CML patients from a collection of United States and European centers (17,18), complete response rates of 70-80% have been obtained for patients treated in early stage relapse (i.e. molecular relapse, cytogenetic relapse, or chronic phase disease) (Table 1). For patients who are treated with disease in the accelerated phase or blast crisis, response rates have been much less averaging 0-30%. Smaller single center studies have reported similar results (19-24). One point which should be emphasized is that some patients relapse with additional acquired karyotypic abnormalities when compared to their initial cytogenetic studies pretransplant, but otherwise have clinical features compatible with chronic phase disease. These patients appear to respond equally well to DLI as those with no karyotypic abnormalities provided there are no other clinical features of accelerated disease (19).

The observation that patients in chronic phase respond better to DLI than those in the more advanced phases of the disease raises the question as to whether DLI would be more effective in patients who are treated when there is only cytogenetic or molecular evidence of disease recurrence. This issue has been addressed by Raanani and colleagues (25) who reported that response rates were higher when patients were treated in cytogenetic or molecular relapse when compared to those patients who were treated in the chronic phase. Specifically, 9 of 10 patients treated in molecular or cytogenetic relapse responded to DLI as compared to only 8 of 20 patients in hematologic relapse. These data suggested that CML patients with early evidence of relapse may respond more favorably than patients with clinically evident disease. Notably, patients in this study also received a wide range of T cell doses. Therefore, it cannot be excluded that this variability in T cell dose may have also contributed in part to the observed differences between groups. A recent study by van Rhee and colleagues (26), however, has similarly found that treatment in early relapse is associated with higher response rates.

Table 1.   Donor leukocyte infusions as treatment for relapsed hematologic malignancies after allogeneic BMT.

	STUDY	
	Kolb	Collins
Number of Patients	135	140
Disease		
CML	84	56
AML	23	46
ALL	22	15
MDS	5	6
MM	0	5
Other	1	12
HLA Donor/Recipient Compatibility		
Related	124 (82%)	128 (91%)
Unrelated	11 (8%)	12 (8%)
Response Rate (CR)		
CML - Cyto Relapse	14/17 (82%)	3/3 (100%)
CP	39/50 (78%)	25/33 (76%)
AP	1/8 (12%)	4/12 (33%)
BC	1/8 (12%)	1/4 (25%)
AML	5/17 (29%)	6/33 (18%)
ALL	0/12 (0%)	2/8 (25%)
MDS	1/4 (25%)	2/5 (40%)

In several studies, patients administered DLI have also been concurrently treated with alpha interferon in order to maximize an antileukemic effect (20,22,23). Conversely, other studies have employed DLI in the absence of alpha interferon and reported equally good response rates (21,25,27). Although there have been no comparative studies, there is currently no evidence that alpha interferon enhances or is necessary for the therapeutic efficacy of DLI in CML.

An important finding of these collective studies is the observation that the GVL effect is a slowly evolving response. In fact, it is not unusual for 4-6 weeks to elapse, in our experience, before one observes a decline in blood counts and the time to reach a molecular remission in the majority of studies has been on the order of 2 to 11 months (10,19,23,25-28) (Table 2). These data suggest that there is a requirement for the prolonged presence of donor-derived antileukemic effector cells in the recipient to achieve remission and has potential implications for alternative therapeutic strategies which are being explored in order to reduce complications from this therapy (see below).

TABLE 2. MEDIAN TIME TO CYTOGENETIC AND MOLECULAR REMISSION AFTER ADMINISTRATION OF DLI FOR RELAPSED CML

Study	Number of Patients	Median Time to Cytogenetic Remission	Median Time to Molecular Remission
Kolb[10]	3	16 weeks	NA
Raanani[25]	17	NA	11 months
Van Rhee[26]	8	16 weeks	6 months
Mackinnon[27*]	16	11 weeks	4 months
Porter[23]	6	NA	2 months
Drobyski[19]	6	31 weeks	9 months
Alyea [28+]	15*	13 weeks	8½ months

* 16 patients were evaluable for cytogenetic remission and 15 for molecular remission
+ 15 patients were evaluable for cytogenetic remission and 12 for molecular remission
NA, Data Not Available

Acute myelogenous leukemia/myelodysplastic syndrome (MDS)

Response rates in patients who relapse with either recurrent AML or MDS have been significantly worse than in CML and have averaged 10 to 40% (17,18,29-31) (Table 1). Interpretation of these data is often confounded by the fact that some patients receive pre-DLI chemotherapy to reduce disease burden and open up a therapeutic window with which to administer DLI. Assessing complete response rates in this latter group of patients is therefore problematic and indirect measurements of the efficacy of DLI can only be inferred from the durability of the responses. Another problem with the use of pre-DLI therapy is that the patient is exposed to a longer degree of pancytopenia necessarily induced by the chemotherapeutic regimen. Since there are few stem cells in unstimulated DLI collections, the infusion per se does not correct this problem and hematopoietic recovery is dependent upon the presence of residual donor stem cells in the patient. One approach to addressing this problem which is being explored is to give the patient growth factor-mobilized stem cells concurrently with donor T cells in an effort to shorten the duration of cytopenia (32). Whether this will prove effective, however, has yet to be determined.

In contrast to use of this therapy in CML, therapy of AML with DLI is made more difficult by a number of factors. First of all, in the majority of AML subtypes, there are no cytogenetic markers of early relapse (as compared to the Philadelphia chromosome in CML). Consequently, it is difficult to institute preemptive therapy for minimal disease burdens. Secondly, in those diseases with characteristic cytogenetic abnormalities, the prognostic value of the abnormality for predicting subsequent disease relapse is often uncertain or unknown. Therefore, whether these patients should even be treated preemptively can be problematic. Thirdly, disease relapse tends to be much more rapid so that the therapeutic window for DLI to be effective is quite narrow which is why pre-DLI chemotherapy is often given. Finally, the AML leukemic cell which is the target of this treatment may be inherently less capable of eliciting a donor-derived antileukemic response (15).

Acute lymphoblastic leukemia

ALL has been the least responsive disease to treatment with DLI of those examined thus far. Complete response rates have generally been only 0-20% with few long term remissions (17,18,33). As noted above for patients with relapsed AML, many patients also receive pre-DLI chemotherapy in order to reduce disease burden. Despite this consolidative effort, there have been few long-term survivors, suggesting that donor T cells are not effective at eradicating ALL leukemia cells. The reason for the lack of response observed in these patients is not clear, although recent studies by Cardoso and colleagues (34) have shown that B7 negative pre B cell ALL in man can induce alloantigen-specific nonresponsiveness. These data suggest that ALL cells may be capable of tolerizing donor T cells in vivo rendering them ineffective at eliminating leukemic cells. If corroborated, then strategies aimed at providing necessary costimulatory signals to these T cells to break tolerance might be efficacious in this group of patients.

Multiple myeloma

Multiple myeloma has recently emerged as a disease entity which may be particularly amenable to DLI therapy (28,35-38). Interest in treating myeloma patients derives from some similarities this disease has to CML. Specifically, patients have a marker for disease recurrence, (elevated serum paraprotein levels or increased urinary light chain excretion), similar to the Philadelphia chromosome, which often antedates clinical disease and therefore can be used as a trigger for early therapy which may render DLI more effective. Secondly, relapsed disease is often indolent in contrast to AML and ALL where the rapidity of relapse often does not allow for a sufficient antileukemia response to be generated. The largest series of multiple myeloma patients treated with DLI has been reported by Lokhorst and colleagues (37) who administered this therapy to thirteen patients who had relapsed after primary BMT. Whether relapse in these patients was characterized as either clinical or biochemical was not specified. All patients in this series received T cell depleted marrow grafts and all but one were transplanted with grafts from HLA-identical siblings. Sixty-two per cent of recipients (8/13) responded with either partial or complete remissions, although 2 of these 8 died of transplant-related complications, specifically due to marrow aplasia. The median response duration, however, was only five months, although 3 patients remain in CR $\geq$ 7 months after DLI. In the study by Alyea and colleagues, 2 of 6 patients have remained in complete remission 12-28 months after DLI, while 3 other patients who had initial responses subsequently progressed. Neither of these studies addressed whether early treatment of patients with residual myeloma after allogeneic BMT will increase response rates. An Eastern Cooperative Oncology Group protocol in which patients with evidence of minimal residual disease post-allogeneic BMT will receive DLI therapy is currently underway and may help to address this issue.

Miscellaneous

A variety of other disease states (non-Hodgkin's lymphoma, Hodgkin's disease, polycythemia vera) have been treated with DLI (18,39-41), but these reports are primarily anecdotal and the efficacy of DLI in these settings is still largely unproven.

COMPLICATIONS OF DLI THERAPY

DLI infusions have generally been well tolerated and at most institutions are administered on an outpatient basis. We routinely premedicate patients in the same manner as for other blood products with antihistamines and acetaminophen before transfusing cells through a standard blood filter to remove cellular microaggregates. In selected cases, when there is an ABO-incompatibility between patient and donor, leukopheresed products may undergo further processing to remove red cells. At our institution, this is done only if there is > 20 cubic centimeters of red blood cells in the product to be infused. In that case, red cells can be removed by ficoll-hypaque density gradient separation or other red cell reduction approaches. Otherwise patients, in our experience, have been able to receive the ABO-mismatched product without incidence.

Graft-versus-host disease (GVHD)

The major complication of DLI therapy has been GVHD. GVHD is caused by mature donor T cells which are capable of recognizing host alloantigens in a similar fashion to what occurs after allogeneic BMT. GVHD has been reported to occur in 50 to 80% of patients treated with DLI and in 10 to 20% of recipients has been fatal (17-24). This problem represents the major non-relapse cause of mortality and is the major limiting factor in preventing the application of this therapy to broader patient populations. The onset of acute GVHD typically occurs within the first 4 to 6 weeks after infusion, although some patients develop GVHD at later timepoints. The skin, liver and intestinal tracts can all be target organs of GVHD similar to what occurs after allogeneic BMT. A prominent difference in our experience, however, has been the disproportionate incidence of GVHD involving the liver as opposed to the intestinal tract. At the Medical College of Wisconsin, a review of patients who developed GVHD after DLI demonstrated that the skin was involved in 85% of these patients, the liver in 55%, the oral cavity in 21% and the intestinal tract in only 15% of the patient population (Table 3). The absence of GI involvement may be in part due to the absence of conditioning therapy which is known to damage GI mucosal surfaces resulting in cytokine release and leakage of lipopolysaccharide across mucosal membranes exacerbating GI damage from donor T cells (42). The reason for the propensity of DLI to preferentially involve the liver is not clear. A characteristic feature of liver GVHD is that the presenting clinical findings are typically elevation of transaminase levels often in the initial absence of elevated serum bilirubin and alkaline phosphatase values in contrast to what occurs after initial BMT (43). A failure to appreciate this presentation can lead to patients being misdiagnosed with hepatitis or other liver disorders and result in the unnecessary delay of effective therapy.

There have been no comparative studies examining the efficacy of various anti-GVHD regimens after DLI. Treatment for GVHD occurring after DLI has typically been similar to what has been employed after allogeneic BMT. Most patients are initially treated with prednisone and/or cyclosporine. Patients who fail front line therapy may then be treated with a variety of salvage regimens (anti-thymocyte globulin, mycophenolic acid, etc), although there are no comparative reports describing GVHD treatment in primary therapy nonresponders.

Table 3. GVHD target organ involvement occurring after 33 DLI treatment cycles

Skin	Intestinal Tract	Liver	Oral Cavity
28/33 (85%)	5/33 (15%)	18/33 (55%)	7/33 (21%)

A total of 53 patients were treated with DLI at the Medical College of Wisconsin between 1991-1998. A treatment cycle was defined as one set of infusions (generally one to four) administered over a one to two week period to reinduce remission. Some patients received more that one set of infusions if no response was observed after the first treatment cycle and therefore are represented twice in the above data. GVHD developed after 33 of these treatment cycles and the site of involvement is noted above in each of these instances.

Marrow Aplasia

The other major complication of DLI therapy has been pancytopenia and marrow aplasia. The mechanism of this complication is thought to be due to donor-derived T cell recognition and subsequent elimination of recipient marrow cells. This is similar to what occurs in transfusion-associated GVHD where transfused lymphocytes recognize not only non-hematopoietic tissues as foreign but marrow cells as well, leading to the development of marrow aplasia (44). In selected cases, if there are not enough residual donor hematopoietic cells to reconstitute the marrow, this can lead to ineffective hematopoiesis and the development of cytopenias. The incidence of marrow aplasia has generally been higher in patients who have complete recipient chimerism, as assessed by cytogenetic analysis, prior to DLI therapy (10,19-22,24,45,46) (Table 4). The inference from these data is that these patients have less donor hematopoietic reserve; consequently once leukemic cells have been eradicated there are an insufficient number of donor hematopoietic cells to reconstitute the recipient. This is further supported by recent studies demonstrating that CD34 chimerism can be informative in determining the likelihood of developing subsequent marrow aplasia (47). These data suggest therefore that one way to minimize this complication from developing is to treat patients when there is still evidence of mixed chimerism.

Table 4. Incidence of pancytopenia/marrow aplasia in recipients of DLI as a function of chimerism status in the bone marrow

Study	Complete Recipient Chimerism	Mixed Chimerism
Kolb[10]	0/2	0/1
Bar[21]	2/2	0/4
Drobyski[19]	4/6	0/0
Herthenstein[20]	5/6	0/0
Leber[44]	0/0	1/1
Cullis[24]	0/1	0/1
Helg[22]	1/2	0/1
	12/19 (63%)	**1/8 (12%)**

Treatment options for these patients who do develop pancytopenia depend upon the severity of this complication. For patients with mild degrees of pancytopenia who are otherwise asymptomatic, conservative approaches can be taken while waiting to determine whether hematopoiesis will improve spontaneously. For patients with more severe pancytopenia, treatment with growth factor therapy (G-CSF or GM-CSF) has been successful in some (17,19,26), while others have required bone marrow boosts from the original donor (17,19,20,26). We typically wait one week to observe whether treatment with growth factors has produced any response. If not, we then begin preparations for a marrow boost which can usually be accomplished within a week if the donor is a family member. For patients with unrelated donors, preparations for a boost need to be anticipated earlier. The latter approach, while being capable of restoring effective donor hematopoiesis, can also contribute to GVHD due to the presence of alloreactive donor T cells in the marrow graft. This problem can be reduced if the donor marrow graft is T cell depleted but this complication is still not entirely eliminated since not all donor T cells can be effectively removed with most T cell depletion approaches. Whether using CD34 selection columns to obtain more purified stem cell populations would be advantageous in this setting by not causing GVHD is an intriguing option but currently untested. Rarely, marrow boosts alone have also failed to reconstitute donor hematopoesis and patients have required conditioning therapy followed by marrow grafting (48).

UNRESOLVED ISSUES

How do donor leukocyte infusions eradicate recurrent or residual malignant cells?

While there have been a plethora of reports on clinical outcomes after DLI, there have been few mechanistic studies on how DLI eradicate malignant cells in man. The temporal association of concurrent GVHD in the majority of patients who have a demonstrable GVL response has provided circumstantial evidence that the primary antileukemic response is directed against host alloantigens and is not leukemia-specific. The fact that some patients have an antileukemic response without demonstrable GVHD is not necessarily evidence for a leukemia-specific response but may be attributable to coexistent but subclinical GVHD. Whether a component of the GVL response is actually leukemia specific remains a possibility but is unknown. Prior studies have demonstrated, at least in CML, that T cells can be generated which recognize the bcr/abl fusion protein (49,50), implying that these cells might contribute to GVL reactivity. Additionally, T cells which recognize alloantigens with restricted tissue expression have also been generated in vitro (51). In the latter case, these cells have the potential to recognize antigens preferentially expressed on hematopoietic cells as opposed to other non-hematopoietic tissues, and appear as relatively leukemia-specific (52-54). This would offer one possible explanation for the occurrence of a GVL response in the absence of clinically significant GVHD in some patients. To that end, Claret and colleagues (55) analyzed the T cell repertoire in four CML patients who went into complete remission after receiving DLI for recurrent disease. GVHD was observed in only one of these four patients. When the T cell receptor repertoire was examined by spectratype analysis, there was an expansion of a Vβ gene family which coincided with disappearance of Philadelphia chromosome positive cells. In at least one patient who failed to experience GVHD, DNA sequence analysis demonstrated that T cell expansion was clonal in origin, suggesting that a T cell clone(s) with GVL but not GVH reactivity existed in vivo after DLI.

The specific cell type(s) which mediate the GVL effect in these patients has not been defined. There are several candidate cells based on in vitro studies using human cell lines. HLA-DR-restricted $CD4^+$ T cells have been generated from normal individuals and found to be capable of specifically lysing CML cells (56). Clinical data indicating that CD8 depleted DLI are able to exert an antileukemic effect in CML patients provides supportive data that $CD4^+$ T cells can eradicate leukemia cells (28,57). Other cells, however, may also play a role in mediating the GVL response. Smit and colleagues identified $CD4^+$, $CD8^+$, and TCR $\gamma\delta^+$ cytotoxic T cells with reactivity against CML cells using a sensitive limiting dilution assay system (58). Finally, NK cells have been shown to be capable of lysing leukemic cells and might be responsible for MHC-nonrestricted cytotoxicity in these patients (59).

An interesting issue which appears to have greatest relevancy in CML has been the role of donor T cells in mediating a GVL effect. Epidemiological studies have confirmed the importance of donor T cells in mediating an antileukemic effect in this disease (4). This premise has been substantiated by data indicating that patients who receive T cell depleted marrow grafts are at increased risk of disease relapse when compared to patients transplanted with unmodified marrow grafts (60). A central biological issue in how DLI eradicates leukemia in CML patients is therefore whether donor T cells from the initial marrow transplant are still present in patients with relapsed disease or whether T cells in these patients are solely recipient in origin prior to DLI. To address this question, we analysed 8 patients with relapsed CML prior to DLI who had been previously transplanted with T cell depleted marrow grafts (19) (Table 5). Using sex mismatching as an indicator of chimerism, we determined that all patients had nearly complete (90-95%) donor T cell chimerism in the peripheral blood prior to DLI. This was in contrast to the other hematopoietic cells in the peripheral blood or bone marrow which were almost exclusively recipient in origin as assessed by restriction fragment length polymorphism (RFLP) analysis. Even though T cells were primarily donor-derived, this was not sufficient to prevent patients from relapsing. The reason for this is unknown, although possibilities include either that these T cells are qualitatively impaired perhaps by being tolerant of host alloantigens rendering them incapable of mediating a GVL response or that these cells are quantitatively deficient (i.e. even though the vast majority of T cells are donor in origin, there are still too few to forestall relapse). How the infusion of naïve mature donor T cells is able to break tolerance and reinduce
remission is uncertain. Further studies are required to define the relevant mechanism(s) with the goal of optimizing the GVL response in both CML and other disease states.

TABLE 5. PREINFUSION DONOR/RECIPIENT CHIMERISM IN PERIPHERAL BLOOD
AND BONE MARROW

	RFLP Studies		Donor/Recipient Sex	T-Lymphocyte Chimerism in Phytohemagglutinin-Stimulated Peripheral Blood Mononuclear Cells by in situ Hybridization*	
UPN	Bone Marrow	Peripheral Blood	Sex	% Male Cells	% Female Cells
225	ND	ND	M / F	ND	ND
364	95% Recipient	95% Recipient	M / F	98.0	2.0
141	90% Recipient	10% Recipient	F / M	1.0	99.0
251	>99% Recipient	95% Recipient	M / F	98.0	2.0
372	98% Recipient	ND	M / M		
357	90% Recipient	80% Recipient	M / F	98.0	2.0
454	90% Recipient	80% Recipient	F / M	2.0	98.0
306	90% Recipient	80% Recipient	M / M		

*Flow cytometric analysis of phytohemagglutinin-stimulated peripheral blood mononuclear cells performed immediately prior to in situ hybridization demonstrated that 80-95% of cells were CD3+.

Abbreviation: RFLP, Restriction Fragment Length Polymorphism

Adapted from reference 19.

Is there an optimal T cell dose for treatment in DLI?

Since T cells appear to be the critical effector cells which both induce a GVL response and also cause GVHD, an important question is whether or not there is an optimal T cell dose which will retain GVL efficacy but minimize GVHD. Few studies have directly addressed this question and in most reports patients have received a wide range of T cell doses. In an effort to address this issue, we examined the efficacy and toxicity of an arbitrarily defined T cell dose ($2.5-5.0$ x 10^8 T cells/kg) in a cohort of patients who had relapsed after HLA-identical sibling marrow transplantation (19). The majority of these patients had recurrent CML. In this study, we demonstrated that this narrow T cell range was capable of mediating an antileukemic response although most patients did develop concurrent GVHD. In a more definitive analysis, Mackinnon and colleagues (27) examined this question by performing a T cell dose escalation study in which CML patients received defined graded doses of T cells at specific intervals if they had not developed an antileukemic response and had no evidence of GVHD. Twenty-two patients were transplanted with graded doses of T cells at 4 to 33 week intervals in 5 fold increments. Patients were initially begun at a dose of 1 x 10^5 T cells/kg but because no responses were observed over the first several dose increments, the last 12 patients in this study were enrolled at a dose of 1 x 10^7 T cells/kg. Nineteen of 22 patients achieved cytogenetic remission and 15 of 17 went into molecular remission. Nine patients developed GVHD. When one examined the relationship between T cell dose and response in this study, patients with hematologic relapse appeared to require higher T cell doses to go into remission than patients in cytogenetic or molecular relapse. The specific T cell dose which elicited remission was difficult to determine in some patients, since dose escalation occurred at short intervals and thus one could have been witnessing overlapping GVL responses. Notably, 7 patients who were treated in molecular or cytogenetic relapse with a single dose of 1 x 10^7 T cells/kg all responded but had no evidence of acute GVHD. Only one of these patients developed chronic GVHD. These data suggested that in selected clinical settings, one may be able to administer a T cell dose which is capable of eliminating recipient leukemia cells without causing clinically significant GVHD.

A related but separate question which pertains to this issue is whether there may be different T cell dose thresholds for particular disease entities. Specifically, are higher T cell doses required for responses in some diseases when compared to other malignant conditions? If so, then one might be able to tailor a particular dose for a specific disease in an attempt to maximize efficacy and minimize toxicity. This question has not been evaluated in a systematic fashion; although, Mackinnon and colleagues did study the relative responses of two diseases present simultaneously in individual patients who were treated with a low dose ($< 10^6$/kg) of donor T cells (61). These investigators reported two patients who had coexistent EBV- lymphoproliferative disease and molecular evidence of CML in the setting of mixed chimerism. Treatment with DLI resulted in eradication of the lymphoproliferative disorder, but both of these patients remained mixed chimeras and subsequently relapsed with CML 45-52 weeks later. These data indicated that in these two patients the dose of T cells sufficient to eliminate EBV lymphoproliferation was not capable of forestalling leukemic relapse suggesting that, at least in these two diseases, there may be differing thresholds for response. Other studies have substantiated that lower T cell doses are effective in treating patients with EBV-lymphoproliferative disorders (16).

Are DLI effective when administered to recipients of unrelated or partially mismatched family marrow grafts?

The vast majority of patients who have been treated with DLI have previously undergone allogeneic BMT from HLA-identical sibling donors. With the increasing emphasis being placed on expanding the donor pool through the use of unrelated and mismatched family donors, a relevant and emerging question is the effectiveness of DLI in the latter settings. Van Rhee and colleagues, in their series of 14 patients treated with DLI for relapsed CML, reported five who had received unrelated marrow grafts (26). Three were in cytogenetic relapse, one in molecular relapse, and one in hematologic relapse at the time of treatment. All five patients attained complete remissions with no fatalities from GVHD, indicating that these patients may also benefit from DLI therapy. A subsequent retrospective study from this group reported similar response rates but no differences in the incidences of acute or chronic GVHD between CML patients who received DLI from either HLA-identical siblings or unrelated marrow donors (62). Results in two patients with relapsed AML who were given DLI from partially mismatched family donors, however, was less encouraging as both patients failed to have durable responses and died of progressive disease, despite developing moderate GVHD (63).

There has been only one large study which has examined the efficacy of DLI in unrelated marrow transplantation. In this report, Porter and colleagues (64) identified 71 patients through the National Marrow Donor Program who had received unrelated marrow grafts and then were treated with DLI for either relapsed leukemia or EBV-associated lymphoproliferative disease. Fifty-eight patients were treated specifically for hematologic relapse (25 CML, 23 AML, 7 ALL, 3 other diseases). The median age of this patient population was 25 years. The median time from BMT to relapse was 28 weeks and the median time from relapse to administration of DLI was 5 weeks. One year survival rates for CML, AML and ALL patients were 39%, 21% and 18%, respectively. With respect to CML, 7 of 12 evaluable patients treated in early relapse (chronic phase disease, cytogenetic or molecular relapse) and 4 of 12 patients treated with advanced disease went into complete remission. Mortality was attributable to DLI-related complications in 31% of patients while 63% of patients died of progressive disease and 6% of other causes. Notably ≥ grade 2 acute GVHD developed in only 34% of patients (24% of patients had ≥ grade III to IV acute GVHD) which was not substantially different from what has been observed in recipients of DLI for HLA-identical siblings. The only variable which was associated with superior survival was administration of a T cell depleted marrow graft at the time of BMT. For patients who received T cell depleted marrow grafts, median survival was 39 weeks versus 10 weeks for patients transplanted with unmodified marrow grafts. Collectively, these data demonstrated that DLI can be administered in the unrelated setting for patients with relapsed hematologic malignancies. CML patients appeared to have the best response rates similar to what has been observed in HLA-identical sibling marrow transplantation. More patients will need to be evaluated before it can be determined which factors predict for response and whether patients with acute leukemia will have an

251

enhanced GVL effect due to the greater HLA disparity between donor and recipient when compared to similar patients receiving DLI from HLA-identical sibling donors.

What is the durability of DLI therapy?

A critical question in the use of DLI to treat relapsed disease is whether patients can actually be cured of their leukemia. Specifically, this questions speaks to the durability of the response induced by DLI. There have been no published studies which have directly addressed this question, although one can infer from data published in a number of small clinical series (18-23) that some patients, predominantly those with CML, have remained in continuing molecular remission for 3 to 5 years. A review of data at the Medical College of Wisconsin on the durability of responses in CML patients treated with DLI is shown in Figure 3. Patients were serially followed using the polymerase chain reaction (PCR) to detect the bcr/abl RNA transcript. Two patients had persistent evidence of molecular disease and subsequently relapsed after having transient hematological responses (UPN 602 and 881). The remaining patients all went into molecular remission as determined by PCR and have remained in remission with follow-ups extending out to 6 years in some patients. Notably, in nearly all of these patients, the duration of remission after DLI has far exceeded the remission duration observed after initial BMT. These data provide strong evidence that many of these patients may in fact be cured of their disease.

Figure 3:   Serial PCR analyses for patients who were treated with donor leukocyte infusions for relapsed CML occurring after allogeneic BMT. Solid circles represent positive PCR assays and open circles negative assays. The symbol "I" denotes the time that the first infusion was administered to each of the respective patients.   The time posttransplant from the initial BMT is indicated at the top and bottom of the figure.

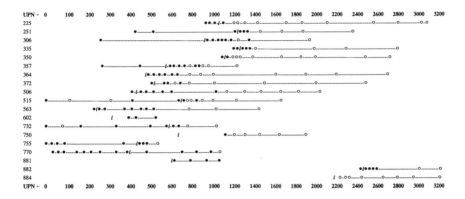

There has been one as of yet unpublished study which has examined long-term outcome in 55 patients who achieved complete remission after DLI (65). This was a multicenter analysis in which approximately 2/3 of patients were treated for recurrent CML while the remainder had either AML (10 patients), ALL (3 patients) or other disease entities. Six of 37 CML patients had either cytogenetic or hematologic relapse after DLI and two additional patients had recurrence documented by molecular evidence of the bcr/abl transcript but have had no evidence of clinical progression. Seven of 37 patients died of transplant-related complications. At a median of 41 months after DLI, 57% of CML patients treated with DLI were alive. Collectively these data indicated that remissions remain durable in the majority of CML patients, although a minority of patients will relapse after DLI. The impact of disease status at the time of DLI, T cell dose, or other factors on remission duration is currently unknown and will require further study. For AML and ALL, the complete remission rate has been too low to allow for a comprehensive assessment of durability of response, although available data suggest that the majority of patients who attain complete remissions after DLI with or without adjunctive chemotherapy are still likely to relapse.

NEW APPROACHES TO INCREASE EFFICACY AND/OR REDUCE TOXICITY FROM DLI

While the durable responses observed in a number of patients treated with DLI for relapsed hematologic malignancies has been encouraging, many patients, in particular those with acute leukemia, do not respond. Alternatively, some patients ultimately succumb to DLI-related complications. A number of approaches are now being investigated in an effort to either improve the antileukemic effect of DLI therapy or reduce the attendant complications which limit the usefulness and applicability of this strategy. Some of these emerging strategies are now detailed.

1. T cell subset depletion.

Animal studies have shown that GVHD posttransplant is generally exacerbated by the cooperative interaction of both $CD4^+$ and $CD8^+$ T cells (66,67). This has led to efforts directed at the selective elimination of one of these T cell subsets with the goal of reducing GVHD without compromising GVL reactivity. Clinical studies in CML patients have shown that depletion of $CD8^+$ T cells from the marrow graft does not appear to compromise GVL reactivity (57). Animal studies have also demonstrated that under certain circumstances specific T cell subsets can differentially mediate GVH/GVL reactivity (68). This premise has recently been extended to recipients of DLI. Giralt and colleagues (69) treated 10 patients with relapsed CML with DLI which had been ex vivo depleted of $CD8^+$ T cells by immunomagnetic separation. This strategy resulted in 97% depletion of $CD8^+$ T cells. Five patients were treated with early stage disease and all sustained complete responses while only one of five patients with advanced disease responded to this form of therapy. The majority of patients also received adjunctive therapy with either interferon alone or in combination with interleukin-2. Notably, GVHD was mild in this cohort of patients occurring in only 3 of 10 patients. This study demonstrated that the depletion of $CD8^+$ T cells did not compromise the GVL response at least in early stage patients, suggesting that $CD4^+$ T cells could mediate an antileukemic effect in CML.

A similar approach was performed by Alyea and colleagues (28) who administered graded doses of $CD4^+$ T cells after ex vivo $CD8^+$ T cell depletion to cohorts of patients who had relapsed with hematologic malignancies after allogeneic BMT. A total of 40 patients received either 0.3, 1.0, or 1.5 x 10^8 $CD4^+$ T cells/kg with individual patients also eligible for dosage escalation if no response was observed at the lower doses. In this study, there was a nonsignificant trend towards higher GVHD rates in patients who were treated at the two higher cell doses when compared to those administered the lowest cell number. Durable remissions were observed in the majority of early stage CML patients (79% molecular remission rate) and also in 2 of 6 patients with relapsed multiple myeloma. Approximately half of patients who obtained CR had no clinical evidence of GVHD. The majority of patients with diseases other than CML or multiple myeloma (AML, ALL, MDS, etc.) failed to respond to DLI similar to what has been reported in other studies. This study substantiated that highly purified $CD4^+$ T cells could exert an antileukemic effect in CML as well as multiple myeloma. The clinical evidence of GVHD was not a prerequisite for an anti-leukemic response. Whether use of specific T cell subsets will be superior to unfractionated DLI, however, was not addressed by either of these reports and will require further study.

2. Incorporation of Suicide Genes into Donor T cells.

This approach is predicated on the premise that the ability to selectively eliminate donor T cells post DLI therapy will allow for more effective control of GVHD. The gene which is currently being utilized in clinical trials is the herpes simplex virus thymidine kinase (TK) gene (70,72). This approach is discussed further in Chapter 16.

3. T Cell Addback Early Posttransplant.

In diseases such as AML and ALL, DLI have had limited efficacy when compared to its application in CML. One of the reasons for this lack of effectiveness is that disease recurrence in these patients is often rapid and therefore does not provide a sufficient therapeutic window. An alternative approach involves the preemptive administration of DLI early after transplant before patients have developed any evidence of relapse. This approach termed "T cell addback" typically involves the administration of graded doses of donor T cells at defined intervals posttransplant (73). Generally, patients have been initially transplanted with T cell depleted marrow grafts and then administered graded doses of donor T cells within a specified number of weeks post BMT. In one such study by Naparstek and colleagues (74), patients received 10^4-10^5 T cells/kg beginning day 1 or alternatively 10^5 T cells/kg beginning day 28 after transplant. The schedule was dependent upon the type of T cell depletion employed for GVHD prophylaxis. Dose escalation was performed at weekly or monthly increments, respectively. The incidence of acute GVHD was 42 to 53% in the two cohorts. While relapse rates in good risk patients were low, the efficacy of this therapy is difficult to evaluate due to the heterogeneity of the patient population and conditioning regimens as well as the absence of a control population. In a subsequent study, Barrett and colleagues (75) administered T cells at one of two dose levels, either 2×10^6 or 1×10^7 T cells/kg beginning on day 30. Patients receiving the lower dose level were eligible for a second dose at 5×10^7/kg at day 45. Of note, all patients also received concurrent cyclosporine GVHD prophylaxis. The incidence of $\geq$ grade two acute GVHD was significantly increased in patients who received the higher T cell dose on day 30 (100% versus 32%). While relapse rates in good risk patients was again relatively low, the efficacy of this therapy could not be ascertained for many of the same above reasons. This study did, however, provide evidence that the severity of GVHD was directly proportional to the dose of T cells.

A modification of this approach which is currently being investigated is to combine the delayed administration of donor T cells posttransplant with a nonmyeloablative conditioning regimen with the goal of reducing early regimen-related toxicity but preserving antileukemic efficacy. Thus far, two studies have employed a nonmyeloablative conditioning regimen and found that durable engraftment is achieved in the vast majority of patients (76,77). In one study (76), regimen-related toxicity was noted to be mild and relapse rates low with limited follow-up. Several patients in this latter study did eventually recur and were then treated with DLI with documented responses in 2/3 patients. The administration of donor T cells posttransplant to recipients of nonmyeloablative regimens, however, has yet to be studied in a systematic fashion and whether this approach will preserve antileukemic efficacy is not known.

4. Generation of Leukemia-Specific Donor T cells.

In an effort to reduce GVHD without compromising GVL reactivity, an alternative strategy has been to attempt to generate either leukemic-specific T cells or T cells with preferential leukemic as opposed to host tissue specificity. Prior studies have shown that cytotoxic T cell lines which recognize leukemic cells but not mitogen-activated normal lymphocytes can be generated from recipients after allogeneic BMT (58,78). Moreover, other studies have demonstrated that some minor histocompatibility antigens are restricted in tissue distribution with preferential expression on cells of the hematopoietic lineage, raising the possibility that targeting these antigens might spare normal tissues from GVHD-induced damage (79). In that regard, Molldrem and coworkers (80) have reported that cytotoxic T cells can be generated which have specificity for a primary granule protein which is overexpressed in leukemic cells. In subsequent studies, these investigators observed that these T cells preferentially inhibited colony forming units from CML but not normal bone marrow, suggesting that an antigen need not necessarily be resticted in expression but might be a useful target if there is differential expression on relevant tissues. The inference from these data is that it may be possible to generate T cell lines which can be used in adoptive immunotherapy trials with the goal of eradicating residual disease without causing collateral normal tissue toxicity. This strategy has yet to undergo formal clinical testing in man but is particularly attractive for use in the DLI setting and awaits clinical application.

CONCLUSIONS

The use of DLI to treat relapsed hematological malignancies has been one of the major advances over the past ten years in the field of allogeneic BMT. This therapy has demonstrated potent antileukemic efficacy and is likely to be curative for a number of patients. Despite this success, mortality, primarily due to GVHD, remains an obstacle to the more widespread application of this treatment. Additionally, disease nonresponsiveness is a particular problem in patients with acute leukemia. The ability to successfully address these challenges will determine whether DLI is ultimately restricted to selected patient populations or can become an effective therapeutic weapon for use in diverse patient populations with a variety of hematologic malignancies.

ACKNOWLEDGMENTS

I would like to thank Ms. Wendy Wozney for assistance in the preparation of the manuscript, and Dr. Marty Hessner for assistance with data analysis.

REFERENCES

1. Gale RP, Champlin RE. How does bone-marrow transplantation cure leukaemia? The Lancet, 1984; 2: 28-30.
2. Bortin MM, Truitt RL, Rimm AA, Bach FH. Graft-versus-leukaemia reactivity induced by alloimmunisation without augmentation of graft-versus-host reactivity. Nature, 1979; 281: 490-491.
3. Truitt RL, Shih CCY, LeFever AV. Manipulation of graft-versus-host disease for a graft-versus-leukemia effect after allogeneic bone marrow transplantation in AKR mice with spontaneous leukemia/lymphoma. Transplantation, 1986; 41: 301-310.

4. Horowitz MM, Gale RP, Sondel PM, Goldman JM, Kersey J, Kolb HJ, Rimm AA, Ringden O, Rozman C, Speck B, Truitt RL, Zwaan FE, Bortin MM. Graft-versus-leukemia reactions after bone marrow transplantation. Blood, 1990; 75: 555-562.
5. Sullivan KM, Weiden PL, Storb R, Witherspoon RP, Fefer A, Fisher L, Buckner CD, Anasetti C, Appelbaum FR, Badger C, Beatty P, Bensinger W, Berenson R, Bigelow C, Cheever MA, Clift R, Deeg HJ, Doney K, Greenberg P, Hansen JA, Hill R, Loughran T, Martin P, Neiman P, Petersen FB, Sanders J, Singer J, Stewart P, Thomas ED. Influence of acute and chronic graft-versus-host disease on relapse and survival after bone marrow transplantation from HLA-identical siblings as treatment of acute and chronic leukemia. Blood, 1989; 73: 1720-1728.
6. Sullivan KM, Storb R, Buckner D, Fefer A, Fisher L, Weiden PL, Witherspoon RP, Appelbaum FR, Banaji M, Hansen J, Martin P, Sanders JE, Singer J, Thomas ED. Graft-versus-host disease as adoptive immunotherapy in patients with advanced hematologic neoplasms. The New England Journal of Medicine, 1989; 320, 13: 828-834.
7. Vos O, Weyzen WWH. "Killing effect" of injected lymph node cells in homologous radiation chimeras. Transplantation Bulletin, 1962; 30: 501.
8. Thompson JS, Simmons EL, Moy RH, Crawford MK. Studies on immunologic unresponsiveness during secondary disease. The Journal of Immunology, 1967; 98, 1: 179-185.
9. Weiden PL, Storb R, Tsoi MS, Graham TC, Lerner KG, Thomas ED. Infusion of donor lymphocytes into stable canine radiation chimeras: implications for mechanism of transplantation tolerance. The Journal of Immunology, 1976; 116, 5: 1212-1219.
10. Kolb HJ, Mittermuller J, Clemm C, Holler E, Ledderose G, Brehm G, Heim M, Wilmanns W. Donor leukocyte transfusions for treatment of recurrent chronic myelogenous leukemia in marrow transplant patients. Blood, 1990; 76, 12: 2462-2465.
11. Slavin S, Or R, Naparstek E, Eckerstein A, Weiss L. Cellular-mediated immunotherapy of leukemia in conjunction with autologous and allogeneic bone marrow transplantation in experiment animals and man. Blood, 1988; 72: 407a.
12. Johnson BD, Drobyski WR, Truitt RL. Delayed infusion of normal donor cells after MHC-matched bone marrow transplantation provides an antileukemia reaction without graft-versus-host disease. Bone Marrow Transplantation, 1993; 11: 329-336.
13. Van Bekkum DW, Kinwel-Bohre EPM. Risk of donor lymphocyte infusions following allogeneic bone marrow transplantation. Experimental Hematology, 1997; 25: 478-480.

14. Johnson BD, Truitt RL. Delayed infusion of immunocompetent donor cells after bone marrow transplantation breaks graft-host tolerance and allows for persistent antileukemic reactivity without severe graft-versus-host disease. Blood, 1995; 85, 11: 3302-3312.

15. Blazar BR, Taylor PA, Boyer MW, Panoskaltsis-Mortari A, Allison JP, Vallera DA.. CD28/B7 interactions are required for sustaining the graft-versus-leukemia effect of delayed post-bone marrow transplantation splenocyte infusion in murine recipients of myeloid or lymphoid leukemia cells. The Journal of Immunology, 1997; 159: 3460-3473.

16. Papadopoulos EB, Ladanyi M, Emanuel D, Mackinnon S, Boulad F, Carabasi MH, Castro-Malaspina H, Childs BH, Gillio AP, Small TN, Young JW, Kernan NA, O'Reilly RJ. Infusions of donor leukocytes to treat Epstein-Barr virus-associated lymphoproliferative disorders after allogeneic bone marrow transplantation. New England Journal of Medicine, 1994; 330: 1185-1191.

17. Collins Jr. RH, Shpilberg O, Drobyski WR, Porter DL, Giralt S, Champlin R, Goodman SA, Wolff SN, Hu W, Verfaillie C, List A, Dalton W, Ognoskie N, Chetrit A, Antin JH, Nemunaitis J. Donor leukocyte infusions in 140 patients with relapsed malignancy after allogeneic bone marrow transplantation. Journal of Clinical Oncology, 1997; 15, 2: 433-444.

18. Kolb HJ, Schattenberg A, Goldman JM, Hertenstein B, Jacobsen N, Arcese W, Ljungman P, Ferrant A, Verdonck L, Niederwieser D, van Rhee F, Mittermueller J, de Witte T, Holler E, Ansari H. Graft-versus-leukemia effect of donor lymphocyte transfusions in marrow grafted patients. Blood, 1995; 86: 2041-2050.

19. Drobyski W, Keever C, Roth M, Koethe S, Hanson G, McFadden P, Gottschall J, Ash R, Van Tuinen P, Horowitz M, Flomenberg N. Salvage immunotherapy using donor leukocyte infusions as treatment for relapsed chronic myelogenous leukemia after allogeneic bone marrow transplantation: Efficacy and toxicity of a defined T-cell dose. Blood, 1993; 82: 2310-2318.

20. Hertenstein B, Wiesneth M, Novotny J, Bunjes D, Stefanic M, Heinze B, Hubner G, Heimpel, H, Arnold R. Interferon-α and donor buffy coat transfusions for treatment of relapsed chronic myeloid leukemia after allogeneic bone marrow transplantation. Transplantation, 1993; 56: 1114-1118.

21. Bar BM, Schattenberg A, Mensink EJBM, Van Kessel G, Smetsers TFCM, Knops GHJN, Linders EHP, De Witte T. Donor leukocyte infusions for chronic myeloid leukemia relapsed after allogeneic bone marrow transplantation. Journal of Clinical Oncology; 1993; 11, 3: 513-519.

22. Helg C, Roux E, Beris P, Cabrol C, Wacker P, Darbellay R, Wyss M, Jeannet M,Chapuis B, Roosnek E: Adoptive immunotherapy for recurrent CML after BMT. Bone Marrow Transplantation, 1993; 12: 125-129.

23. Porter DL, Roth MS, McGarigle C, Ferrara JLM, Antin JH. Induction of graft-versus-host disease as immunotherapy for relapsed chronic myeloid leukemia. The New England Journal of Medicine, 1994; 330, 2: 100-106.

24. Cullis JO, Jiang YZ, Schwarer AP, Hughes TP, Barrett AJ, Goldman JM. Donor leukocyte infusions for chronic myeloid leukemia in relapse after allogeneic bone marrow transplantation. Blood, 1992;79: 1379-1381.

25. Raanani P, Dazzi F, Sohal J, Szydlo RM, van Rhee F, Reiter A, Lin F, Goldman JM, Cross NCP. The rate and kinetics of molecular response to donor leucocyte transfusions in chronic myeloid leukaemia patients treated for relapse after allogeneic bone marrow transplantation. British Journal of Haematology, 1997; 99: 945-950.

26. van Rhee F, Lin F, Cullis JO, Spencer A, Cross NCP, Chase A, Garicochea B, Bungey J, Barrett J, Goldman JM. Relapse of chronic myeloid leukemia after allogeneic bone marrow transplant: The case for giving donor leukocyte transfusions before the onset of hematologic relapse. Blood, 1994, 83: 3377-3383.

27. Mackinnon S, Papadopoulos EB, Carabasi MH, Reich L, Collins NH, Boulad F, Castro-Malaspina H, Childs BH, Gillio AP, Kernan NA, Small TN, Young JW, O'Reilly RJ. Adoptive immunotherapy evaluating escalating doses of donor leukocytes for relapse of chronic myeloid leukemia after bone marrow transplantation: separation of graft-versus-leukemia responses from graft-versus-host disease. Blood, 1995; 86: 1261-1268.

28. Alyea EP, Soiffer RJ, Canning C, Neuberg D, Schlossman R, Pickett C, Collins H, Wang Y, Anderson KC, Ritz J. Toxicity and efficacy of defined doses of CD4+ donor lymphocytes for treatment of relapse after allogeneic bone marrow transplant. Blood; 91: 3671-3680.

29. Mehta J, Powles R, Singhal S, Tait D, Swansbury J, Treleaven J. Cytokine-mediated immunotherapy with or without donor leukocytes for poor-risk acute myeloid leukemia relapsing after allogeneic bone marrow transplantation. Bone Marrow Transplantation, 1995; 16: 133-137.

30. Porter DL, Roth MS, Lee SJ, McGarigle C, Ferrara JLM, Antin JH. Adoptive immunotherapy with donor mononuclear cell infusions to treat relapse of acute leukemia or myelodysplasia after allogeneic bone marrow transplantation. Bone Marrow Transplantation, 1996; 18: 975-980.

31. Mehta J, Powles R, Kulkarni S, Treleaven J, Singhal S. Induction of graft-versus-host disease as immunotherapy of leukemia relapsing after allogeneic transplantation: single-center experience of adult patients. Bone Marrow Transplantation, 1997; 20: 129-135.

32. Glass B, Majolino I, Dreger P, Scime R, Santoro A, Vasta S, Suttorp M, Haferlach T, Schmitz N. Allogeneic peripheral blood progenitor cells for treatment of relapse after bone marrow transplantation. Bone Marrow Transplantation, 1997; 20: 533-541.

33. Atra A, Millar B, Shepherd V, Shankar A, Wilson K, Treleaven J, Pritchard-Jones K, Meller ST, Pinkerton CR. Donor lymphocyte infusion for childhood acute lymphoblastic leukaemia relapsing after bone marrow transplantation. British Journal of Haematology, 1997; 97: 165-168.

34. Cardoso AA, Schultze JL, Boussiotis VA, Freeman GJ, Seamon MJ, Laszlo S, Billet A, Sallan SE, Gribben JG, Nadler LM. Pre-B acute lymphoblastic leukemia cells may induce T-cell anergy to alloantigen. Blood, 1996; 88: 41-48.

35. Verdonck LF, Lokhorst HM, Dekker AW, Nieuwenhuis HK, Petersen EJ. Graft-versus-myeloma effect in two cases. The Lancet, 1996; 347: 800-801.

36. Tricot G, Vesole DH, Jagannath S, Hilton J, Munshi N, Barlogie B. Graft-versus-myeloma effect: Proof of principle. Blood, 1996; 87: 1196-1198.

37. Lokhorst MH, Schattenberg A, Cornelissen JJ, Thomas LLM, Verdonck LF. Donor leukocyte infusions are effective in relapsed multiple myeloma after allogeneic bone marrow transplantation. Blood, 1997; 90: 4206-4211.

38. Bertz H, Burger JA, Kunzmann R, Mertelsmann R, Finke J. Adoptive immunotherapy for relapsed multiple myeloma after allogeneic bone marrow transplantation (BMT): evidence for a graft-versus-myeloma effect. Leukemia, 1997; 11; 281-283.

39. Van Besien KW, De Lima M, Giralt SA, Moore Jr DF, Khouri IF, Rondon G, Mehra R, Andersson BS, Dyer C, Cleary K, Przepiorka D, Gajewski JL, Champlin RE. Management of lymphoma recurrence after allogeneic transplantation: the relevance of graft-versus-lymphoma effect. Bone Marrow Transplantation, 1997; 19: 977-982.

40. Russell LA, Jacobsen N, Heilmann C, Simonsen AC, Christensen LD, Vindelov LL. Treatment of relapse after allogeneic BMT with donor leukocyte infusions in 16 patients. Bone Marrow Transplantation, 1996; 18: 411-414.

41. Slavin S, Naparstek E, Nagler A, Ackerstein A, Samuel S, Kapelushnik J, Brautbar C, Or R.. Allogeneic cell therapy with donor peripheral blood cells and recombinant interleukin-2 to treat leukemia relapse after allogeneic bone marrow transplantation. Blood 1996; 87: 2195-2204.

42. Hill GR, Crawford JM, Cooke KR, Brinson YS, Pan L, Ferrara JLM. Total body irradiation and acute graft-versus-host disease: The role of gastrointestinal damage and inflammatory cytokines. Blood, 1997; 90: 3204-3213.

43. Bacigalupo A, Soracco M, Vassallo F, Abate M, Van Lint MT, Gualandi F, Lamparelli T, Occhini D, Mordini N, Bregante S, Figari O, Benvenuto F, Sessarego M, Fugazza G, Carlier P, Valbonesi M. Donor lymphocyte infusions (DLI) in patients with chronic myeloid leukemia following allogeneic bone marrow transplantation. Bone Marrow Transplantation, 1997; 927-932.

44. Anderson KC, Weinstein HJ. Transfusion-associated graft-versus-host disease. New England Journal of Medicine, 1990; 323: 315-321.

45. Leber B, Walker IR, Rodriguez A, McBride JA, Carter R, Brain MC. Reinduction of remission of chronic myeloid leukemia by donor leukocyte transfusion following relapse after bone marrow transplantation: recovery complicated by initial pancytopenia and late dermatomyositis. Bone Marrow Transplantation, 1993; 12: 405-407.

46. Rapanotti MC, Arcese W, Buffolino S, Lori AP, Mengarelli A, De Cuia MR, Cardillo A, Cimino, G. Sequential molecular monitoring of chimerism in chronic myeloid leukemia patients receiving donor lymphocyte transfusion for relapse after bone marrow transplantation. Bone Marrow Transplantation, 1997; 19: 703-707.

47. Keil F, Haas OA, Fritsch G, Kalhs P, Lechner K, Mannhalter C, Reiter E, Niederwieser D, Hoecker P, Greinix HT. Donor leukocyte infusion for leukemic relapse after allogeneic marrow transplantation: Lack of residual donor hematopoiesis predicts aplasia. Blood; 89: 3113-3117.

48. Keil F, Kalhs P, Haas OA, Fritsch G, Mitterbauer G, Brugger S, Lechner K, Schwarzinger I, Mannhalter C, Linkesch W, Kurz M, Greinix HT. Graft failure after donor leucocyte infusion in relapsed chronic myeloid leukaemia: successful treatment with cyclophosphamide and antithymocyte globulin followed by peripheral blood stem cell infusion. British Journal of Haematology, 1996; 94: 120-122.

49. Chen W, Peace DJ, Rovira DK, You SG, Cheever MA. T-cell immunity to the joining region of p210[BCR-ABL] protein. Proceedings of National Academy and Sciences, 1992; 89: 1468-1472.

50. Bocchia M, Korontsvit T, Xu Q, Mackinnon S, Yang SY, Sette A, Scheinberg DA. Specific human cellular immunity to bcr-abl oncogene-derived peptides. Blood, 1996; 87: 3587-3592.

51. Warren EH, Greenberg PD, Riddell SR. Cytotoxic T-lymphocyte-defined human minor histocompatibility antigens with a restricted tissue distribution. Blood, 1998; 91: 2197-2207.

52. Voogt PJ, Goulmy ELS, Veenhof WFJ, Hamilton M, Fibbe WE, Van Rood JJ, Falkenburg JHF. Cellularly defined minor histocompatibility antigens are differentially expressed on human hematopoietic progenitor cells. Journal of Experimental Medicine, 1988; 168: 2337-2347.

53. Faber LM, van Luxemburg-Heijs SAP, Willemze R, Falkenburg JHF. Generation of leukemia-reactive cytotoxic T lymphocyte clones from the HLA-identical bone marrow donor of a patient with leukemia. Journal of Experimental Medicine, 1992; 176: 1283-1289.

54. Marijt WA, Veenhof WFJ, Brand A, Goulmy E, Fibbe WE, Willemze R, Van Rood JJ, Falkenburg JHF. Minor histocompatibility antigen-specific cytotoxic T cell lines, capable of lysing human hematopoietic progenitor cells, can be generated in vitro by stimulation with HLA-identical bone marrow cells. Journal of Experimental Medicine, 1991; 173: 101-109.

55. Claret EJ, Alyea EP, Orsini E, Pickett CC, Collins H, Wang Y, Neuberg D, Soiffer RJ, Ritz J. Characterization of T cell repertoire in patients with graft-versus-leukemia after donor lymphocyte infusion. Journal of Clinical Investigation, 1997; 100: 855-866.

56. Jiang YZ, Barrett AJ. Cellular and cytokine-mediated effects of CD4-positive lymphocyte lines generated in vitro against chronic myelogenous leukemia. Experimental Hematology, 1995; 23: 1167-1172.

57. Champlin R, Ho W, Gajewski J, Feig S, Burnison M, Holley G, Greenberg P, Lee K, Schmid I, Giorgi J, Yam P, Petz, L, Winston D, Warner N, Reichert T. Selective depletion of CD8$^+$ T lymphocytes for prevention of graft-versus-host disease after allogeneic bone marrow transplantation. Blood, 1990; 76: 418-423.

58. Smit WM, Rijnbeek M, Van Bergen CAM, Willemze R, Falkenburg JHF. Generation of leukemia-reactive cytotoxic T lymphocytes from HLA-identical donors of patients with chronic myeloid leukemia using modifications of a limiting dilution assay. Bone Marrow Transplantation, 1998; 21: 553-560.

59. Jiang YZ, Cullis JO, Kanfer EJ, Goldman JM, Barrett AJ. T cell and NK cell mediated graft-versus-leukaemia reactivity following donor buffy coat transfusion to treat relapse after marrow transplantation for chronic myeloid leukaemia. Bone Marrow Transplantation, 1993; 11: 133-138.

60. Goldman JM, Gale RP, Horowitz MM, Biggs JC, Champlin RE, Gluckman E, Hoffmann, RG, Jacobsen SJ, Marmont AM, McGlave PB, Messner HA, Rimm AA, Rozman C, Speck B, Tura S, Weiner RS, Bortin MM. Bone marrow transplantation for chronic myelogenous leukemia in chronic phase: Increased risk of relapse associated with T-cell depletion. Annals Internal Medicine, 1988; 108: 806-814.

61. Mackinnon S, Papadopoulos EB, Carabasi MH, Reich L, Collins NH, O'Reilly RJ. Adoptive immunotherapy using donor leukocytes following bone marrow transplantation for chronic myeloid leukemia: is T cell dose important in determining biological response? Bone Marrow Transplantation, 1995; 15: 591-594.
62. Van Rhee F, Savage D, Blackwell J, Orchard K, Dazzi F, Lin F, Chase A, Bungey J, Cross NCP, Apperley J, Szydlo R, Goldman JM. Adoptive immunotherapy for relapse of chronic myeloid leukemia after allogeneic bone marrow transplant: equal efficacy of lymphocytes from sibling and matched unrelated donors. Bone Marrow Transplantation, 1998; 21: 1055-1061.
63. Pati AR, Godder K, Lamb L, Gee A, Henslee-Downey PJ. Immunotherapy with donor leukocyte infusions for patients with relapsed acute myeloid leukemia following partially mismatched related donor bone marrow transplantation. Bone Marrow Transplantation, 1995; 15: 979-981.
64. Porter D, Collins R, Mick R, Kernan N, Giralt S, Flowers M, Casper J, Drobyski W, Leahey A, Parker P, Bates B, King R, Antin J. Unrelated donor leukocyte infusions to treat relapse or EBV-lymphoproliferative disease after unrelated donor bone marrow transplantation. Blood 1998; 90: 590a.
65. Porter DL, Collins R, Drobyski W, Connors JM, Van Hoef M, Antin J. Long term follow up of 55 patients who received complete remission after donor leukocyte infusions for relapse after allogeneic bone marrow transplantation. Blood 1997; 90: 549a.
66. Korngold R, Sprent J. Variable capacity of L3T4$^+$ T cells to cause lethal graft-versus-host disease across minor histocompatibility barriers in mice. Journal of Experimental Medicine, 1987; 165: 1552-1564.
67. Drobyski WR, Majewski D, Ozker K, Hanson G. Ex vivo anti-CD3 antibody-activated donor T cells have a reduced ability to cause lethal murine graft-versus-host disease but retain their ability to facilitate alloengraftment. Journal of Immunology, 1998; 161(5): 2610-2619.
68. Truitt RL, Atasoylu AA. Contribution of CD4$^+$ and CD8$^+$ T cells to graft-versus-host disease and graft-versus-leukemia reactivity after transplantation of MHC-compatible bone marrow. Bone Marrow Transplantation, 1991; 8: 51-58.
69. Giralt S, Hester J, Huh Y, Hirsch-Ginsberg C, Rondon G, Seong D, Lee M, Gajewski J, Van Besien K, Khouri I, Mehra R, Przepiorka D, Korbling M, Talpaz M, Kantarjian H, Fischer H, Deisseroth A, Champlin R. CD8-depleted donor lymphocyte infusion as treatment for relapsed chronic myelogenous leukemia after allogeneic bone marrow transplantation. Blood, 1995; 86, 11: 4337-4343.

70. Helene M, Lake-Bullock V, Bryson JS, Jennings CD, Kaplan AM. Inhibition of graft-versus-host disease: Use of a T cell-controlled suicide gene. Journal of Immunology, 1997; 158: 5079-5082.

71. Cohen JL, Boyer O, Salomon B, Onclercq R, Charlotte F, Bruel S, Boisserie G, Klatzmann D. Prevention of graft-versus-host disease in mice using a suicide gene expressed in T lymphocytes. Blood, 1997; 89: 4636-4645.

72. Bonini C, Ferrari G, Verzeletti S, Servida P, Zappone E, Ruggieri L, Ponzoni M, Rossini S, Mavilio F, Traversari C, Bordignon C. HSV-TK gene transfer into donor lymphocytes for control of allogeneic graft-versus-leukemia. Science, 1997; 276: 1719-1724.

73. Slavin S, Naparstek E, Nagler A, Ackerstein A, Kapelushnik J, Or R. Allogeneic cell therapy for relapsed leukemia after bone marrow transplantation with donor peripheral blood lymphocytes. Experimental Hematology, 1995; 23: 1553-1562.

74. Naparstek E, Or R, Nagler A, Cividalli G, Engelhard D, Aker M, Gimon Z, Manny N, Sacks T, Tochner Z, Weiss L, Samuel S, Brautbar C, Hale G, Waldmann H, Steinberg SM, Slavin S. T-cell-depleted allogeneic bone marrow transplantation for acute leukaemia using campath-1 antibodies and post-transplant administration of donor's peripheral blood lymphocytes for prevention of relapse. British Journal of Haematology, 1995; 89: 506-515.

75. Barrett AJ, Mavroudis D, Tisdale J, Molldrem J, Clave E, Dunbar C, Cottler-Fax M, Phang S, Carter C, Okunnieff P, Young NS, Read EJ. T cell-depleted bone marrow transplantation and delayed T cell add-back to control acute GVHD and conserve a graft-versus-leukemia effect. Bone Marrow Transplantation, 1998; 21: 543-551.

76. Giralt S, Estey E, Albitar M, van Besien K, Rondon G, Anderlini P, O'Brien S, Khouri I, Gajewski J, Mehra R, Claxton D, Andersson B, Beran M, Przepiorka D, Koller C, Kornblau S, Korbling M, Keating M, Kantarjian H, Champlin R. Engraftment of allogeneic hematopoietic progenitor cells with purine analog-containing chemotherapy: Harnessing graft-versus-leukemia without myeloablative therapy. Blood 1997; 89: 4531-4536.

77. Slavin S, Nagler A, Naparstek E, Kapelushnik Y, Aker M, Cividalli, Varadi G, Kirschbaum M, Ackerstein A, Samuel S, Amar A, Brautbar C, Ben-Tal O, Eldor A, Or R. Nonmyeloablative stem cell transplantation and cell therapy as an alternative to conventional bone marrow transplantation with lethal cytoreduction for the treatment of malignant and nonmalignant hematologic diseases. Blood, 1998; 91: 756-763.

78. Datta AR, Barrett AJ, Jiang YZ, Guimaraes A, Mavroudis DA, van Rhee F, Gordon AA, Madrigal A. Distinct T cell populations distinguish chronic myeloid leukaemia cells from lymphocytes in the same individual: a model for separating GVHD from GVL reactions. Bone Marrow Transplantation, 1994; 14: 517-524.

79. De Bueger M, Bakker A, Van Rood JJ, Van Der Woude F, Goulmy E. Tissue distribution of human minor histocompatibility antigens. Ubiquitous versus restricted tissue distribution indicates heterogeneity among human cytotoxic T lymphocyte-defined non-MHC antigens.   Journal of Immunology, 1992; 149: 1788-1794.

80. Molldrem JJ, Clave E, Jiang YZ, Mavroudis D, Raptis A, Hensel N, Agarwala V, Barrett AJ. Cytotoxic T lymphocytes specific for a nonpolymorphic proteinase 3 peptide preferentially inhibit chronic myeloid leukemia colony-forming units. Blood, 1997; 90, 7: 2529-2534.

12

CLINICAL USE OF IRRADIATED DONOR LYMPHOCYTES IN BONE MARROW TRANSPLANTATION

Alan M. Ship, M.D. C.M., and Edmund K. Waller, M.D. Ph.D., FACP

Emory University School of Medicine, Atlanta GA 30322 USA

INTRODUCTION

Only 25% of patients presenting for allogeneic bone marrow transplantation will have a sibling who is an antigenically matched potential donor (1). The use of alternative stem cell sources such as volunteer unrelated donors, mismatched related donors, cord blood, and placental blood has increased to meet the demands imposed by the limited number of matched sibling donors (2-4). As antigenic diversity between donor and host increases, so does the risk of graft versus host disease (GvHD) and graft rejection. Manipulations of the stem cells to reduce the risk of GvHD, such as T-cell depletion, lead to increased graft rejection and relapse among patients with malignancies (5-9). The risk of GvHD or rejection increases from 20% with a matched sibling donor to as high as 60% for a matched unrelated donor or over 70% for a mismatched unrelated donor (10-12). An important goal in extending the range of alternative donor is to achieve immunologic balance between donor and host T-cells and produce stable donor-derived hematopoiesis post-transplant.

THE RATIONALE FOR CELLULAR IMMUNOTHERAPY

The phenomena of GvHD, graft versus leukemia (GvL) and graft rejection, are immunologically mediated side effects of the antigenic diversity between donor and recipient. GvHD is an immune response of the graft donors T-cells against the host cells and tissues, whereas graft rejection is an immune response of chemo- and radio-resistant recipient T-cells against the graft. Engraftment is related to the relative number of host and donor T-cells. When the balance falls in favor of an excess of donor T-cells the strength of the GvHD vector is enhanced; when the balance is shifted toward excess host T-cells the graft rejection vector is increased and there is an increased incidence of relapse (Figure 1).

Figure 1. Achieving the Proper Balance in Allogeneic Transplantation

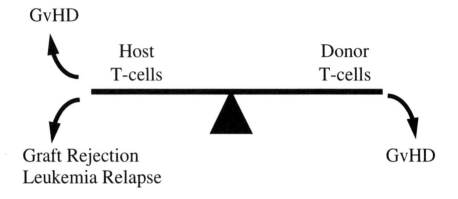

One approach to prevent GvHD in allogeneic bone marrow transplantation has been to remove immunocompetent T-cells from the graft by various means including: using elutriation, absorption to lectin, application of specific monoclonal antibodies with complement or immuno toxin, or by specific selection of CD34[+] donor stem cells (5, 9, 13-17). Removing T cells from the bone marrow allograft resulted in a decreased incidence of serious GvHD, but a significantly increased incidence of graft rejection and leukemia relapse (18). More sophisticated methods of graft engineering, such as transducing donor T-cells with a "suicide gene" (such as thymidine kinase) and returning them to a T-cell depleted graft are currently being developed (see chapter 16).

The existence of the undesirable immunologic side effects related to host and donor T-cells has also directed researchers to modulate host and donor immunity by selective add-back of donor immune cells to achieve a GvL effect (21-28) (see chapter 11).

The mononuclear fraction of human peripheral blood was prepared by Ficoll-Hypaque centrifugation treated with 0, 2.5, 7.5, 10 or 20 Gy ionizing radiation. Irradiated cells were cultured in RPMI media containing 10% v/v autologous plasma, 100 units/ml IL2, and 10 ng/ml OKT3. Fresh media containing IL2 was added weekly. Following 2, 4, 7 and 20 days of culture, aliquots were counted for the number of viable cells and analyzed by FACS for the presence of CD3$^+$ T-cells and CD3-, CD56$^+$ NK cells. The total number of T-cells and NK cells in culture at various times is shown by the height of the vertical bars.

RATIONALE FOR THE USE OF IRRADIATED DONOR LYMPHOCYTES IN BMT

A method of preserving the GvL potential of donor lymphocytes while inhibiting their ability to induce GvHD would be of significant benefit in allogeneic transplantation. The rationale for the irradiation of donor T-cells derives from effects of radiation on lymphocytes and animal experiments. Exposure to ionizing radiation limits the ability for long-term proliferation of lymphocytes in vivo while preserving their ability for cytotoxic activity against tumor cells (29) or as veto cells against host cytolytic cells (30). A human T-cell line (TALL-104), irradiated to a dose of 20 Gy, has recently been shown to be effective in eliminating clonogenic human leukemic cells when co-cultures of irradiated T-cells and leukemia cells were infused into human bone xenografts in immunodeficient SCID-hu mice (31). In theory, irradiated donor lymphocytes could have all of the desirable short-term effects of donor T-cells infusions without causing GvHD.

Figure 2. Survival of human PBMC in vitro after different doses of ionizing radiation.

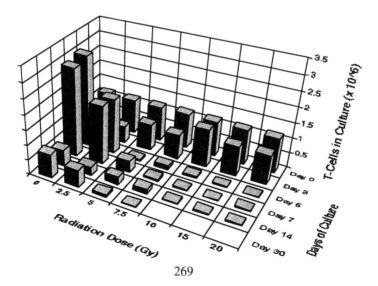

EFFECTS OF IRRADIATION ON THE LYMPHOCYTE

The growth inhibitory and pro apoptotic effects on resting and growing lymphocytes have been well documented in the literature. Lymphocytes have been shown to be sensitive to radiation doses of 5 Gy or higher in vivo (32-35) and in vitro (36, 37). The survival of human T-cells exposed to radiation doses between 0 and 10 Gy and then cultured in the presence of IL2 is shown in Figure 2. Taliaferro, Dixon, and Anderson performed the most extensive studies on radiation-induced suppression and augmentation of the immune response in which >5 Gy whole body radiation delayed the primary immune response to allogeneic skin graft rejection (38,39). Paradoxically, low dose radiation (<3 Gy) enhanced the immune response, presumably by selecting for antigen-primed lymphocytes that proliferated in the absence of more radiosensitive suppresser cells (33, 40). A number of studies have shown that activated T-cells can survive doses of radiation that are cytotoxic to resting T-cells. Stimulation with phytohemagluttinin (PHA) transforms lymphocytes into blasts and protects them against the cytotoxic effect of 8 Gy of radiation (36,37,41). A dose-dependent inhibition of thymidine incorporation in response to PHA stimulation in vitro was noted when cells were treated with radiation doses in the range of 2.5 to 20 Gy (40, 42). When lymphocytes were exposed to radiation doses of 4-6 Gy T helper cell activity was augmented, suppresser cell activity was inhibited, and the ability of parental lymphocytes to produce GvHD in neonatal recipients was inhibited (43-45). Exposure of peripheral blood lymphocytes to 2-10 Gy of gamma radiation has also been shown to produce enhanced cytotoxic activity against tumor cells (46-48). The proliferative potential of non-sensitized lymphocytes in a mixed lymphocyte culture (MLC) was blocked by exposure to radiation doses of 6 Gy or more, while allo-sensitized human T lymphocytes continued to proliferate in MLR following exposure of up to 20 Gy (49). Nichols also demonstrated that exposure of allo-sensitized effector human T cells to a wide range of radiation doses, from 1 to 10 Gy, resulted in enhanced cytolytic activity against ^{51}Cr labeled allo-targets (49). CD28 costimulation has been shown to block radiation-induced apoptosis by enhancing the expression of Bcl-X_L (50). T-cells activated by ligation of the CD3 complex with monoclonal antibody died over a 4 day period if secreted IL2 was removed from the culture media; the pro-apoptotic effect of removing IL2 was blocked by the addition of anti-CD28 monoclonal antibodies. Analysis of intracellular levels of Bcl-X_L and Bcl-2 mRNA levels revealed significant synergistic up-regulation of Bcl-X_L mRNA by anti-CD3 and anti-CD28 antibodies without changes in the level of Bcl-2 mRNA (50). These data, that radiation activates the cytolytic activity of T-cells, and that T-cell activation via CD3 and CD28 blocks the apoptotic pathway support the potential role of irradiated allogeneic donor T-cells in

BMT based upon the differential effect of radiation on activated T-cells versus non-activated T-cells (50, 51).

PRECLINICAL DATA THAT IRRADIATED DONOR LYMPHOCYTES FACILITATE ENGRAFTMENT IN ANIMAL MODELS OF BMT

The literature on the use of irradiated allogeneic lymphocytes in animal models of bone marrow transplantation is limited to date (52,53). Doses of 15-20 Gy were used in these studies to treat the allogeneic donor cells, and these cells were administered concomitantly with allogeneic bone marrow cells or many days following the bone marrow graft. A series of five infusions of irradiated (15 Gy) donor lymphocytes was used by Gratwohl et al, one to ten days following the infusions of allogeneic bone marrow cells to facilitate transplantation between genetically unrelated rabbits (52). Irradiated autologous bone marrow cells were also infused into these animals. The addition of irradiated donor lymphocytes alone did not prevent graft rejection when they were added to allogeneic bone marrow, but the addition of cyclosporine immuno-suppression to a separate group of rabbits receiving a combination of TCD allogeneic BM, irradiated autologous BM and irradiated allogeneic buffy coat cells increased the rate of engraftment to 80%. However, 40% of the recipients of this latter combination died of GvHD (52). The Seattle group found that bone marrow transplantation between dog leukocyte antigen (DLA) mis-matched donor-recipient pairs led to fatal graft rejection, and that the addition of viable donor lymphocytes to DLA mis-matched bone marrow grafts increased hematopoietic engraftment, but produced uniformly fatal GvHD (54). Infusions of irradiated (20 Gy) donor lymphocytes to DLA mis-matched bone marrow transplants did not prevent fatal graft failure (53). In the same dog model, gamma irradiation (20 Gy) of whole blood products transfused prior to DLA-mis-matched allogeneic bone marrow transplantation in dogs prevented sensitization to alloantigens in recipients, but did not induce allo-specific tolerance, suggesting a limited role for irradiated donor leukocytes in clinical marrow transplantation (55).

We have tested whether irradiation of donor allogeneic lymphocytes would preserve their graft-enhancing activity while inhibiting their potential for GvHD in a mouse model of BMT (56). Irradiation of mouse T-cells to 7.5 Gy inhibited their proliferative capacity *in vitro* and *in vivo* and prevented GvHD in parent → F1 mouse BMT recipients. Irradiated donor T-cells survived transiently for up to 3 days in the bone marrow of MHC mismatched recipients. Daily injections of irradiated allogeneic splenocytes in the peri-transplant period in combination with a limited number of allogeneic bone marrow cells significantly increased the sixty day survival among MHC mis-matched transplant recipients from 2%

271

(bone marrow alone) to 60% (recipients of bone marrow plus 75 x 10^6 irradiated splenocytes); p<1 x 10^{-6}. Recipients of an equal number of non-irradiated donor splenocytes uniformly died of hyper-acute GvHD. The graft facilitating activity of irradiated allogeneic splenocytes depended on the schedule and number of cells injected, with optimal results obtained using 50-75 x 10^6 irradiated donor splenocytes in multiple injections from day -1 to day +1 after bone marrow transplantation. Recipients of irradiated allogeneic splenocytes and allogeneic bone marrow had stable donor-derived hematopoiesis without a significant contribution of irradiated donor cells to the T-cell compartment.

CLINICAL EXPERIENCE USING IRRADIATED DONOR LYMPHOCYTE INFUSIONS IN BMT

The literature on the use of irradiated donor leukocytes in humans has been limited to date. Irradiated donor lymphocytes have been given to patients with aplastic anemia in an attempt to prevent graft rejection after allogeneic bone marrow transplantation (57). Recipients of donor leukocytes irradiated to 20 Gy had a risk of graft rejection that was 14% compared to an incidence of graft rejection of 22% among non-randomized control patients who received bone marrow cells alone (57) . However, both groups of patients experienced a 20% incidence of fatal GvHD. Gratwohl et al. treated recipients of T-cell depleted allogeneic bone marrow transplantation with five infusions of irradiated (15 Gy) donor lymphocytes post-transplant, and reported no cases of graft failure, but noted an overall incidence of GvHD of 85%, and a 15% incidence of fatal GvHD (58). Reisner et. al. reported the use of irradiated (20 Gy) allogeneic donor lymphocytes from the Soy Bean Agglutinin (SBA) positive cell fraction of bone marrow in combination with T-cell depleted (SBA negative) haplo-identical bone marrow cells to treat patients with severe combined immunodeficiency (15). In this study, no evidence of hyperacute GvHD was seen, but the contribution of the irradiated donor lymphocytes to hematopoietic engraftment or clinical GvHD was unclear since there was no way to distinguish the irradiated lymphocytes from the variable number of non-irradiated lymphocytes contained within the bone marrow graft.

Figure 3. Treatment Schema for Patients Receiving Donor Leukocyte Infusions.

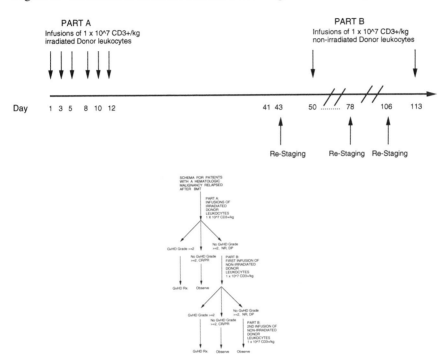

PHASE I/II TRIAL USING IRRADIATED DONOR LYMPHOCYTES FOR TREATMENT OF LEUKEMIA RELAPSE FOLLOWING ALLOGENEIC BMT

Based upon the promising results for our preclinical murine studies, we have initiated a Phase I/II clinical trial to evaluate the safety and efficacy of multiple infusions of irradiated donor lymphocytes. Eligible study subjects include any patient who has a hematologic malignancy that has relapsed following allogeneic BMT, and who is not experiencing active GvHD. Eleven patients have been enrolled to-date. In the study design patients have received 6 infusions of 1×10^7 CD3$^+$ donor T-cells/kg over a two week period (Figure 3), and were then followed with monthly re-staging. Patients whose disease did not respond to the irradiated donor lymphocytes went on to receive non-irradiated donor lymphocytes as the standard of care (27). Of 11 patients treated to-date on this study, three have shown objective complete responses to multiple infusions of irradiated donor lymphocytes: 2 patients with CML and one patient with low grade non-Hodgkin's lymphoma. These three patients achieved complete cytogenetic or radiographic remissions without any additional chemo or radiotherapy, and were treated when they had not been receiving immuno-

273

suppressive therapy for at least 1 year. Response of one patient with CML who achieved a transient molecular and stable cytogenetic CR is shown in Figure 4. Three patients with acute leukemia have died while on this study; two patients died of pneumonia and one patient died of a thromboembolic event. Of six patients with CML in cytogenetic or hematologic relapse, five patients remain alive, two in cytogenetic CR. One CML patient died of hemoptysis after she failed to respond to irradiated DLI and developed aGvHD after receiving 4 separate infusions of non-irradiated allogeneic lymphocytes. No acute toxicity related to the infusions of irradiated donor lymphocytes has been seen in any patient. Data from this trial as well as producing a demonstrable anti-leukemic activity in some patients suggests that multiple infusions of irradiated cells are safe and well tolerated.

Figure 4. Cytogenetic and Molecular Response of a Patient with Relapsed CML Treated with Multiple Infusions of Irradiated Allogeneic Lymphocytes. Serial bone marrow aspirates from a patient with chronic phase CML were obtained 1 month before and at a yearly interval after an allogeneic bone marrow transplant. Bone marrow samples were analyzed for the presence of CML leukemia cells by standard cytogenetics, Flourescent in situ hybridization (FISH) and polymerase chain amplification of the bcr/abl cDNA (PCR). The percentage of bone marrow cells showing the t(9;22) translocation by cytogenetics or FISH is shown using the left hand ordinate; the relative PCR signal (as assessed by comparing the patient signals to the bcr/abl signals generated from a series of 10-fold dilutions of K562 cDNA) is shown on the right hand ordinate. This assay can detect an equivalent of 1/100,000 bcr/abl positive cells (a value of 10^{-5}); samples in which the bcr/abl gene product was not detected are shown with relative values of 10^{-6} on the LOG scale to the left.

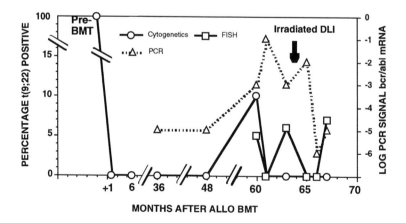

FUTURE LABORATORY AND CLINICAL INVESTIGATIONS

Correlative laboratory studies of the effect of low-dose radiation on human lymphocytes have been performed. Radiation exposure enhanced NF kappa B levels and increased the cytotoxicity of T-cells against allogeneic leukemia targets in a LDH release assay. (Figure 5) These data on the effect of radiation of human cells corroborates earlier work using murine model system and supports the idea that low-dose radiation activates T-cells while inhibiting their potential for long-term proliferation.

Figure 5. Lysis of CD34$^+$ Selected Acute Myeloid Leukemia Cells by Irradiated HLA-matched Allogeneic Donor Lymphocytes. CD34$^+$ leukemia cells were selected using the Mini-MACS CD34$^+$ selection system from the bone marrow aspirate of a patient (RB) whose disease had relapsed 80 days after allogeneic bone marrow transplantation. Lymphocytes were collected by apheresis from his sister and irradiated to 7.5 Gy with a Cs^{137} source. The irradiated and non-irradiated effector cells were incubated with non-irradiated CD34$^+$ leukemia target cells and specific cytotoxicity of the cells was measured using the CytoTox 96$^®$ Cytotoxicity Assay from Promega (Madison, WI). The mean (+/- S.D.) of specific cytotoxicity for quadruplicate sample is shown for E:T ratios 0.3:1 to 10:1.

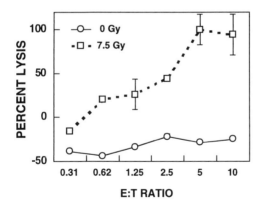

The exact mechanism of action of irradiated donor leukocytes is still unclear. Three hypotheses could explain the graft facilitating and anti-leukemia activity of irradiated allogeneic leukocytes that we have observed in mouse BMT recipients: 1) that irradiated leukocytes retain a direct contact-dependent cytotoxic effect against allogeneic leukemia cells; 2) that irradiated leukocytes elaborate cytokines that mediate an anti-proliferative or cytopathic effect against allogeneic host (leukemia) cells (59, 60); and 3) that administration of irradiated leukocytes enhances the activity of co-existing non-irradiated or radio-resistant donor leukocytes (61) (Figure 6). Ongoing work is focused on defining the cellular and molecular mechanism(s) for this novel approach as well as testing whether infusions of irradiated allogeneic donor cells facilitate engraftment in patients receiving allogeneic PBSC transplants following non-myeloablative conditioning regimens.

Figure 6. Models for the Anti-leukemic Effect of Irradiated Allogeneic Lymphocytes. Solid lines represent cytolytic activity; dashed lines represent release of growth-inhibitory and cytotoxic cytokines.

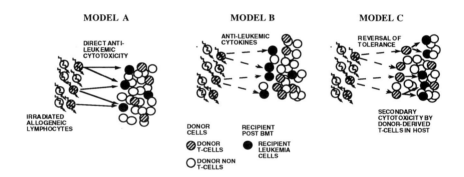

REFERENCES:

1. Storb R. "Marrow transplantation in the treatment of malignant diseases." Progress in transplantation. Morris and Tilney ed. 1984 Churchill Livingstone. New York.
2. Kernan NA, Bartsch G, Ash R, Beatty PG, Champlin R, Filipovich A, Gajewski J, Hansen J, Henslee-Downey J, McCullough Jea. Analysis of 462 transplantations from unrelated donors facilitated by the National Marrow Donor Program. New England Journal of Medicine. 1993; 328:593-602.

3. Bishop MR, Henslee-Downey PJ, Anderson JR, Romond EH, Marciniak E, Yankey R, Reeves M, Thompson JS. Long-term survival in advanced chronic myelogenous leukemia following bone marrow transplantation from haploidentical related donors. Bone Marrow Transplantation. 1996; 18:747-753.

4. Fleming DR, Henslee-Downey PJ, Romond EH, Harder EJ, Marciniak E, Munn RK, Messino MJ, Macdonald JS, Bishop M, Rayens MK, Thompson JS. Allogeneic bone marrow transplantation with T cell-depleted partially matched related donors for advanced acute lymphoblastic leukemia in children and adults: a comparative matched cohort study. Bone Marrow Transplantation 1996; 17:917-922.

5. Filipovich AH, Vallera DA, Youle RJ, Haake R, Blazar BR, Arthur D, Neville DM, N.K.C. R, McGlave P, Kersey JH. Graft-versus-host disease prevention in allogeneic bone marrow transplanation from histocompatible siblings. Transplantation 1987; 44:62-69.

6. Meagler RC, Lowder JN, Herzig RH. "Aspects of bone marrow transplantation in the treament of hematologic malignancies." Neoplastic Diseases of the Blood. Wiernick, Canellos, Kyle and Schiffer eds. 1991 Churchill Livingstone. New York.

7. O'Reilly R. Allogenic bone marrow transplantation: Current status and future directions. Blood 1983; 62:941-964.

8. Goldman JM, Gale RP, Horowitz MM, Biggs JC, Champlin RE, Gluckman E, Hoffman RG, Jacobsen SJ, Marmont AM, McGlave PB, Messner HA, Rimm AA, Rozman C, Speck B, Tura S, Weiner RS, Bortin MM. Bone marrow transplantation for chronic myelogenous leukemia in chronic phase. Increased risk of relapse associated with T-cell depletion. Annals of Internal Medicine 1988; 108:806-814.

9. Delain M, Cahn JY, Racadot E, Flesch M, Plouvier E, Mercier M, Tiberghien P, Pavy JJ, Deschaseaux M, Deconick E, Couteret Y, Brion A, Herve P. Graft failure after T cell depleted HLA identical allogeneic bone marrow transplantation: risk factors in leukemic patients. Leukemia and Lymphoma 1993; 11:359-368.

10. McGlave P, Bartsch G, Anasetti C, Ash R, Beatty P, Gajewski., Kernan NA. Unrelated donor bone marrow transplantation therapy for chronic myelogenous leukemia: Initial experience of the National Marrow Donor Program. Blood 1993; 81:543-550.

11. Petersdorf EW, Longton GM, Anasetti C, Martin PJ, Mickelson EM, Smith AG, Hansen J. The significance of HLA-DRB1 matching on clinical outcome after HLA-A, B, DR identical unrelated donor marrow transplantation. Blood 1995; 86:1606-1613.

12. Gingrich RD, Ginder GD, Goeken NE, Howe CW, Wen BC, Hussey DH, Fyfe MA. Allogeneic marrow grafting with partially mismatched unrelated marrow donors. Blood 1988; 71:1375-1381.
13. Wagner JE, Zahurak M, Piantadosi S, Geller RB, Vogelsang GB, Wingard JR, Saral R, Griffin C, Shah N, Zehnbauer BA et al. Bone marrow transplantation of chronic myelogenous leukemia in chronic phase: evaluation of risks and benefits. J Clin Oncol. 1992; 10:779-789.
14. Almici C, Donnenberg AD, Rizzoli V. Counterflow centrifugal elutriation: experimental and clinical applications. J Hematother. 1992; 1:279-288.
15. Reisner Y, Kapoor N, Kirkpatrick D, Pollack MS, Cunningham-Rundles S, Dupont B, Hodesm MZ, Good RA, O'Reilley RJ. Transplantation for severe combined immunodeficiency with HLA-A, B, D, DR imcompatible marrow cells fractionated by soybean agglutinin and sheep red blood cells. Blood 1983; 61:341-348.
16. Champlin R, Ho W, Gajeski J, Feig S, Burnison M, Holley G, Greenbergh P, Lee K, Schmid I, Giorgi J, Yam P, Petz L, D. W, Warner N, Reichert T. Selective depletion of CD8[+] T lymphocytes for prevention of graft-versus-host disease after allogeneic bone marrow transplantation. Blood 1990; 76:418-423.
17. Bensinger WI, Buckner CD, Shannon-Dorcy K, Rowley S, Appelbaum FR, Benyunes M, Clift R, Martin P, Demirer T, Storb R, Lee M, Schiller G. Transplantation of allogeneic CD34[+] peripheral blood stem cells in patients with advanced hematologic malignancy. Blood 1996; 88:4132-4138.
18. O'Reilly RJ, Keever C, Kernan NA, Brochstein J, Collins N, Flomenberg N, Laver J, Emanuel D, Dupon B, Cunningham I, et al. HLA non-identical T cell depleted bone marrow transplants: a comparison of results in patients treated for leukemia and severe combined immunodeficiency disease. Transplantation Proceedings 1987; 19:55-60.
19. Tiberghien P, Reynolds CW, Keller J, Spence S, Deschaseaux M, Certoux JM, Contassot E, Murphy WJ, Lyons R, Chiang Y, Herve P, Longo D, Ruscetti FW. Ganciclovir treatment of herpes simplex thymidine kinase-transduced primary T lymphocytes: an approach for specific in vivo donor T-cell depletion after bone marrow transplantation? Blood 1994; 84:1333-1341.
20. Bordignon C, Bonini C, Verzeletti S, Nobili N, Maggioni D, Traversari C, Giavazzi R, Servida P, Zappone E, Benazzi E, et al. Transfer of the HSV-tk gene into donor peripheral blood lymphocytes for in vivo modulation of donor anti-tumor immunity after allogeneic bone marrow transplantation. Human Gene Therapy 1995; 6:813-819.

21. Truitt RL, LeFever AV, Shih C-Y, Jeske J, Martin TM. "Graft vs. Leukemia effect." Graft-Versus-Host Disease: Immunology, Pathophysiology, and Treatment. Burakoff, Deeg, Ferrara and Atkinson eds. 1990 Marcel Dekker. New York.
22. Barnes DWH, Loutit JF. Treatment of murine leukemia with X-rays and hemologous bone marrow. Br. J. Haematology 1957; 3:241-252.
23. Horowitz MM, Gale RP, Sondel PM, et al. Graft-versus-leukemia reactions after bone marrow transplanation. Blood 1990; 75:555-562.
24. Sullivan KM, Weiden PL, Storb R, Witherspoon RP, Fefer A, Fisher L, Buckner CD, Anasetti C, Appelbaum FR, Badger C, et al. Influence of acute and chronic graft-versus-host disease on relapse and survival after bone marrow transplantation from HLA-identical siblings as treatment of acute and chronic leukemia. Blood 1989; 73:1720-1728.
25. Kolb HJ, Mittermuller J, Clemm C, Holler E, Ledderose G, Brehm G, Heim M, Wilmanns W. Donor leukocyte transfusions for treatment of recurrent chronic myelogenous leukemia in marrow transplant patients. Blood 1990; 76:2462-2465.
26. Kolb H, Schattenberg A, Goldman J, Hertenstein B, Jacobsen N, Arcese W, Ljungman P, Ferrant A, Verdonck L, Niederwieser D, et al. Graft-versus-leukemia effect of donor lymphocyte transfusions in marrow grafted patients. European Group for Blood and Marrow Transplantation Working Party Chronic Leukemia. Blood. 1995; 86:2041-2050.
27. Collins RH, Shpilberg O, Drobyski WR, Porter DL, Giralt S, Champlin R, Goodman SA, Wolff SN, Hu W, Verfaille C, List A, Dalton W, Ognoskie N, Chetrit A, Antin JH, Nemunaitis J. Donor leukocyte infusions in 140 patients with relapsed malignancy after allogeneic bone marrow transplantation. Journal of Clinical Oncology 1997; 15:(2)433-444.
28. Zeder K, Waller EK, Yeager A, Redei I, S.M. D. Impact of donor-lymphocyte infusion for relapsed hematological malignancy. submitted to Bone Marrow Transplantation 1998.
29. Lu PH, Negrin RS. A novel population of expanded human $CD3^+CD56^+$ cells derived from T cells with potent in vivo antitumor activity in mice with severe combined immunoideficiency. Journal of Immunology 1994; 153:1687-1696.
30. Muraoka S, Miller RG. Cells in murine fetal liver and in lymphoid colonies grown from fetal liver can suppress generation of cytotoxic T lymphocytes directed against their self antigens. Journal of Immunology 1983; 131:45-49.
31. Cesano A, Pearson G, Visonneau S, Migliaccio AR, Santoli D. Use of a lethally irradiated major histocompatibility complex nonrestricted cytotoxic T-cell line for effective purging of marrows containing lysis-sensitive or -resistant leukemic targets. Blood 1996; 87:(1)393-403.

32. Sutter GM. "Response of hematopoietic systems to X-rays." USAEC Doc. MDDC-824. 1947 U.S Atomic Energy Commission. Oakridge, TN.

33. Dixon FJ, Talmage DW, Maurer PH. Radiosensitive and radioresistent phases in the antibody response. J. Immunology 1952; 68:693-700.

34. Osgood EE. Radiobiologic observations on human hemic cells in vivo and in vitro. Ann. N. Y. Acad. Sci. 1961; 95:828-838.

35. Schrek R. In vitro sensitivity of normal human lymphocytes to x-rays and radiomimetic agents. J Lab. Clin. Med. 1958; 51: 904-915.

36. Schrek R, Stefani S. Radioresistence of phitohemagglutinin-treated normal and leukemic lymphocytes. J. of National Cancer Institute 1964; 32:507-517.

37. Fleidner TM, Kretchmer V, Hillen M, Wandt F. DNS und RNS in mit Phytohamagglutinin stimulierten Lymphocyten. Schweiz. Med. Wschr 1965; 95:1499.

38. Taliaferro WH, Taliaferro LG. Effects of irradiation on initial and anamnestic hemolysin responses in rabbits. Antigen injection before x-rays. J. Immunol. 1970; 104(6): 1364-1376.

39. Anderson RE, Williams WL. Radiosensitivity of T and B lymphocytes. V. Effects of whole-body irradiation on numbers of recirculating T cells and sensitization to primary skin grafts in mice. Am. J. Pathol. 1977; 89:367-378.

40. Dixon FJ, McConahey PJ. Enhancement of antibody formation by whole body x-radiation. J. Exp. Med. 1963; 117:833.

41. Conrad RA. Quantitative study of radiation effects in phytohematoagglutinin-stimulated leukocyte cultures. Int. J. Radiat. Biol. 1969; 16:157-165.

42. Rickinson AB, Ilbery PLT. The effect of radiation upon lymphocyte response to PHA. Cell tissue Kinet. 1971; 4:549-562.

43. Sprent J, Anderson RE, Miller JF. Radiosensitivity of T and B lymphocytes. II. Effect of irradiation on response of T cells to alloantigens. European Journal of Immunology 1974; 4:204-210.

44. Lawrence DA, Eastman A, Weigle WD. Murine T-cells preparations: Radiosensitivity of helper activity. Cell. Immunology 1978; 36:97-114.

45. Eardley DD, Gershon RK. Induction of specific suppressor T cells in vitro. J. Immunol. 1976; 117:313-318.

46. Dean DM, Pross HF, Kennedy JC. Spontaneous human lymphocyte-mediated cytotoxicity against tumor target cells.III. Stimulatory and inhibitory effects of ionizing radiation. Int. J. Rad. Onc. Biol. Phys. 1978; 4:633-641.

47. Hellstrom KE, Hellstrom I, Kant JA, Tamerius JD. Regression and Inhibition of sarcoma growth by interference with a radiosensitive T-cell population. J. Exp.Med. 1978; 148:799-804.

48. Rotter V, Trainin N. Inhibition of tumor growth in syngeneic chimeric mice mediated by a depletion of suppressor T cells. Transplantation 1975; 20:68.

49. Nichols WS, Troup GM, Anderson RE. Radiosensitivity of sensitized and nonsensitized human lymphocytes evaluated in vitro. American Journal of Pathology 1975; 79:499-508.
50. Boise LH, Minn AJ, Noel PJ, June CH, Accavitti MA, Lindsten T, Thompson CB. CD28 costimulation can promote T cell survival by enhancing te expression of Bcl-xl. Immunity 1996; 3:87-98.
51. Strober S, Weissman IL. "Immunosuppressive and tolerogenic effects of whole-body, total lymphoid, and regional radiation." The Current Status of Modern Therapy. Salaman ed. 1981 MTP Press. Lancaster, England.
52. Gratwohl A, Baldomero H, Nissen C, Speck B. Engraftment of T-cell depleted rabbit bone marrow. Acta Haematol. 1987; 77:208-214.
53. Deeg HJ, Storb R, Weiden PL, Shulman HM, Graham TC, Torok-Storb BJ, Thomas ED. Abrogation of resistance to and enhancement of DLA-nonidentical unrelated marrow grafts in lethally irradiated dogs by thoracic duct lymphocytes. Blood 1979; 53:552-587..
54. Storb R, Epstein RB, Bryant J, Ragde H, Thomas ED. Marrow grafts by combined marrow and leukocyte infusions in unrelated dogs selected by histocompatability typing. Transplantation 1968; 6:587-593..
55. Bean MA, Graham T, Appelbaum FR, Deeg HJ, Scheuning F, Sale GE, Leisenring W, Pepe M, Storb R. Gamma irradiation of blood products prevents rejection of subsequent DLA-identical marrow grafts. Transplantation 1996; 61:334-335.
56. Waller EK, Ship AM, Murray TW, Holden J, Boyer M. Irradiated allogeneic lymphocytes: a novel strategy of immunotherapy. Biology of Blood and Bone Marrow Transplantation 1998; 2:(3)150 (abs.).
57. Storb R, Doney KC, Thomas ED, Applebaum F, Buckner CD, Clift RA, Deeg HJ, Goodell BW, Hackman R, Hansen JA, Sanders J, Sullivan K, Weicker PL, Witherspoon RP. Marrow transplantation with or without donor buffy coat cells for 65 transfused aplastic anemia patients. Blood 1982; 59:236-246.
58. Gratwohl A, Tichelli A, Wursch A, Dieterle A, Lori A, Thomssen C, Baldomero H, de Witte T, Nissen C, Speck B. Irradiated buffy coat following T-cell depleted bone marrow transplants. Bone Marrrow Transplantation 1988; 3:577-582.
59. Hallahan DE, Spriggs DR, Beckett MA, Kufe DW, Weichselbaum RR. Increased tumor necrosis factor a mRNA after cellular exposure to ionizing radiation. Proc. Nat. Acad. Sci. 1989; 86:10104-10107.
60. Martin PJ. Influence of alloreactive T cells on initial hematopoietic reconstitution after marrow transplantation. Experimental Hematology 1995; 23:174-179.

61. Drobyski W, Thibodeau S, Truitt R, Baxter-Lowe LA, Gorski J, Jenkins R, Gottschall J, Ash RC. Third-party-mediated graft rejection and graft-versus-host disease after T-cell-depleted bone marrow transplantation, as demonstrated by hypervariable DNA probes and HLA-DR polymorphism. Blood 1989; 74:2285-2294.

13

DENDRITIC CELLS AND THEIR CLINICAL APPLICATIONS

D.N.J. Hart and G.J. Clark

Mater Medical Research Institute. South Brisbane 4101, Queensland, Australia

The key role dendritic cells (DC) play in initiating primary (and probably secondary) immune responses is now well recognised. There is still much uncertainty as to how to define DC, as it now appears that there may be several different DC differentiation pathways giving rise to subsets of DC, which have different phenotypic and functional properties (1). Thus, there are epithelial and interstitial associated subsets of DC (2). The monocyte derived DC (Mo-DC) is distinguished from these DC types on both molecular and functional criteria (3). There is also data derived from mouse studies to indicate that DC may be derived from both myeloid and lymphoid precursors (4) and that the former cells are generally immunostimulatory, whereas the lymphoid precursor-derived DC may exert an alternative negative regulatory function. The molecular bases whereby the myeloid DC responds to danger signals and takes up antigen, prior to migrating to the lymph nodes to interact with T lymphocytes, is slowly being unravelled. Undoubtedly, DC play a major role in immunological events. Indeed, there is data to suggest that abnormal DC function contributes to the progress of human malignancies (5) and now some of the encouraging animal data using DC based vaccines for clinical cancer immunotherapy.

BASIC DC PHYSIOLOGY

Most information to date relates to the "gold standard" myeloid differentiation pathway of DC. Myeloid DC were identified originally as having unique morphological features and remarkable potency as antigen presenting cells (APC). They lack most of the markers typical of other leucocyte populations but express MHC molecules in high density and some DC-associated differentiation/activation markers after appropriate stimulation (Table 1). DC have unique migratory properties and the capacity to take up, process and then present antigen in association with appropriate accessory signals to T lymphocytes. Their APC function has been assessed in the main by using the allogeneic mixed leucocyte reaction (MLR), but there is now a greater appreciation that the full antigen processing pathway needs to be tested with specific antigen.

Table 1. Dendritic Cell Phenotype.

MYELOID	CD33	Low
	CD13	Positive
	CD4	Positive
	CD11b	Negative (? Positive in mice)
	CD83	Positive
	CMRF-44	Positive
	CMRF-56	Positive
	M-CSFR	Negative
	IL-3R	Negative
	FcRs	Low/negative
	DEC-205	Positive
	MMR	Negative
	HLA – class I	High
	class II	High
	CD1a	High (epidermal)
LYMPHOID (mouse)	CD33	Negative
	CD13	Negative
	CD8	Positive
	CD11b	Negative
	DEC-205	Positive

DC develop from bone marrow-derived precursors (6), and enter the circulation in an immature form, which can readily be distinguished from monocytes (7). These blood DC were initially separated by a negative selection procedure but the recent availability of the CMRF-44 reagent has allowed direct comparison of the DC population with monocytes and only the former stimulate an allogeneic MLR and primary antigen response (8). These myeloid DC precursors then migrate into the tissues and establish sentinal networks of epithelial associated and interstitial tissue located DC. Recent data has emphasized that these two populations might be distinct from each other in relation to the special requirements related to their anatomical location. This appears to manifest itself most obviously as a phenotypic difference in the level of CD1 molecules expressed (2). Some elegant studies have now shown that these two DC populations may diverge at the CD34 stage of commitment (9). A third potential myeloid DC differentiation pathway may also be important. Thus monocytes cultured *in vitro* in the presence of GM-CSF and IL-4 generate a number of DC-like properties (3), and differentiate further after exposure to TNFα, LPS or monocyte conditioned media to become a complex mixture of highly allostimulatory cells (10). We have suggested that this may be an inflammatory boost pathway for recruiting APC and that these cells may have more of a role in secondary responses. It is by no means clear what combination of growth factors and cytokines drive DC haematopoiesis but it seems that all three types of myeloid DC emerge from human bone marrow, mobilized CD34 blood cells or cord blood CD34 cells. Stem cell factor (SCF),FLT-3 ligand, IL3, GM-CSF, IL-4, IL-7, TNF-α and IFN-γ have all been used *in vitro* to support DC growth (11,12,13,14). Of particular interest TGF-β appears to influence commitment to the epithelial pathway ie Langerhans type cell production, depending on the time it is added to cultures (15).

The peripheral DC turn over at highly different frequencies, depending on their localization (16). Tissue produced chemokines probably account for DC migration from capillaries into the tissues, a process mediated by rolling, adherence and transmigration across endothelial surfaces (17). At the epithelial surfaces DC form an apparently contiguous network of cells, which are best revealed by en face sections (18). It appears that the majority of these cells are in a resting or "immature" state. After exposure to danger signals, consisting of either bacterial, viral or possibly tumour-related compounds or alternatively, other inflammatory mediators, such as LPS, IL-1 and TNFα, these DC migrate into the draining lymphatics (19). This is clearly an active process and further migration into the T lymphocyte areas of lymph nodes is again under the influence of a chemokine gradient (20). Originally it was assumed that the DC expressed innate antigen receptors or that they ingested antigen by pinocytosis in much the same way as macrophages. It is now clear that this is a fundamental control point in DC physiology (Table 2) and that certain signalling events are mandatory before DC express antigen uptake receptors, such as the lectin like compound DEC-205 (21). It is also probable that DC also use Fc receptors and complement receptors to effect antigen uptake (22).

Table 2. Control Points in DC Activity.

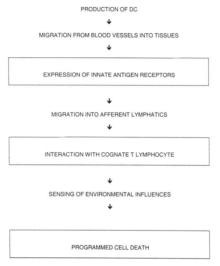

The migration of an antigen exposed DC to the draining lymph node is accompanied by major phenotypic and morphological changes. Antigen processing leads to upregulation of MHC molecules on the surface of DC and the MHC/antigenic peptide complexes have a long half life of up to 48hr. Coincidental with this is the upregulation of other DC differentiation/activation molecules such as CMRF-44 (8), CD83 (23) and CMRF-56 (24). The expression of the critical costimulator molecules CD80 and CD86 on the DC may be a later event; indeed there is reason to believe that this first requires the DC to interact with antigen specific T lymphocytes. Again the DC appears to play a role in this interaction as well as secreting chemokines, notably DC-CK1 which recruit naive T lymphocytes (25). The cognate recognition of antigen on the DC surface leads to a T lymphocyte response inducing CD40L that delivers signals into DC via CD40 on the surface (26). The density and kinetics of CD80 and CD86 surface expression on the DC may influence the type of immune response that follows ie TH1 or TH2. Highly relevant too in this process is the upregulation of cytokine gene expression by DC. Thus DC produce IL-12 (27) and IL-7 (28) amongst other cytokines essential to drive T lymphocyte proliferation. DC activated by helper cells stimulate cytotoxic T lymphocytes via CD40 (29), and helper T lymphocytes also interact with B lymphocytes to drive an antibody mediated response. Direct interaction between DC and B lymphocytes has been demonstrated *in vitro* (30) and DC have been identified in B follicules (31). It appears that not all DC in the draining lymph node undergo activation. It is interesting to note that the DC, which do not cluster with T lymphocytes, undergo significant downregulation of their function (McLellan et al., in preparation). This represents a second major control point in DC activity (Table 2). Finally, regulated cell death of DC is likely as part of the process of controlling the initial phase of antigen stimulation, but experimental validation of this third control point for DC activity is only just beginning.

The identification of a CD8 positive DC within mouse thymic cell preparations led, in time, to the identification of the lymphoid precursor derived DC, which is thought to have a down regulatory function. These cells require a different mix of growth factors and cytokines to grow them *in vitro* but some plasticity in their differentiation may also be a feature. Lymphoid DC were suggested to deliver a Fas mediated inhibitory signal to CD4 T lymphocytes (32), and another mechanism was suggested to inhibit CD8 T lymphocytes (33). Several investigators have searched diligently in man for an equivalent lymphoid population but as yet clear evidence has not been forthcoming (34). A CD10 positive precursor which gave rise to DC *in vitro* and lymphoid DC populations has been described but these have been CD4 positive as is the myeloid DC (35). The recent description of an IL-3R positive DC has enticed some to use this as an indicator of a lymphoid origin but the original description allocated the expression of IL-3R to the circulating myeloid blood DC population. The population of DC in the tonsil, which lack myeloid markers and express CD4 but not CD11c have also been offered as a possible human lymphoid DC contender (31, 36,37), but recent data (Summers et al, in preparation) suggests that these are more likely to be myeloid DC, which have a relatively unactivated phenotype.

THE CONTRIBUTION DC MAKE TO TOLERANCE

There are several possible mechanisms whereby DC (either lymphoid or myeloid precusor derived) might be postulated to perform an alternative down regulatory function. This might involve deleting T lymphocytes, anergizing them or actively suppressing them.

Perhaps the most established information relates to the characterization of thymic DC, which are located at the cortico-medullary junction (38). These have until recently always been assumed to have a myeloid origin. Early thymocytes receive a negative, apoptotic signal if the evolving T lymphocyte TCR binds with high affinity to self antigenic peptide plus MHC on APC within the thymus. Thus it appears that DC are essential to central deletional tolerance

(39). It has proved surprising just how available peripheral self antigens are for self presentation in the thymus – perhaps a tribute to the DC ability to sift its environment and to present more than one antigen (40). It is thought that the critical issue is the relative T lymphocyte immaturity and susceptibility to signalling. Indeed, splenic DC can induce tolerance when introduced into thymic lobes (41). However, there may also be an ongoing process involving activated T lymphocytes recirculating via the thymus, a fact particularly relevant to allogeneic BMT. Thus, thymic DC pulsed with immunogenic peptide of myelin basic protein produced tolerance following intravenous innoculation into normal but not thymectomized rats in whom experimental allergic encephalomyelitis is induced by vaccination with myelin-basic protein (42).

The peripheral resting or immature myeloid DC has the phenotype of a cell, which may fail to provide all the signals required for full T lymphocyte activation. Indeed, it was hypothesized some time ago that these cells would *in vivo* have the potential to deliver signal one ie self antigenic peptides and self MHC to the T lymphocyte receptor in the absence of signal two – the co-stimulator molecules (43). This would lead to anergy. For example, in the NOD mouse, the injection of DC derived from draining pancreatic lymph prevents the onset of autoimmune diabetes (44). The co-culture of bone marrow-derived DC with allogeneic T lymphocytes results in alloantigen hypo-responsiveness (45). *In vitro* data suggests that low density expression of the co-stimulator molecules on APC results in an anergic response specific to the stimulator but a specific response to third party is still seen (46). These types of experiments argue in favour of the capacity of DC to induce some form of peripheral tolerance, which is not mediated by T lymphocyte deletion. DC that are treated with UV or heat to destroy their antigen presenting potential yet retain allogeneic activity, do have an immunosuppressive effect (47).

The DC may also contribute by skewing the type of immune response significantly towards a TH2 response, and this may be particularly true of gut derived DC (48). It is clear that a DC may, as a result of the influences it receives from the environment, evolve a variety of costimulator phenotypes not only in terms of the cell surface molecules that it expresses but also in terms of the cytokine repertoire expressed. Thus, high expression of IL-12 is associated with a TH1 response but low levels of IL-2 and some IL-8 may be associated with DC induction of a TH2 response (49). The latter may of course be responsible for a significantly different clinical outcome.

The possibility that another subset of lymphoid derived DC may have the specialized function of down regulating T lymphocyte function is very attractive. Thus, the suggestion that the tolerizing DC and the naive T lymphocyte are produced in a co-ordinated way from a common thymic lymphoid precursor has been made. The myeloid but not the lymphoid DC is compromised in mice lacking the rel-B transcription factor and this will provide a useful model for dissecting the relative contributions of the two types of cell (50,51).

DC IN TRANSPLANTATION

The original description of the interstitial DC identified these cells in kidney and heart (52,53). Experiments soon established that these cells were the "passenger" leucocyte that was responsible for part of the acute rejection response (54). A critical feature of this response probably involves an activation of the DC into a high allogeneic stimulator state driven by the stress of ischaemia etc. If resting DC are used to prime allogeneic recipients then the opposite effect may be possible, namely, an abrogation of the strength of the immune response resulting in prolonged graft acceptance (55). These effects may not be so evident at a CD4 proliferative level but may be reflected more in the reduced help provided for T cytotoxic and B lymphocyte derived antibody responses (56).

Consistent with the view above – namely that an unstimulated DC may tolerize - an alternative set of results evolved from experiments associated with liver transplantation (57). Here it was initially postulated that the liver DC was delivering a negative signal responsible for the prolonged graft acceptance noted to occur with this organ. However, it seems now that it may be more likely that the haematopoietic precursors within the liver give rise to circulating allogeneic cells possibly including DC. It is these cells in the tissues which appear to mediate some form of peripheral tolerance. Attempts to exploit this phenomena using donor bone marrow have not been successful but this might have been predicted on the basis of the marrows content of differentiated DC.

An analogous set of events has been postulated to operate in bone marrow transplantation (1). Thus, because marrow contains preformed mature DC (6), it can stimulate a strong allogeneic response which may activate sufficient residual host T lymphocyte responses to mediate rejection. It is worth noting that the responding T lymphocytes are almost certainly memory T lymphocytes, which have evolved a cross-reactive allogeneic specificity as a result of another sensitizing event (58). Long term graft rejection seems unlikely to involve a host derived DC based mechanism.

Graft versus host disease (GVHD) on the other hand almost certainly involves DC in both acute and chronic disease. In acute GVHD two different mechanisms have been postulated (1). The first suggests that recipient DC survive the conditioning to some extent and that these cells stimulate a strong and immediate donor T lymphocyte response (59). The site of this sensitisation may be either peripheral donor T lymphocytes trafficking through skin or central ie migration of recipient DC from the peripheries is driven by the stimuli resulting from the conditioning process. Endotoxin known to be released during conditioning is likely to stimulate residual DC release from the gut (60). These recipient DC stimulate an allogeneic response when they meet donor T lymphocytes trafficking through the draining lymph nodes. This equates to the direct sensitization seen in solid organ transplantation and this perhaps indicates the relative contribution that interfering in this process might make clinically. Alloresponsive T lymphocytes, in the absence of recipient DC, may in certain circumstances eg lack of help, undergo antigen induced cell activation and death.

It is also certain that, once engrafted, the donor marrow will give rise to donor derived DC and that these will take up, process and present recipient antigens. These will in turn be presented to donor derived T lymphocytes. Of course, these T lymphocytes consist of a mixture of cells: those that matured originally in the donor and the cells that have been derived from donor lymphoid progenitors within the recipient environment. If the latter cells have had the opportunity to develop in an appropriate environment, for example, the recipient thymus, in the presence of donor derived thymic DC then an increased degree of T lymphocyte tolerance of the host might be predicted. However, imperfections in this process are likely and it is these that may generate the T lymphocyte precursors, which then mediate the GVHD reaction. This indirect mechanism is likely to contribute significantly to acute GVHD but it is also likely to be the prime mechanism involved in chronic GVHD. It is tempting to speculate that there may be a temporal separation of these events and that acute GVHD relates to T lymphocytes that have been derived at a post thymic differentiation stage from the donor. Chronic GVHD on the other hand is likely to involve T lymphocytes that have undergone the key maturation events in T lymphopoiesis within the host (Figure 1).

Figure 1. The potential interactions between recipient and donor DC are illustrated. The naïve T-lymphocytes which differentiate in the new host will have a different repertoire of allospecificities from the memory of T-lymphocytes preformed in the donor which are likely to have a higher precursor frequency.

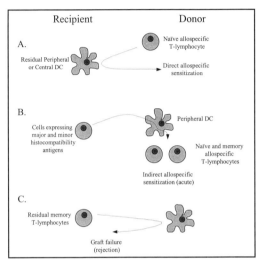

RECONSTITUTION OF DC AFTER BMT

Conditioning in the form of myeloablative treatment virtually arrests ongoing donor DC haematopoiesis (52). It is probable that some DC persist but these are likely to migrate rapidly out of the peripheral tissues as a result of the plethora of signals produced during conditioning, notably those associated with the cytokine storm (61). It is important to realize that there may be major differences in these processes for each DC subset and microenvironment. In man, Langerhans cells have been observed to decline at a rate which is somewhat slower than for other interstitial associated DC (62, 63). It is also possible that the relatively radio-resistant monocytes may persist and undergo subsequent differentiation into Mo-DC.

The reconstitution of myeloid derived interstitial DC seems to be relatively rapid in animal models (52). Reconstitution of Langerhans cells appears to take longer and in man the full reconstitution of the epidermal network with donor derived cells may take up to a year (62). It appears that DC hematopoiesis per se is relatively normal after transplantation (64). It may well be that DC migration, homing and localization are more subtlely compromised. Indeed, there is good data to suggest that the T lymphocyte influences these events (65) and the immunosuppressive drugs used may well have an indirect effect on this aspect of DC function. The probability that other DC functions will be compromised directly by immunosuppressive drugs or indirectly via their effects on T lymphocyte function is also relevant. Whilst there has been little opportunity to study the DC after allogeneic transplantation it seems logical to predict that deficiencies in the function of DC will be major contributors to the compromised immune function that occurs post allo-transplantation (66).

The recent availability of a method for counting human DC reliably in the blood has generated an opportunity for getting some essential preliminary human data (64). The method, based on the monoclonal antibody CMRF-44, identifies the population of blood DC as consisting of around 0.42% of peripheral blood mononuclear cells or in absolute terms approximately 10×10^6/L. Following autologous engraftment, this blood DC population appears to recover rapidly with similar kinetics to the other myeloid populations – detailed studies to clarify this are underway. The situation following allogeneic transplantation is much less clear. The first preliminary data suggests that acute GVHD is associated with a decrease in circulating DC counts. Whether this is a consequence, relating to the allogeneic interactions, or whether it is an indirect effect of a general inflammatory response remains an intriguing question.

CANCER AND DC FUNCTION

Many cancers express tumour associated antigens (TAA) which can be recognized by host T lymphocytes. The DC might, as the cell monitoring the environment, be expected to play a significant role in initiating the anti cancer response. Whether tumours trigger DC recruitment, antigen uptake and migration is clearly important and is likely to contribute to the prognosis in individual cases (5).

The first studies examining DC in tumours used antibodies to S-100 to stain and identify DC. There are difficulties with this approach but the data from several cancer types suggests that the number of S-100 cells correlated with the outcome (5). The availability of the CMRF-44 monoclonal antibody allowed activated DC to be followed in several human cancers. In renal cell carcinoma it was clear that DC were not recruited into the malignant tissue in increased numbers and that no more were activated than in the adjacent normal tissue

(67). Similar results have also been obtained in other cancers including prostate (68), bladder (69), breast and bowel cancer (Gibbs et al, in preparation). Furthermore, the DC isolated from renal cell carcinomas appeared to have compromised allostimulatory activity compared to normal blood DC (68) suggesting that the cancers were in some way down-regulating DC function.

Potential mechanisms for the defects in DC function in tumours are being explored. Vascular endothelial growth factor, which is produced by most solid tumours, has been identified as directly responsible for inhibiting maturation of DC from precursors (70). IL-10 also produced by many tumours, inhibits upregulation of the CD80/86 costimulatory molecules on APC (71), and their expression is essential for effective DC-T lymphocyte interaction. Activation of T lymphocytes in the presence of IL-10, leads to long term anergy of the T lymphocyte. TGF-β has also been shown to have indirect effects on DC function by its effects on T lymphocytes (72). Intriguing data was presented recently to suggest that malignant cells may trigger apoptosis of DC.

A malignancy may also have systemic effects on DC. Mature blood DC from tumour bearing animals are ineffective at inducing anti-tumour cytotoxic T lymphocytes, whereas DC generated from BM precursors were fully functional (73). Breast cancer patients have also been suggested to have lower numbers of mature DC and these cells showed reduced ability to stimulate autologous and allogeneic MLRs (74). However, cytokine generated DC from patients with renal cell carcinoma (75) and prostate cancer (76) have also been shown to be fully functional.

The administration of GM-CSF subcutaneously appears to recruit DC effectively within tumour bearing hosts for priming to tumour antigens (Pardoll review). FLT-3 ligand has activity on haematopoietic progenitors and stimulates DC production *in vivo* (14). Again it seems to be efficacious in tumour bearing animals (77).

Table 3. Potential TAA for DC Immunotherapy.

Viral antigens	EBV
	HTLV-1
	Papilloma virus
	HSV-6
Recombined proteins	BCR-ABL (chronic myeloid leukaemia)
	NPM/ALK (large cell NHL)
	DEK/CAN (acute myeloid leukaemia)
	PML/RARα (promyelocytic leukaemia)
	TLS-FUS/ERG (acute myeloid leukaemia)
	IL-2/BCM (T-NHL)
Mutated Oncogenes	H-ras
	K-ras
	P53
Oncofetal Oncogenes	MAGE-1 (melanoma)
	MAGE-2 (melanoma)
	CAE (bowel)
Molecules abnormally expressed	MUC.1 (breast and other)
Idiotype	Ig (B-NHL, myeloma)
	TCR (T-NHL)
Tissue Specific Antigen	PSM (prostate)
	MART-1 (melanoma)
	Gp100 (melanoma)
	Gp75 (melanoma)
	CD33 (acute myeloid leukaemia)

DC PRODUCTION FOR IMMUNOTHERAPY

Serious investigative endeavour has established an ever increasing list of potential tumour associated antigens for targeting in immunotherapy strategies (Table 3). These involve viral antigens, tumour specific antigens and tissue specific antigens (5). The data above has vindicated the hypothesis that DC presentation of tumour antigen may be compromised in a number of ways. Indeed, we now hypothesize further that different tumours, just like viruses, will have multiple different ways of subverting DC function to frustrate the immune response. Thus, it becomes extremely logical to try and bypass this block in DC presentation of tumour antigens. There are various strategies to do this.

The first to be investigated clinically has been the "accidental" recruitment of DC in the host by gene therapy protocols. The inoculation of animals and humans with GM-CSF transduced tumour cells is accompanied by an "inflammatory' infiltrate which includes DC (78). Subsequent experiments have confirmed that DC play a vital role in the GM-CSF mediated antigen priming. The use of naked DNA to vaccinate against tumour antigens particularly via the intramuscular and subcutaneous routes has attracted attention. This too seems to operate via DC as the vehicle for absorbing the secreted protein and presenting the antigen (79,80). It may be that certain vectors are adsorbed directly to DC and transported intracellularly via DNA receptors. Certain poorly understood characteristics of the vector sequences appear to contribute to DC activation and trafficking.

It is clear that FLT-3 ligand has a potent anti-tumour effect when administered to mice (77). Physiologically, the compound has a number of effects including supporting stem cell proliferation, monocyte and DC production as well as effects on NK function. The effect on DC production in mice is dramatic with a marked increase in spleen cellularity associated with a tenfold increase in DC counts (14). It seems that the majority of the increase is associated with a rise in the lymphoid DC counts but myeloid DC are also increased. Although in theory this might create some concerns regarding the balance of stimulatory versus tolerogenic effects, the overall result is stimulatory. The administration of FLT-3 ligand to humans is also associated with a marked increase in DC in the blood (Maraskovsky et al, in press). It has yet to be established whether this is therapeutic in its own right against cancer as an immune adjuvant. Equally FLT-3 ligand administration may become a very attractive way of mobilizing DC to be harvested for *in vitro* priming. The FLT-3 ligand-G-CSF chimeric product may also prove useful in this regard. There is also some early data to suggest that there may be a spontaneous rise in DC after cyclophosphamide induced CD34 stem cell mobilization (64) and harvesting of the DC could fit on the back of this procedure.

Whilst it seems preferable, if possible, to use the natural circulating DC precursor for immunotherapy (81) the fact that DC circulate in low numbers has encouraged the majority of other investigators to use cultured DC. One source is cultured CD34$^+$ blood cells, which in the presence of various combinations of growth factors/cytokines, differentiate into DC-like cells. Combinations of SCF/FLT-3 ligand and GM-CSF/IL-4 have been used (12,82). Both IL-7 and IFN (83) have been added to some cocktails. These cultures in general produce about a ten-fold cell yield of which only 10% or so are thought to be DC, and yields are much lower in the absence of exogenous serum. An alternative has been to use a combination of GM-CSF and TNF-α to differentiate the CD34 cell directly into a DC without a proliferative step (Monji et al submitted). These cells seem to be at a stage of maturity which makes them suitable for antigen loading. Furthermore, the shorter period of culture required and the absence of a need to purify the cells further makes the latter method the most attractive of these preparative options.

The differentiation of monocytes into DC ie Mo-DC has been the most popular approach. Peripheral blood mononuclear cells are obtained and these are cultured in the presence of GM-CSF/IL-4 and matured in TNF–α (3) or monocyte conditioned medium (84). These populations are not homogeneous (10) and the presence or absence of T lymphocytes in the starting population may influence the final phenotype and function of the Mo-DC. It was a major concern as to whether these cells would maintain a stable phenotype and could migrate effectively once returned to the patient. It appears that they do in a monkey model (85).

Having obtained a satisfactory DC yield the next issue is to load them with antigen effectively (5). The choice of tumour antigen is a major issue. This may be so called "gamesh" ie whole tumour homogenate or a TAA protein, acid eluted (86) or synthetic peptide(s) (87,88). Other approaches have used DNA encoded antigens (89,90) or RNA isolated from the tumour. Optimal loading may involve targeting nonspecific receptors eg DEC-205, or using liposomes (91) to load material into DC. Once DC are loaded with antigen then their administration has been via the IV , SC, dermal and intra-nodal routes. It is suggested that dermal vaccination may prove to be the optimum: there are some arguments against the IV route as this may induce tolerance in certain circumstances.

THERAPEUTIC EFFECTS OF DC VACCINATION

Studies using mouse models have established the efficacy of using DC pulsed with TAA for the rejection of tumours (5). The results predicably vary according to the model. Artificial antigens eg viral proteins, transfected ovalbumin and -galactosidase stimulate an active high precursor T lymphocyte response and excellent tumour control. Even more impressive is the response seen with more aggressive tumour models eg fibrosarcomas (92) and a more typical TAA eg p53 (74). These models will be crucial for learning the basic biology of cancer vaccination. Some important cautionary data suggests that in certain circumstances it is possible to tolerize for a TAA.

Human DC have been reported to stimulate primary T lymphocyte responses to KLH and HIV proteins *in vitro*. The ability of DC to prime for other true primary antigens eg pigeon cytochrome C or sperm whale myoglobin appears to be dominated by the responding T lymphocyte precursor frequency (81). Anti melanoma specific CTLs have been generated using DC pulsed with the melanocyte differentiation antigens MART-1, gp100 and tyrosinase. Reeves et al retrovirally transduced DC with MART-1 cDNA and were able to stimulate a MART-1 specific T cell line (89). It has also been possible to transfect human DC with the MUC-1 gene leading to its expression (90). DC incubated with bcr-abl peptide stimulate bcr-abl specific T lymphocytes (93). DC can also present prostate specific peptides (94). DC generated from CML patients (95) and AML patients appear to stimulate leukaemia specific T lymphocyte responses *in vivo*.

Percoll gradient immunoselected blood DC have been used to vaccinate patients with idiotype protein derived from their low grade B cell lymphomas (96). T lymphocyte responses have been observed in the patients to the idiotype - a result not achieved with other vaccination systems. Late relapses perhaps emphasize the need to continue vaccinations to maintain immunological memory. Another group are actively investigating the use of DC pulsed with PSM to generate an immunological response to prostate cancer (97). Clinical trials using MUC-1 as an antigen are just commencing in breast cancer. Several investigators are now initiating DC vaccination protocols using myeloma idiotype protein. Other haematological diseases are seen as attractive targets and these include CML and Hodgkins disease. The latter is particularly interesting as it seems likely that at least some cases of the disease involve malignancies in the DC lineage (98).

It is malignant melanoma that has attracted the most attention because of the availability of several defined melanoma TAA and the awful prognosis of advanced melanoma. In the first study reported, cytokine generated DC were pulsed with a cocktail of melanoma specific peptides and injected directly into the patient's lymph nodes (99). There were some good clinical responses in 5 of 16 patients treated but in the other instances the disease escaped from immunological control by one mechanism or another, highlighting the importance of this issue. At least another four trials in this disease have commenced and soon there will be enough phase one data to decide the issues for the phase two studies. The data accruing from the plethora of alternative vaccination studies (Table 4) will also be invaluable in directing the way forward.

Table 4. Clinical Trials.

INVESTIGATOR	PREPARATION (route)	ANTIGEN
Engelman & Levy	Blood DC (subcutaneous)	Ig Idiotype
Urdal	Blood DC (subcutaneous)	Prostate Ag
Nestle	GM-CSF/IL-4 Mo-DC	Peptide lysate
Murphy	Mo-DC (intravenous)	Prostate S membrane
Mertelsmann	CD34$^+$ DC (intravenous)	Melan-A and other pe₁
Schuler	Mo-DC (subcutaneous)	MAGE-3 peptide
Lotze	GM-CSF/IL-4 Mo-DC (subcut)	Mart 1
	or CD34$^+$ DC (subcut)	gp100
Titzer	CD34$^+$	Ig idiotype
	GM-CSF/TNFα Mo-DC	
Champlin	Leukaemic	
	GM-CSF/IL-4 Mo-DC	
Banchereau	CD34$^+$ DC	
Brenner	GM-CSF/IL-4 Mo-DC	EBV

DC MANIPULATION IN ALLOGENEIC BMT

Recognizing that the DC primes the all important allogeneic response makes it possible to contemplate several possibilities for exploiting this knowledge in allogeneic transplantation. Targeting the DC to prevent the allogeneic response may allow control of acute GVHD (Figure 2). Likewise, it may be that problems with DC function contribute to the immunosuppression and vulnerability to infection seen post transplant. One of the fundamental assumptions in regard to tumour immunotherapy is that it will operate best in a minimal disease environment. Thus, DC immunotherapy is likely to be applied after both auto and allo transplantation.

Figure 2.   An   approach to   the cellular   engineering of   an   allogeneic transplant is presented. Initial effective myeloid engraftment in the absence of complex   allogeneic interactions is the first aim. Subsequently, grafting of the immune   system (T-lymphocytes) is proposed   at   the time when GVHD is controllable. The application of TK "suicide gene technology" is a potential possibility. Vaccination with donor DC exposed to TAA is aimed at boosting a sustained specific anti-cancer response *in vivo*. Expansion of TAA specific T lymphocytes *in vitro*   and their administration to the recipient may also be necessary for an adequate   response   to   certain malignancies.   Finally,   donor T lymphocyte infusions in the absence of immunosuppression for uncontrolled relaspe (risk of GVHD) may be necessary.

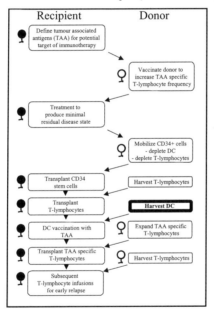

The ability to target DC and influence their function may well contribute significantly to facilitating transplantation across greater antigenic disparities. Thus, we would envisage immunosuppressive therapies targeted on the DC to control the critical allogeneic priming in both HVG and GVH directions. This earlier control of the immune response should pay dividends in avoiding amplification of the reactive allo T lymphocyte response. At a practical level this may include antibody targeted destruction of residual host DC which survive conditioning. This might usefully be combined with treatment such as CD45 reagents targeted on other residual leukaemic cells. More importantly, reagents such as CMRF-44 or CD83 or pharmacological compounds aimed at blocking DC function are likely to reduce the risk of acute GVHD. Such therapy if combined with T lymphocyte depletion should result in a profound immunological paralysis, which would ensure engraftment without significant GVHD. Subsequent T lymphocyte reconstitution would be delayed until full engraftment was established and the immediate post transplant complications resolved. At this point, thymidine kinase (TK) gene technology would be used to ensure control of the infused T lymphocytes (100). The greater histocompatibility differences allowed in this scenario should allow further infusions of donor lymphocytes for immunotherapy particularly under the control of the TK gene technology. It is even conceivable that recipient DC might be stored with a view to maximizing the intensity of this therapeutic controlled GVHD.

Immune therapy after allogeneic transplantation has two advantages not available in the autologous option. Firstly, a healthy immune system is infused, although this may subsequently be compromised by immunosuppressive drugs, and secondly, there are a number of alloantigens that might be exploited as tumour targets. The ability to mobilize DC and harvest them is likely to be achieved soon and these will be the preferred preparations for the future. It is not yet clear just how much purification will be required until the question of the subsets is resolved. The DC will probably require controlled stimulation eg with CD40 to ensure upregulation of antigen receptors and processing machinery (81). After introduction of the antigen in an optimal form, further cytokine treatment may be required to drive the most effective T lymphocyte response. A combination of helper epitopes will be required and CD40 expression is essential to drive cytotoxic T lymphocyte differentiation. Vaccination is likely to be most effective if scheduled outside the periods of significant immunosuppression.

An alternative to DC vaccination *in vivo* is to use donor DC and T lymphocytes *in vitro* to generate significant expansions of TAA specific T cells for reinfusion. This approach is already being applied to post-transplant EBV lymphomas (101). Subsequent *in vivo* vaccination with DC may be an economic method for maintaining memory beyond this point. Theoretically, there would be few ethical objections even to priming motivated donors with their own DC and TAA *in vivo* in a bid to expand the lymphocyte precursor frequency.

Whilst the anti-tumour effect of DC priming has been discussed above it should be acknowledged that, if the methods become routine, then the facility to use DC to drive strong protective responses against micro-organisms will also become most appealing. Finally, it is possible that DC fixed by some means in a resting state will be used to generate tolerance. Given the paucity of animal data in this area it will be some time before this comes to clinical fruition.

CONCLUSION

DC are critical to the initiation of an immune response both to allo antigens and to TAA. Manipulation of DC both *in vivo* and *in vitro* represents the next frontier for improving the results of allogeneic transplantation. DC directed immunosuppression will be particularly helpful in transplanting across greater histocompatibility barriers.

ACKNOWLEDGEMENTS

The authors would like to thank the many colleagues who contributed to the discussions associated with some of the concepts in this Chapter. We also wish to thank Ms Vicky Lancaster and Ms Lisa Whyte for their assistance with its preparation.

REFERENCES

1. Hart DN. Dendritic cells: unique leucocyte populations which control the primary immune response. Blood 1997;90:3245-3287.
2. McLellan AD, Heiser A, Sorg RV, Fearnley DB, Hart DNJ. Dermal dendritic cells associated with T lymphocytes in normal human skin display an activated phenotype. J.Invest.Dermatol 1998; 11 (5): 841-849.
3. Sallusto F, Lanzavecchia A. Efficient presentation of soluble antigen by cultured human dendritic cells is maintained by granulocyte/macrophage colony- stimulating factor plus interleukin 4 and downregulated by tumour necrosis factor. J Exp.Med. 1994;179:1109-1118.
4. Ardavin C, Shortman K. Thymic dendritic cells and T cells develop simultaneously in the thymus from a common precursor population. Nature 1993;362:761-763.
5. Troy AJ, Hart DNJ. Dendritic cells in cancer: progress towards a new cellular therapy. Journal of Hematotherapy 1997;6:523-533.
6. Egner W, McKenzie JL, Smith SM, Beard MEJ, Hart DNJ. Identification of potent mixed leucocyte reaction-stimulatory cells in human bone marrow. J Immunol. 1993;150:3043-3053.

7. Egner W, Andreesen R, Hart DNJ. Allostimulatory cells in fresh human blood: heterogeneity in antigen presenting cell populations. Transplantation 1993;56:945-950.
8. Fearnley DB, McLellan AD, Mannering SI, Hock BD, Hart DNJ. Isolation of human blood dendritic cells using the CMRF-44 monoclonal antibody: implications for studies on antigen presenting cell function and immunotherapy. Blood 1997;89:3708-3716.
9. Strunk D, Rappersberger K, Egger C, Strobl H, Kromer E, Elbe A, Maurer D, Stingl G. Generation of human dendritic cell/Langerhans cells from circulating CD34$^+$ hematopoietic progenitor cells. Blood 1996;87:1292-1302.
10. Vuckovic S, Fearnley DB, Mannering SI, Dekker LF, Whyte L, Hart DNJ. Generation of CMRF-44$^+$ monocyte derived dendritic cells: Insights into phenotype and function. Exp.Hematol. 1998;26 (13):1255-1264.
11. Young JW, Szabolcs P, Moore MAS. Identification of dendritic cell colony-forming units among normal human CD34$^+$ bone marrow progenitors that are expanded by c-kit ligand and yield pure dendritic cell colonies in the presence of granulocyte/macrophage colony-stimulating factor and tumor necrosis factor alpha. J Exp.Med. 1995;182(4):1111-1119.
12. Siena S, Di Nicola M, Bregni M, Mortarini R, Anichini A, Lombardi L, Ravagnani F, Parmiani G, Gianni AM. Massive ex vivo generation of functional dendritic cells from mobilized CD34$^+$ blood progenitors for anticancer therapy. Exp.Hematol. 1995;23:1463-1471.
13. Szabolcs P, Avigan D, Gezelter S, Ciocon DH, Moore MAS, Steinman RM, Young JW. Dendritic cells and macrophages can mature independently from a human bone marrow-derived, post-colony-forming unit intermediate. Blood 1996;87:4520-4530.
14. Maraskovsky E, Brasel K, Teepe M, Roux ER, Lyman SD, Shortman K, McKenna HJ. Dramatic increase in the numbers of functionally mature dendritic cells in Flt3 ligand-treated mice: multiple dendritic cell subpopulations identified. J Exp.Med. 1996;184:1953-1962.
15. Geissman F, Prost C, Monnet J-P, Dy M, Brousse N, Hermine O. Transforming growth factor 1, in the presence of granulocyte/macrophage colony stimulating factor and interleukin 4, induces differentiation of human peripheral blood monocytes into dendritic Langerhans Cells. J Exp Med. 1998;187:961-966.
16. Kaplan G, Nusrat A, Witmer MD, Nath I, Cohn ZA. Distribution and turnover of Langerhans cells during delayed immune responses in human skin. J Exp.Med. 1987;165:763-776.

17. Sozzani S, Luini W, Borsatti A, Polentarutti N, Zhou D, Piemonti L, D'Amico G, Power CA, Wells TNC, Gobbi M, Allavena P, Mantovani A. Receptor expression and responsiveness of human dendritic cells to a defined set of CC and CXC chemokines. J Immunol. 1997;159:1993-2000.
18. Romani N, Schuler G. The immunologic properties of epidermal Langerhans cells as a part of the dendritic cell system. Springer Semin.Immunopathol. 1992;13:265-279.
19. Roake JA, Rao AS, Morris PJ, Larsen CP, Hankins DF, Austyn JM. . Dendritic cell loss from nonlymphoid tissues after systemic administration of lipopolysaccharide, tumour necrosis factor and interleukin 1. J Exp Med1995;181:2237-2247.
20. Sozzani S, Sallusto F, Luini W, Zhou D, Piemonti L, Allavena P, Van Damme J, Valitutti S, Lanzavecchia A, Mantovani A. Migration of dendritic cells in response to formyl peptides, C5a, and a distinct set of chemokines. J Immunol. 1995;155:3292-3295.
21. Kato M, Neil T, Clark G, Morris C, Sorg R, Hart DNJ. cDNA cloning of human DEC-205, a putative antigen-uptake receptor on dendritic cells. Immunogenetics 1998;47:442-450.
22. Fanger NA, Voigtlaender D, Liu C, Swink S, Wardwell K, Fisher J, Graziano RF, Pfefferkorn LC, Guyre PM. Characterization of expression, cytokine regulation, and effector function of the high affinity IgG receptor FcyRI (CD64) expressed on human blood dendritic cells. J Immunol. 1997;158:3090-3098.
23. Zhou LJ, Tedder TF. Human blood dendritic cells selectively express CD83, a member of the immunoglobulin superfamily. J Immunol. 1995;154:3821-3835.
24. Hock BD, Fearnley D, Boyce A, Sorg RV, McLellan AD, Hart DNJ, Kato M. Characterisation of CMRF-56, a selective marker for differentiated/activated human dendritic cell populations. (in preparation) 1998.
25. Adema GJ, Hartgers F, Verstraten R, de Vries E, Marland G, Menon S, Foster J, Xu Y, Nooyen P, McClanahan T, Bacon KB, Figdor CG. A dendritic-cell-derived C-C chemokine that preferentially attracts naive T cells. Nature 1997;387:713-717.
26. McLellan AD, Sorg RV, Williams LA, Hart DNJ. Human dendritic cells activate T lymphocytes via a CD40:CD40 ligand-dependent pathway. Eur.J Immunol. 1996;26:1204-1210.
27. Yawalkar N, Brand CU, Braathen LR. IL-12 gene expression in human skin-erived CD1a (+) dendritic lymph cells. Arch.Dermatol. 1996;288:79-84.

28. Sorg RV, McLellan AD, Hock BD, Fearnley DB, Hart DNJ. Human dendritic cells express functional interleukin -7. Immunobiology 1998;198(5): 514-526.
29. Bennett SR, Carbone FR, Karamalis F, Flavell RA, Miller JF, Heath WR. Help for cytotoxic T-cell responses is mediated by CD40 signalling. Nature 1998;393:478-480.
30. Dubois B, Massacrier C, Vanbervliet B, Fayette J, Briere F, Banchereau J, Caux C. Critical role of IL-12 in dendritic cell-induced differentiation of naive B lymphocytes. Immunol 1998;1161:2223-2231.
31. Grouard G, Durand I, Filgueira L, Banchereau J, Liu Y-J. Dendritic cells capable of stimulating T cells in germinal centres. Nature 1996;384:364-367.
32. Suss G, Shortman K. A subclass of dendritic cells kills CD4 T cells via Fas/fas-ligand-induced apoptosis. J Exp.Med. 1996;183:1789-1796.
33. Kronin V, Winkel K, Suss G, Kelso A, Heath W, Kirberg J, von Boehmer H, Shortman K. A subclass of dendritic cells regulates the response of naive CD8 T cells by limiting their IL-2 production. J Immunol. 1996;157:3819-3827.
34. Res P, Martinezcaceres E, Jaleco AC, Staal F, Noteboom E, Weijer K, Spits H. CD34(+) CD38 (dim) cells in the human thymus can differentiate into T, natural killer, and dendritic cells but are distinct from pluripotent stem cells. Blood 1996;87:5196-5206.
35. Galy A, Travis M, Cen D, Chen B. Human T, B, natural killer and dendritic cells arise from a common bone marrow progenitor cell subset. Immunity 1995;3:459-473.
36. Olweus J, BitMansour A, Warnke R, Thompson PA, Carballido J, Picker LJ, Lund-Johansen F. Dendritic cell ontogeny: A human dendritic cell lineage of myeloid origin. Proc Natl Acad Sci. 1997;94:12551-12556.
37. Grouard G, Rissoan M-C, Filgueira L, Durand I, Banchereau J, Liu Y-J. The enigmatic plasmacytoid T cells develop into dendritic cells with interleukin (IL)-3 and CD40-ligand. J Exp.Med. 1997;185:1101-1111.
38. Ardavin C. Thymic dendritic cells (see comments). Immunol Today 1997;18:350-361.
39. Brocker T, Riedinger M, Karjalainen K. Targeted expression of major histocompatibility complex (MHC) class II molecules demonstrates that dendritic cells can induce negative but not positive selection of thymocytes in vivo. J Exp Med 1997;185:541-550.
40. Kyewski BA, Fathman CG, Rouse RV. Intrathymic presentation of circulating non-MHC antigens by medullary dendritic cells. An antigen-dependent microenvironment for T cell differentiation. J Exp.Med. 1986;163:231-246.

41. Matzinger P, Guerder S. Does T-cell tolerance require a dedicated antigen-presenting cell? Nature 1989;338:74-76.

42. Khoury SJ, Gallon L, Chen W, Betres K, Russell ME, Hancock WW, Carpenter CB, Sayegh MH, Weiner HL. Mechanisms of acquired thymic tolerance in experimental autoimmune encephalomyelitis: thymic dendritic-enriched cells induce specific peripheral T cell unresponsiveness in vivo. J Exp Med 1995;183:357-366.

43. Hart DNJ, Calder VL. Human dendritic cells: function and cytokine production. Immunopharmacology of macrophages and other antigen-presenting cells. In: Bruijnzeel-Loomen D, ed. Handbook of Immunopharmacology, 1994:63-91.

44. Clare-Salzier MJ, Brooks J, Chai A, Van Herle K, Anderson C. Prevention of diabetes in nonobese diabetic mice by dendritic cell transfer. J Clin.Invest. 1992;90:741-748.

45. Lu L, McCaslin D, Starzl TE. Bone marrow-derived dendritic cell progenitors (NLDC145+, MHC class II+,B7-1dim,B7-2-) induce alloantigen-specific hyporesponsiveness in murine T lymphocytes. Transplantation 1995;60:1539-1545.

46. Tan P, Anasetti C, Hansen JA, Melrose J, Brunvand M, Bradshaw J, Ledbetter JA, Linsley PS. Induction of alloantigen-specific hyporesponsiveness in human T lymphocytes by blocking interaction of CD28 with its natural ligand B7/BB1. J Exp.Med. 1993;177:165-173.

47. Freeman AJ, Baird MA. Immunosuppression mediated by heat-treated cells: suppression or anergy? Transplantation 1992;55:1439-1442.

48. Everson MP, McDuffie DS, Lemak DG, Koopman WJ, McGhee JR, Beagley KW. Dendritic cells from different tissues induce production of different T cell cytokine profiles. J Leuk.Biol. 1996;59:494-498.

49. Vezzio N, Sarfati M, Yang L-P, Demeure CE, Delespesse G. Human T$_h$2-like cell clones induce IL-12 production by dendritic cells and may express several cytokine profiles. Int.Immunol. 1996;8:1963-1970.

50. Weih F, Carrasco D, Durham SK, Barton DS, Rizzso CA, Ryseck R-P, Lira SA, Bravo R. Multiorgan inflammation and hematopoietic abnormalities in mice with a targeted disruption of RelB, a member of the NF-kB/Rel family. Cell 1995;80:331-340.

51. Burkly L, Hession C, Ogata L, Reilly C, Marconi LA, Olson D, Tizard R, Cate R, Lo D. Expression of relB is required for the development of thymic medulla and dendritic cells. Nature 1995;373:531-536.

52. Hart DN, Fabre JW. Demonstration and characterization of Ia-positive dendritic cells in the interstitial connective tissues of rat heart and other tissues, not brain. J Exp.Med. 1981;153:347-361.

53. Hart DNJ, Fuggle SV, Williams KA, Fabre JW, Ting A, Morris PJ. Localization of HLA-ABC and DR antigens in human kidney. Transplantation 1981;31:428-433.
54. McKenzie JL, Beard MEJ, Hart DNJ. Depletion of donor kidney dendritic cells prolongs graft survival. Transplant.Proc. 1984;16:948-951.
55. Fu F, Li Y, Qian S, Lu L, Chambers F, Starzl TE, Fung JJ, Thomson AW. Costimulatory molecule-deficient dendritic cell progenitors (MHC class II+, CD80dim, CD86-) prolong cardiac allograft survival in nonimmunosuppressed recipients. Transplantation 1996;62:659-665.
56. Hart DN, Fabre JW. Localization of MHC antigens in long surviving rat renal allografts: probable implication of passenger leucocytes in graft adaption. Transplant.Proc. 1981;13:95-99.
57. Thomson AW, Lu L, Subbotin VM, Li S, Qian S, Rao AS, Fung JJ, Starzl TE. In vitro propagation and homing of liver-derived dendritic cell progenitors to lymphoid tissues of allogeneic recipients. Transplantation 1995;59:544-551.
58. Sherman LW, Chattopadhyay S. The molecular basis of allorecognition. Annu.Rev.Immunol. 1993;11:385-402.
59. van Lochem E, van der Keur M, Mommaas AM, de Gast GC, Goulmy E. Functional expression of minor histocompatibility antigens on human peripheral blood dendritic cells and epidermal Langerhans cells. Transpl.Immunol. 1996;4:151-157.
60. MacPherson GG, Jenkins CD, Stein MJ, Edwards C. Endotoxin-mediated dendritic cell release from the intestine: characterisation of released dendritic cells and TNF dependence. J Immunol. 1995;159:1317-1322.
61. Ferrara JL. Paradigm shift for graft-versus-host disease. Bone.Marrow.Transplant. 1994;14:183-184.
62. Perreault C, Pelletier M, Belanger R, Boileau J, Bonny Y, David M, Gyger M, Landry D, Montplaisir S. Persistence of host Langerhans cells following allogeneic bone marrow transplantation: possible relationship with acute graft-versus-host disease. Br.J Haematol. 1985;60:253-260.
63. Perreault C, Pelletier M, Landry D, Gyger M. Study of Langerhans cells after allogeneic bone marrow transplantation. Blood 1984;63:807-811.
64. Fearnley DB, Whyte LF, Carnoutsos SA, Cook AH, Hart DNJ. Monitoring human blood dendritic cell numbers in normal individuals and in stem cell transplantation. Blood 1998; 93 (2):728-736.
65. Austyn JM, Larsen CP. Migration patterns of dendritic leukocytes. Transplantation 1990;49:1-7.

66. Talmadge J, Reed K, Ino K, Kuszynski C, Heimann D, Varney M, Jackson J, Vose JM, Bierman PJ. Rapid immunologic reconstitution following transplantation with mobilized peripheral blood stem cells as compared to bone marrow. Bone Marrow Transplantation 1997;19:161-172.

67. Troy AJ, Summers KL, Davidson PJT, Atkinson CA, Hart DNJ. Minimal recruitment and activation of dendritic cells within renal cell carcinoma. Clinical Cancer Research 1998;4:585-593.

68. Troy AJ, Davidson P, Atkinson C, Hart D. Phenotypic characterization of the dendritic cell infiltrate in prostate cancer. J Urol. 1998;160:214-219.

69. Troy AJ, Davidson PJT, Atkinson CH, Hart DNJ. CD1a dendritic cells predominate in transitional cell carcinoma of bladder and kidney but are minimally activated. J Urol 1998;Submitted.

70. Gabrilovich DI, Chen HL, Girgis KR, Cunningham HT, Meny GM, Nadaf S, Kavanaugh D, Carbone DP. Production of vascular endothelial growth factor by human tumors inhibits the functional maturation of dendritic cells. Nat.Med. 1996;2:1096.

71. Koch F, Stanzl U, Jennewein P, Janke K, Heufler C, Kampgen E, Romani N, Schuler G. High level IL-12 production by murine dendritic cells: upregulation via MHC class II and CD40 molecules and downregulation by IL-4 and IL-10. J Exp.Med. 1996;184:741-746.

72. Summers KL, O'Donnell JL, Highton J, Hart DNJ. Rheumatoid synovial fluid TGF- inhibits dendritic cell-T lymphocyte interactions. Arthritis and Rheumatism 1998;Resubmitted.

73. Gabrilovich DI, Ciernik F, Carbone DP. Dendritic cells in antitumor immune responses. I. Defective antigen presentation in tumor-bearing hosts. Cell.Immunol. 1996;170:101-110.

74. Gabrilovich DI, Corak J, Ciernik IF, Kavanaugh D, Carbone DP. Decreased antigen presentation by dendritic cells in patients with breast cancer. Clinical Cancer Research 1997;3:483-490.

75. Radmayr C, Bock G, Hobisch A, Klocker H, Bartsch G, Thurnher M. Dendritic antigen-presenting cells from the periphal blood of renal-cell-carcinoma patients. Int.J Cancer 1995;63:627-632.

76. Tjoa B, Erickson S, Barren R, Ragde H, Kenny G, Boynton A, Murphy G. In vitro propagated dendritic cells from prostate cancer patients as a component of prostate cancer immunotherapy. Prostate 1995;27:63-69.

77. Lynch DH, Andreasen A, Maraskovsky E, Whitmore J, Miller RE, Schuh JCL. Flt3 ligand induces tumor regression and antitumor immune responses *in vivo*. Nat.Med. 1997;3:625-631.

78. Pardoll DM. Cancer Vaccines. Nat Med 1998;5 Suppl:525-531.

79. Casares S, Inaba K, Brumeanu T, Steinman RM, Bona CA. Antigen presentation by dendritic cells following immunization with DNA encoding a class II-restricted viral epitope. J. Exp. Med 186, 1481-1486 1997.

80. Colonna M. Specificity and function of immunoglobulin superfamily NK cell inhibitory and stimulatory receptors. Immunol.Rev. 1997;155:127-133.

81. Mannering SI, McKenzie JL, Hart DNJ. Optimisation of the conditions for generating human DC initiated primary antigen specific T lymphocyte lines in vitro. J Immunol Methods 1998; 219 (1-2): 69-83.

82. Mackensen A, Herbst B, Kohlter G, Wolff-Vorbeck G, Rosenthal F, Veelken H, Kulmburg P, Schaefer HE, Mertelsmann R, Lindemann A. Delineation of the dendritic cell lineage by generating large numbers of birbeck granule-positive Langerhans cells from human peripheral blood progenitor cells in vitro. Blood 1995;86:2699-2707.

83. Luft T, Pang KC, Thomas E, Hertzog P, Hart DNJ, Trapani J, Cebon J. Type I IFNs enhance the terminal differentiation of dendritic cells. J Immunol 1998;161:1947-1953.

84. Romani N, Reider D, Heuer M, Ebner S, Kampgen E, Eibl B, Niederwieser D, Schuler G. Generation of mature dendritic cells from human blood: an improved method with special regard to clinical applicability. J Immunol Methods 1996;196:137-151.

85. Barratt-Boyes SM, Watkins SC, Finn OJ. In vivo migration of dendritic cells differentiated in vitro. J Immunol. 1997;158:4543-4547.

86. Zitvogel L, Mayordomo JI, Tjandrawan T, DeLeo AB. Therapy of murine tumors with tumor peptide-pulsed dendritic cells: dependence on T cells, B7 costimulation and T helper cell 1-associated cytokines. J Exp.Med. 1996;183:87-97.

87. van Elsas A, van der Burg SH, van der Minne C, Borghi M, Mourer JS, Melief CJM, Schrier PI. Peptide-pulsed dendritic cells induce tumoricidal cytotoxic T lymphocytes from healthy donors against stably HLA-A*0201-binding peptides from the Melan-A/MART-1 self antigen. Eur.J Immunol. 1996;26:1683-1689.

88. Bakker AB, Marland G, de Boer AJ, Huijbens RJF, Danen EHJ, Adema GJ, Figdor CG. Generation of antimelanoma cytotoxic T lymphocytes from healthy donors after presentation of melanoma-associated antigen-derived epitopes by dendritic cells in vitro. Cancer Res. 1995;55:5330-5334.

89. Reeves ME, Royal RE, Lam JS, Rosenberg SA, Hwu P. Retroviral transduction of human dendritic cells with a tumor-associated antigen gene. Cancer Res. 1996;56:5672-5677.

90. Henderson RA, Nimgaonkar MT, Watkins SC, Robbins PD, Ball ED, Finn OJ. Human dendritic cells genetically engineered to express high levels of the human epithelial tumour antigen mucin (MUC-1). Cancer Res. 1996;56:3763-3770.
91. Nair S, Zhou F, Reddy R, Huang L, Rouse BT. Soluble proteins delivered to dendritic cells via pH-sensitive liposomes induce primary cytotoxic T lymphocyte responses in vitro. J Exp.Med. 1992;175:609-612.
92. Grabbe S, Bruvers S, Gallo RL, Knisely TL, Nazareno R, Granstein RD. Tumor antigen presentation by murine epidermal cells. J Immunol. 1991;146:3656-3661.
93. Mannering SI, McKenzie JL, Fearnley DB, Hart DNJ. HLA-DR1-restricted bcr-abl (b3a2)-specific CD4$^+$ T lymphocytes respond to dendritic cells pulsed with b3a2 peptide and antigen-presenting cells exposed to b3a2 containing cell lysates. Blood 1997;90:290-297.
94. Tjoa B, Boynton A, Kenny G, Ragde H, Misrock SL, Murphy G. Presentation of prostate tumor antigens by dendritic cells stimulates T-cell proliferation and cytotoxicity. Prostate 1996;28:65-69.
95. Choudhury A, Gajewski JL, Liang JC, Popat U, Claxton DF, Kliche K-O, Andreeff M, Champlin RE. Use of leukemic dendritic cells for the generation of antileukemic cellular cytotoxicity against Philadelphia chromosome-positive chronic myelogenous leukemia. Blood 1997;89:1133-1142.
96. Hsu FJ, Benike C, Fagnoni F, Liles TM, Czerwinski D, Taidi B, Engelman EG, Levy R. Vaccination of patients with B-cell lymphoma using autologous antigen-pulsed dendritic cells. Nat.Med. 1996;2:52-57.
97. Murphy G, Tjoa B, Ragde H, Kenny G, Boynton A. Phase I clinical trial: T-cell therapy for prostate cancer using autologous dendritic cells pulsed with HLA-A0201-specific peptides from prostate-specific membrane antigen. Prostate 1996;29:371-380.
98. Sorg UR, Morse TM, Patton WN, Hock BD, Angus HB, Robinson BA, Colls BM, Hart DNJ. Hodgkin's cells express CD83, a dendritic cell lineage associated marker. Pathology 1997;29:294-299.
99. Nestle FO, Alijagic S, Gilliet M, Sun Y, Grabbe S, Dummer R, Burg G, Schadendorf D. Vaccination of melanoma patients with peptide- or tumour lysate-pulsed dendritic cells. Nat.Med. 1998;4:328-332.
100. Bordignon C, Bonini C, Ferrari G, Verzeletti S, Servida P, Zappone E, Ruggieri L, Ponzoni M, Rossini S, Mavilio F, Traversari C. HSV-TK gene transfer into donor lymphocytes for control of allogeneic grant-versus-leukemia. Science 1997;276:1719-1724.

101.Heslop HE, Ng CYC, Li C, Smith CA, Loftin SK, Krance RA, Brenner MK, Rooney CM. Long-term restoration of immunity against Epstein-Barr virus infection by adoptive transfer of gene-modified virus-specific T lymphocytes. Nat.Med. 1996; 2:551-555.

14

ENGINEERING HEMATOPOIETIC GRAFTS USING ELUTRIATION AND POSITIVE CELL SELECTION TO REDUCE GVHD

Stephen J. Noga, M.D., Ph.D.

The Johns Hopkins Oncology Center, Rm 804, 550 N. Broadway Avenue, Baltimore, MD 21205 USA

INTRODUCTION

Over the last two decades, allogeneic bone marrow transplantation (BMT) has provided a means of delivering potentially curative therapy to patients with hematologic malignancies (1). Unfortunately, approximately 70% of allogeneic BMT patients receiving unmodified (wherein marrow is immediately infused) grafts develop acute graft-vs-host disease (GVHD) with one third of these patients rapidly succumbing to this complication (2,3). Of patients surviving more than 100 days, half will later develop chronic GVHD which has an attendant mortality of almost 50% (4). This incidence increases still further for those individuals who receive an HLA mismatched or unrelated donor graft. It was initially believed that the use of allogeneic peripheral blood stem cells (PBSC) would reduce the incidence of GVHD. Unfortunately, both acute and chronic GVHD are as prevalent (or even greater in the case of chronic GVHD) with PBSC as that seen with bone marrow as the stem cell source (5,6). The lack of suitable donors and high morbidity has popularized other high dose chemotherapy/ stem cell rescue approaches such as autologous BMT and peripheral blood stem cell (PBSC) transplantation. To date, allogeneic BMT still generates the highest cure rates, largely due to its inherent anti-tumor [or graft-vs-leukemia (GVL)] properties which results in low relapse rates (7,8). The dilemma often facing the transplant physician is whether to suggest that a patient undergo a less morbid transplant approach with a higher relapse risk or accept the greater mortality risk of allogeneic BMT in hopes of achieving a cure. Improvements in supportive care and

Similar advances must be achieved in the allogeneic setting for this to remain a viable option, regardless of it's curative potential.

T cell depletion (TCD) of donor marrow was initially perceived as accomplishing these goals: both animal and human studies implicated T cells as the primary mediators of GVHD (9). Clinical studies demonstrated that radical (3 to 4 $\log_{10}$) TCD successfully reduced the incidence of acute GVHD (10,11). Surprisingly, the few randomized TCD trials did not show improved overall disease free survival (DFS) over those patients receiving an unmanipulated graft (12,13). While GVHD caused high mortality in the latter, TCD marrow recipients were dying from graft failure, leukemic relapse and B cell lymphoproliferative disease: all previously low incidence complications (14,15).

Subsequent studies have confirmed that ancillary marrow (other than pluripotent stem) cell populations do mediate GVHD, but they and/or other cells also facilitate engraftment and possess anti-leukemic properties (4,9,16-18). Many of the TCD techniques radically deplete ancillary cell populations (including committed progenitor cells) via non-specific loss (19-21). Thus, trial design must incorporate a means of comparing the target goals (GVHD) with other outcome parameters (engraftment, blood product utilization, relapse, cost, etc) to determine the overall impact on quality of life for that particular graft manipulation procedure. Our approach (termed "graft engineering") involved using a series of sequential, interdependent phase I and I/II clinical trials to systematically alter the lymphohematopoietic characteristics of the graft and/or the host to improve long term survival (22). Animal models were utilized, where possible, to guide the preclinical development of new approaches. At times, this actually occurred in reverse order where animal studies were used to evaluate an unexpected clinical outcome. This design also facilitated the incorporation of new technology (investigational devices) whose performance characteristics could be easily evaluated and compared to the previous study that did not include this step. Various graft characteristics (stem cell content, lymphocyte subsets, NK activity, etc) were tracked and correlated with specified "performance" characteristics such as those listed above. This approach would allow total flexibility including the eventual incorporation of genetic engineering strategies. However, for the present, the available tools for graft engineering comprise bulk manipulation of cell populations, immuno/pharmacologic modulation of the donor/host or graft and the use of "first generation" genetically engineered products. This chapter will summarize our experience in allogeneic graft engineering - with particular emphasis placed on the reduction of acute and chronic GVHD. This will be followed by a discussion of the current status of graft engineering and outline the future directions and clinical trials that could further improve patient outcome using this approach.

Using Elutriation for TCD

Lymphocyte modified grafts. Although the long term complications of TCD outweighed its beneficial effects, it was extraordinarily successful in abrogating the early post-BMT morbidity associated with acute GVHD (12,16). Rather than abandon TCD altogether, we hypothesized that long term complications could be minimized by "dosing back" a predetermined number of lymphocytes into the TCD graft. Preclinical studies suggested that the physical separation technology of elutriation was well suited for this approach. Elutriation can rapidly and reliably separate bulk cell populations differing in sedimentation coefficient (size and density) into distinct cellular fractions with virtually no loss in either recovery or viability (23-25). An entire marrow graft could be consistently depleted of T cells (2.0 to 2.5 $\log_{10}$) in 40 minutes. The only surrogate marker that was available to assess engraftment during these initial studies was the colony-forming unit (CFU). Over 90% of the CFU-granulocyte/ macrophage (CFU-GM) or granulocyte/ erythroid/ macrophage/ megakaryocyte (CFU-GEMM or Mix) were recovered in this large-sized TCD fraction (23). Patients received an HLA (6/6) matched sibling TCD graft fraction as well as a second product derived from the lymphoid-rich fractions to construct a graft containing either 1×10^6 or 5×10^5 lymphocytes/ kg recipient ideal body weight (26,27). Limiting dilution analysis demonstrated that this correlated with a functional T cell dose of 4×10^5 or 2×10^5 cells/kg, respectively (28). The functional T cells were almost totally derived from the second lymphoid-rich product. Cyclosporine A (CSA) was administered for 180 days for GVHD prophylaxis because of the intentional inclusion of T cells. There was little reduction in clinically significant (stage ≥ 2) acute GVHD using modified grafts containing 1×10^6 lymphocytes/kg (46% historical, matched controls to 38% with the elutriated grafts). However, patients receiving grafts constructed with 5×10^5 lymphocytes/kg had only an 11% incidence of acute GVHD (27). In addition, the 5-year probability of developing chronic GVHD was also decreased from 56% to 6%, respectively (29). Early graft failure was documented in 10% of the patients. Perhaps more worrisome was the overall delayed effect of elutriation on engraftment kinetics. The median day to an absolute neutrophil count (ANC) >500 was 22 days and to an untransfused platelet count of $\geq 50,000/\mu l$ was 44 days (27). An additional 4% of patients eventually showed complete loss of the donor graft while mixed hematopoietic chimerism could be documented in an additional 32% (30). In contrast to patients with diagnoses of lymphoma, multiple myeloma (MM) or acute leukemia, 79% of patients transplanted with TCD grafts for CML relapsed within 2 years (31). These patients had nearly a 100% probability of relapse at 30 months as compared to <10% for non-TCD patients.

Over a 6-year period (1986-1992), 106 patients received lymphocyte-modified, elutriated grafts. Patients with CML were excluded from elutriation protocols between 1988 and 1994 (Figure 1). Benefits derived from this procedure included decreased morbidity from acute and chronic GVHD and the inclusion of patients up to age 45 (and later, 55) for allogeneic BMT. With the exception of patients with CML, the GVL effect of allogeneic BMT was not compromised by this graft modification technique. Secondary B cell malignancies have not proven to be a complication of elutriated grafts and the risk of infection was not increased (32). There were still several outcome parameters that had a negative impact with this approach. Although there was a low graft failure rate (10%), the delayed engraftment kinetics was worrisome. The persistence of mixed hematopoietic chimerism that could be documented for more than 4 years post-transplant was also an issue. It was reassuring that the Nijmegen group had also reported similar findings with elutriation. In agreement with our patient cohort, it was not associated, long term, with relapse (33). Also, this approach was not acceptable for CML, thus excluding a fairly large transplant population. Lastly, one phase I study utilized elutriation without CSA prophylaxis. This study was terminated after enrolling 4 patients due to a 100% incidence of graft failure (34). Apparently, this form of TCD had an absolute CSA requirement to ensure durable engraftment in addition to CSA's role in suppressing GVHD. Laboratory investigation was then directed towards improving engraftment kinetics and in determining what conditions, if any, would allow elutriation to be used again in CML.

Figure 1. This schema outlines the Hopkins approach to allogeneic hematopoietic graft engineering over the past 12 years. Prior to this time, whole or erythrocyte depleted donor marrow was infused. The primary or "first generation" procedures employed the physical separation method of elutriation to effect T cell depletion along with a designated "add-back" of lymphoid cells at BMT day 0. Later protocols employed CD34[+] salvage along with elutriation to augment the stem cell dose. Future protocols will employ prophylactic add-back of sequentially positive selected lymphoid cells to further combat relapse.

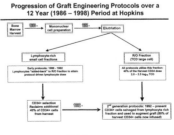

CD34⁺ STEM CELL AUGMENTATION

A murine model of elutriation was developed and indicated that a small sized, lineage undefined cell residing in the lymphoid-rich elutriation fraction was responsible for long term durable engraftment (35). This cell population was distinct from the larger-sized lineage defined cell population found in the TCD fraction that generated 14-day hematopoietic colonies. In man, the development of the anti-CD34 monoclonal antibody, which defined early hematopoietic progenitor cell populations, and more sophisticated flow cytometric systems which could easily discern rare events permitted a detailed evaluation of the clinical elutriation fractions. This data indicated that two-thirds of the CD34⁺ cells were small in size and co-eluted with the lymphocytes that were not included in the graft (36).

If these smaller-sized CD34⁺ cells (which did not give rise to appreciable 14 day colonies) were similar to the long term phenotype^{neg} repopulating cells in the mouse, then their loss from the graft could account for the delayed engraftment kinetics seen with elutriated marrow. Furthermore, animal data also suggested that higher stem cell doses may also out-compete malignant stem cells during repopulation, thus reducing the probability of relapse (37). This could be particularly important in CML where most patients are transplanted in chronic phase and have a significant tumor burden at the time of transplant. DeWitte et al. (38) used incremental flow rates to separate these smaller sized stem cells away from their lymphoid counterparts. Unfortunately, this resulted in variable CD34⁺ cell recoveries and lymphocyte contamination.

Shortly after the human progenitor/stem cell epitopes were characterized, several clinical devices were developed to capture and isolate these CD34⁺ cells from marrow (39,40). While high purity (>90%) could be achieved using the pre-clinical devices along with marrow aspirate-sized samples, use of whole marrows with clinical scale devices yielded purities between 50-70% (41). For an allogeneic graft, this inferred a variable level of T cell contamination in the CD34⁺ selected graft raising the probability of increased GVHD rates. Alternatively, if the marrow graft is elutriated first, this will result in a well defined TCD fraction containing almost all the committed progenitor cells and it will also provide well-defined smaller sized fraction(s) which contain cells of uniform size, with significantly less platelets and mature erythrocytes than whole marrow. Since the lymphoid-rich small cell fractions were previously discarded, they were available for large-scale CD34⁺ cell selection procedures. These fractions were pooled, incubated with biotinylated anti-CD34 monoclonal antibody and washed. Passing them over an avidin gel column could then capture the labeled cells. Use of the CellPro

CEPRATE© SC Stem Cell Concentrator system resulted in a median CD34$^+$ purity and yield of 80% and 60%, respectively. This adsorbed fraction represented only 2% of the cells loaded unto the column. T cell contamination was 5% of the positively selected cells; $<1 \times 10^5$ T cells/kg would be derived from this fraction if it were infused. Furthermore, the total graft CD34$^+$ cell dose could be effectively doubled if this product were to be given along with the elutriated TCD fraction (36).

Matched related trials using CD34$^+$ augmentation/elutriation

Phase I trial. If engraftment kinetics are affected by stem (CD34$^+$) cell dose, especially in the TCD setting, then the ability to recover twice as many CD34$^+$ cells should impact on this outcome. The initial phase I trial (N=10) elutriation trials along with the CD34$^+$ selected product derived from the pooled small lymphoid fractions (42). Post BMT CSA prophylaxis for HLA matched, related, TCD graft was maintained for 180 days. Use of the CD34$^+$ selected product effectively doubled the graft's CD34$^+$ cell dose to 3.4×10^6/kg while total T cell content averaged 6×10^5/kg (42). The enriched CD34$^+$ small cell fraction represented 0.4% of the initially harvested cells, but contained 50% of the combined graft CD34$^+$ cells. As with elutriation alone, the CD34$^+$ fraction contributed very few committed progenitor cells (only 10% of the CFU-GMs), but the majority of the cells capable of initiating long term hematopoiesis on marrow stromal layers resided in this fraction. Granulocyte and platelet engraftment was rapid and durable with a median of 19 and 24 days, post BMT, respectively. No patient had stage 3 or 4 acute GVHD; one patient had stage 2 which resolved and no patient developed chronic GVHD (Table 1).

Phase II trials. Several phase II trials were then conducted to explore the durability and kinetics of engraftment using this approach. Since CSA was an absolute requirement with elutriation alone, different post-transplant intervals were investigated. CSA has several deleterious side effects such as hypertension, nephro/neurotoxicity, immune suppression and increased relapse risk, which significantly affect post-transplant morbidity. It was argued that long term outcome may be improved by CSA reduction post BMT. In this case, the ability to reproducibly engineer the hematopoietic graft combined with the use of standardized preparative and supportive care regimens could permit the investigation of single variables such as CSA duration. Therefore, CSA effect on transplant outcome (engraftment, GVHD, morbidity, costs, etc) could be determined.

Effect of CSA duration on engraftment. Animal data suggested that 30 to 60 days of CSA were required to ensure durable TCD allogeneic engraftment (Hess AD, unpublished data, 1990). Three concurrent phase II graft engineering studies were used to determine the effects of post-BMT CSA duration (43,44). The daily dosing schedule was constant; CSA was administered for 180 (CSA180, N=28), 30 (CSA30, N=30) and 80 (CSA80, N=52) days. In terms of graft composition, the results for all 3 studies were pooled since there were no statistical differences detected in the engineered graft product. In this series, the average engineered graft had a CD34$^+$ cell dose of 3.3x10^6/kg. The majority (96.5%) of patients demonstrated prompt granulocyte and platelet engraftment: the median days to reach an ANC >500/ul and platelet count >50,000/ul were 16 and 24 days on the CSA30 study and 17 and 26 days for the CSA80/180 trials (44). It should also be noted that no hematopoietic growth factors were given to these patients during the post transplant period. These results are significantly improved over the kinetics of granulocyte and platelet engraftment seen with elutriated marrow only (20 and 41 days, respectively) and compare favorably with historical controls that received unmanipulated marrow [17 and 22 days, respectively (12,19,29)]. Four patients (3.6%) failed to engraft (FTE) (2 in CSA80, 2 in CSA180 cohort). This is less than the incidence of FTE seen with elutriation alone (10% incidence) or with other forms of TCD. However, it is still higher than the <1% incidence reported for unmanipulated marrow grafts (16). Two of the 4 patients (AML CR2, CR3) were highly alloimmunized and had received platelet products from their respective donors during induction therapy (prior to BMT). The third patient had AML arising out of MDS and the fourth had MDS arising after aplastic anemia. The disease status of these patients suggests the possibility of an underlying micro environmental marrow disorder predisposing to graft failure. All 4 patients received an optimal engineered graft product. The total number of mononuclear cells, CD34$^+$ cells and CFU-GM per graft were all within the 95% confidence intervals for these graft parameters (Table 1).

As discussed previously, the use of elutriated grafts has been associated with high rates of mixed hematopoietic chimerism. While apparently not influencing the relapse rate in acute leukemia or lymphoma, it is conceivable that diseases that have strong marrow micro environmental components such as CML or MDS may require higher CD34$^+$ cell doses to establish normal hematopoiesis. Southern blot analysis of restriction fragment length polymorphisms (RFLP) or sex chromosome differences were used to evaluate hematopoietic chimerism in the 78 patients who survived beyond the peri-transplant period. There was no evidence of persistent, mixed chimerism (>20% host BM cells >60 days post-BMT). A shift to mixed chimerism from 100% donor engraftment was seen in 16 patients (20%) but 14 of these patients had documented relapse (44). The duration of CSA had no impact on mixed hematopoietic chimerism. Therefore, CD34$^+$ augmentation of elutriated grafts resulted in rapid and durable engraftment and the disappearance of mixed hematopoietic chimerism when compared to elutriation alone. Similarly, it appeared that the absolute requirement for post-BMT CSA had been abrogated. Either doubling the CD34$^+$ cell dose or the inclusion of previously discarded stem cell populations had eliminated this complication of elutriation/TCD.

Table 1. Graft Engineering Trials Conducted at Johns Hopkins (1986-1998). These results represent trials involving >450 manipulated MRD (matched related donor) grafts and a similar number of unmanipulated marrows during this time period. R/O is the TCD large cell fraction obtained following elutriation. CD34$^+$ augmented grafts also contain the concentrated CD34$^+$ cells salvaged from the lymphocyte-rich small cell elutriation fractions. CSA duration is in post-transplant days. T cells were initially measured by limiting dilution analysis and later by flow cytometry (CD3). Early graft failure and TRM (transplant related mortality) is defined as that occurring within the first 100 days post transplant. The incidence of GVHD represents all stages of acute (1-4) and chronic (limited + extensive) disease.

Engineered graft type	CD34/kg (x10^6)	CSA duration (days)	T cells/kg (x10^5)	Early Graft failure (%)	GVHD (%) (acute)	GVHD (%) (chronic)	TRM (%)
R/O: (lymphocyte adjusted)	1.5	180	5.0	10	45	11	40
R/O: (lymphocyte adjusted)	1.5	180	2.5	20	22	4	12
R/O: (lymphocyte adjusted)	1.5	0	5.0	100	NE	NE	50
R/O plus CD34+ augment	3.2	>80	5.0	4	19	11	20
R/O plus CD34+ augment	3.2	30	5.0	0	52	24	60
Unmanipulated marrow graft	4.0	180	>1000	<1	50	25	50

The impact of CSA duration on GVHD. It was uncertain whether CSA duration would influence the incidence of GVHD. With all groups combined, the overall incidence of clinically significant acute GVHD (>Stage I) for all CSA dosing schedules combined (N=104 evaluable patients) was 11% (19% grades 1-4; Table 1). This was similar to the previous elutriation studies using elutriation alone combined with 180 days of CSA (27,28). However, the overall incidence of >Stage I acute GVHD differed significantly between 30 and 80 days of CSA (p=0.002) and between 30 and 180 days of CSA (p=0.02) but there was no difference observed between 80 and 180 days (p=0.67). For this discussion, the results of CSA prophylaxis can be discussed in terms of 30 vs. >30 days duration. The incidence of >stage I acute GVHD was 23% for the CSA30 group vs. 5% (p=0.012) for those receiving >30 days of CSA (44). The incidence of chronic GVHD also approached but did not achieve statistical significance between the CSA groups. The overall incidence of chronic GVHD was higher than that observed with elutriation/CSA180 (15% vs. 6%, respectively). However, there was a 23% incidence in the CSA30 group compared to an 11% incidence in the >CSA30 group (p=0.10). More importantly, there was a significant difference between the groups in the number of patients with chronic GVHD who had prior acute GVHD (80% in the CSA30 group vs. 25% in the >CSA30 group, p=0.019). The latter observation gives support to the hypothesis that acute and chronic GVHD may be independent immune phenomena which are separable only in settings where the incidence of acute GVHD is minimal, such as the >CSA30 cohort (43,44) or regimens employing allogeneic peripheral blood stem cells.

CSA duration and morbidity. Overall post-BMT infectious complications accounted for 5% mortality for all studies combined. Peri-transplant mortality was significantly higher in the group of patients receiving 30 days of CSA prophylaxis (10% vs. 2%, p=0.013) with the excess mortality due to infection and acute GVHD. The 3 deaths from GVHD (2 from acute, 1 from chronic) also were restricted to the CSA30 group (44). Patients succumbing to infectious complications all had antecedent GVHD requiring corticosteroid therapy. The majority of these deaths were complicated by opportunistic infections (CMV, PCP, and Aspergillosis). There did not appear to be any disease-specific effect on mortality which was distributed approximately equally among the various diagnoses (AML, ALL, MDS/AML, NHL, HD, MM). The causes of mortality differed between the peri-transplant and late-transplant (>100 days post-BMT) periods. Incidence of infectious deaths was about equal. In the peri-transplant period 64% of mortality was due to veno-occlusive disease, graft failure, acute GVHD, and organ failure while in the late-transplant period 67% of mortality was due to relapse-related causes.

Age influences transplant related mortality. Younger aged adults (21-49 years of age) had lower TRM rates (16%) than the older patient (50-65 yrs) cohort did (36%, p=0.027). When the patient population was stratified at 40 years of age there was no significant difference between mortality in the two groups (15% vs. 24%, respectively; p=0.25). These data are important since only a few patients aged 40 or over were transplanted at Hopkins prior to elutriation due to high post-BMT mortality. Mortality in the late-transplant period (>100 days post-BMT) in the <50 year and >50 year age groups approached but did not achieve statistical significance at a median follow-up period of 296 days (range 3-1284 days).

Overall assessment in the matched, related setting. An unexpected benefit of these phase II studies was that the rapid engraftment, lack of significant GVHD, decreased febrile episodes, decreased blood product and antibiotic utilization, reduced GI complications and improved oral intake. These led to shorter in patient hospitalization stays (median 12 day reduction) and a concomitant 40% reduction in patient charges (45,46). This provided the impetus for performing allogeneic BMT (using engineered grafts) in an intensive ambulatory setting in carefully selected individuals; a third of whom never have a febrile episode or have an in patient admission during their initial transplant course.

It appears that the intentional inclusion of even low numbers of T cells necessitates the use of moderate post-transplant immuno-suppression (i.e. CSA) to control GVHD. However, augmenting the allograft with salvaged $CD34^+$ cells has resulted in durable engraftment that is no longer dependent on immunosuppression. These studies would indicate that at least two to three months of CSA are required to prevent excess morbidity in the post-transplant period. If additional cell populations are to be administered (i.e. $CD56^+$ NK cells, donor leukocytes) at intervals post-BMT to augment anti-tumor activity, it may be necessary to extend immunosuppressive coverage to beyond the last treatment cycle to minimize complications. The results of the above studies prompted the extension of this engineered graft approach to the matched unrelated and mismatched related setting since high complication rates have always thwarted the more wide-spread use of these modalities.

Engineering grafts in the unrelated and mismatched setting

Risks and benefits of using alternative donor grafts.
The HLA barrier still limits the utility of allogeneic BMT. The above improvements apply only to those receiving an HLA matched sibling transplant. Extension of these graft engineering techniques to alternative donor sources would significantly increase the utility of this approach. The use of matched unrelated donors (MUDs) or partially matched related donors (PMRDs) is fraught with serious obstacles. Use of these unmanipulated grafts, even with intense immunosuppression results in high morbidity and mortality from acute and chronic GVHD, opportunistic infection and even graft failure (which is rarely seen with HLA matched sibling grafts). The incidence of post-transplant B cell lymphoproliferative disorders is also increased (17). Initial studies using T cell

depletion did show a moderate decrease in the incidence of GVHD, but all of the above complications were greatly increased by marrow manipulation. Despite these problems, survivors of alternative donor transplant have high cure rates, presumably related to augmented anti-tumor effect conveyed by HLA disparity (47,48). For many patients, this may be their only option due to resistant disease and/or the lack of a fully matched sibling donor.

Elutriation/CD34$^+$ augmentation of alternative donor grafts.   Given the amplification of deleterious outcomes observed with previous TCD studies, we elected to use a similar approach to that used in the matched related donor (MRD) setting. It was hoped that an engineered graft containing a defined T cell dose and CD34$^+$ stem cell complement would overcome many of these hurdles. It would be necessary to bolster immunosuppression, but intensive, maximal therapy was avoided. The initial trial enrolled patients from 0 to 55 years of age identified with a MUD or PMRD (1 or 2 antigen mismatch). Patients received cyclophosphamide [200 mg/kg ideal body weight (IBW)] and fractionated total body irradiation (TBI, 1200 cGY), methyprednisolone starting on day –5 and slowly tapering off by day 60 and CSA from day –2 to day +180. Patients received an elutriated/CD34$^+$ augmented graft if the initial marrow harvest was ≥ 2.5 x 10^8 mononuclear cells/kg. As of June 1997, 33 patients were enrolled on this protocol (49): 27 received MUD and 6 received PRMD grafts. Only 28 patients received manipulated grafts because 5 MUD grafts did not meet harvest cell number criteria. These patients received an unmanipulated graft using the same preparative regimen along with ATG and methotrexate for additional GVHD prophylaxis. Graft characteristics were slightly different from those obtained in the MRD setting. Both the median CD34$^+$ stem cell (5.6 x 10^6/kg) and T cell (1.2 x10^6/kg) dose were higher (Table 2). All patients receiving an engineered graft had prompt and durable engraftment whereas 66% of patients who received unmanipulated marrows showed delayed engraftment, especially for platelet recovery. The incidence of GVHD was attenuated but not as low as that seen with engineered MRD grafts. The incidence of acute (>stage 1) and chronic GVHD was 9% and 9%, respectively. The incidence of GVHD did not differ between MUD and PMRD recipients or between those less than or greater than 16 years of age.

Table 2. Hopkins Experience with Engineered Grafts in the MUD/PMRD Setting.

| Graft manipulaton: | N | CD34/kg (x106) | T cells/kg (x105) | Delayed or graft failure (%) | GVHD (%)[1] | | 1 YR mortality (%) |
					Acute	Chronic	
R/O plus CD34+ augment	28	5.6	12.0	0	40	20	83%>18yrs 43%<18yrs
Unmanipulated marrow graft	5	3.0	>1000	66%	75	58	59%

These results constitute the previous high risk graft engineering trial for MUD/PMRD transplant at Hopkins which ended in mid 1998. The R/O product is the TCD large cell fraction obtained following elutriation. $CD34^+$ augmented grafts also contain the concentrated $CD34^+$ cells salvaged from the lymphocyte-rich small cell elutriation fractions. Engraftment is defined as delayed if granulocyte (>500/ul) or platelet (>50,000/ul) recovery is not achieved by days 28 and 35, respectively.

[1] Incidence of >stage 1 acute GVHD

Outcome of engineered alternative donor grafts.   The overall survival did not differ between the source of the graft. Overall and disease free survival was 44% at 5 years (Table 2). However, further inspection of the data showed an abrupt difference in survival between adults (>18 yrs) and children ($\leq$ 18 years; Figure 2). The major causes of death for all patients were GVHD, CMV disease and opportunistic infection but the majority of GVHD and infectious deaths (most likely resulting from prolonged treatment of GVHD) were in the adult cohort. It appears that the reduction in GVHD is sufficient for the younger age group while it is still deleterious for the older population. Anti-tumor effect is preserved in all groups as evidenced by a plateaued relapse rate of approximately 20%. Further modifications will be necessary to improve survival in those over age 16.

Modifications in the adult alternative donor regimen. There was concern that the lack of control over the collection of MUD grafts could have affected the separation procedures. This is no more clearly demonstrated than in the 5 MUD grafts which were used, unmodified, due to very low initial mononuclear cell numbers in the harvest. Also, increased contamination with peripheral blood (poor graft quality) could lead to increased T cell numbers in the final product. Will doubling the T cell dose have that much impact on GVHD and its attendant morbidity? Clearly, doubling the $CD34^+$ stem cell dose abrogated engraftment problems with engineered grafts. Initial elutriation trials using twice ($1x10^6$/kg) the number of lymphocytes than is currently used had acute and chronic GVHD rates (45%, 11%, respectively) comparable to unmanipulated marrow (27). The fact that this patient cohort has double the T cell number of MRD grafts may be cause for concern. We have currently adopted a more aggressive GVHD prophylaxis regimen in our adult population. It is similar to that used at the University of South Carolina for high-risk alternative donor transplants – given the unparalleled level of success with their approach. We are currently evaluating the use of an additional anti-CD2 positive selection step to more thoroughly deplete mature T cells from the $CD34^+$ graft product if the GVHD incidence and morbidity continue to be higher than in the MRD setting.

Figure 2. Alternative donor survival using engineered unrelated, or partially-matched related allografts. There is a clear long term survival advantage in patients under the age of 18 years, despite a similar incidence and severity of GVHD.

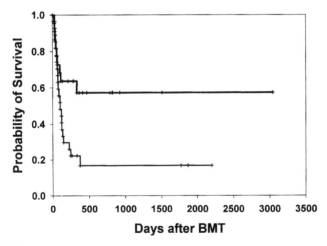

SUMMARY

A systematic approach to hematopoietic graft manipulation has minimized several of the variables inherent to allogeneic BMT. Through this approach, we have been able to significantly impact on morbidity and quality of life following allogeneic transplantation. Acute and chronic GVHD, blood product and antibiotic usage, in patient hospitalization, acuity, costs and survival (especially in patients older than

40) have been improved. The HLA barrier still presents a formidable obstacle to achieving a more widespread use of this therapy. The complications encountered in HLA matched/TCD grafts occur with even greater magnitude in the HLA-mismatched or unrelated donor setting. Several centers are now engaged in studies using TCD grafts that are augmented with high doses of CD34$^+$ cells to ensure engraftment while reducing the incidence of GVHD (50-53).

Mobilized allogeneic PBSC appear to be an excellent source of stem cells for BMT (5,6). The earlier reports showed decreased rates of GVHD, despite having T cell burdens 10 times higher than those found in unmanipulated bone marrow. However, several of these centers now report an unacceptably high incidence of chronic GVHD (along with its attendant morbidity) following allogeneic PBSC transplantation (54-55). Initial results of TCD in these PBSC grafts using CD34$^+$ selection are disappointing in that recipients developed unexpectedly high incidences of both acute and chronic GVHD (56). No doubt, significant differences exist between marrow and PBSC ancillary cell populations. For example, two laboratories now report the presence of natural suppressor cells in these allogeneic PBSC products in both mice (57) and humans (58). Thus, the same, step-wise approach would be expected to improve graft performance when using PBSC, cord blood, fetal tissue, xenografts or genetically engineered products as a stem cell source. Indeed, there are new reports of improved clinical outcome (especially in the incidence of GVHD) in the PMRD setting using both CD34$^+$ selected (59) and sequential CD34$^+$/CD2$^+$ selected (60) PBSC grafts. It is hoped that future graft engineering approaches will be as successful as previous studies and will extend this form of therapy to an even larger patient population.

ACKNOWLEDGMENTS

I wish to thank the members of the Graft Engineering Laboratory and the BMT physicians and nurses for their dedication and devotion to the patients enrolled in these studies. This work is supported in part through funding from the NIH (CA 15396, CA67787, and HL 46533).

REFERENCES

1. Santos G.W. Bone Marrow Transplantation in Hematologic Malignancies. Cancer 1990; 65:786-791.
2. Noga, S.J. and Hess, A.D. Lymphocyte Depletion in Bone Marrow Transplantation: Will Modulation of Graft-versus-Host Disease Prove to be Superior to Prevention? Seminars in Oncology 1993; 20:28-33.

3. Vogelsang, G.B. Acute and Chronic Graft-vs-Host Disease. Current Opinions in Oncology 1993; 5:276-281.
4. Vogelsang, G.B., Hess, A.D., and Santos, G.W. Acute Graft-versus-Host Disease: Clinical Characteristics in the Cyclosporine Era. Medicine 1988; 67:163-174.
5. Bensinger, W.I., Clift, R., Martin, P., Appelbaum, F.R., Demirer, T., Gooley, T., Lilleby, K., Rowley, S., Sanders, J., Storb, R., and Buckner, C.D. Allogeneic peripheral blood stem cell transplantation in patients with advanced hematologic malignancies: A retrospective comparison with marrow transplantation. Blood 1996; 88:2794-2800.
6. Schmitz, N., Dreger, P., Suttorp, M., Rohwedder, E.B., Haferlach, T., Loffler, H., Hunter, A., and Russell, N,H. Primary transplantation of allogeneic peripheral blood progenitor cells mobilized by filgrastim (granulocyte colony-stimulating factor). Blood 1995; 85:1666-1672.
7. Horowitz, M.M., Gale, R.P., Sondel, P.M., Goldman, J.M., Kersey, J., Kolb, Rimm A.A., Ringden, O., Rozman, C., Speck, B., Truitt, R.L., Zwaan, F.E., Bortin, M.M. Graft-versus-leukemia reactions after bone marrow transplantation. Blood 1990; 75:555-562.
8. Ringden O., Horowitz, M. Graft-versus-leukemia reactions in humans. Transplant Proceedings 1989; 21:2989-2992.
9. Noga, S.J. and Hess, A.D. Lymphocyte Depletion in Bone Marrow Transplantation: Will Modulation of Graft-versus-Host Disease Prove to be Superior to Prevention? Seminars in Oncology 1993; 20:28-33.
10. Filipovich, A.H., McGlave, P.B., Ramsay, N.K. Ex-vivo Treatment of Donor Bone Marrow with Monoclonal Antibody OKT3 for Prevention of Acute Graft-vs-Host Disease in Allogeneic Histocompatible Bone Marrow Transplantation. Lancet 1984; i:469-472.
11. Antin, J., Bierer, B., Smith, B., et al. Selective Depletion of Bone Marrow T Lymphocytes with Anti-CD5 Monoclonal Antibodies: Effective Prophylaxis for Graft-versus-Host Disease in Patients with Hematologic Malignancies. Blood 1991; 78:2139-2149.
12. Mitsuyasu, R.T., Champlin, R., Gale, R.P. Treatment of Donor Bone Marrow with Monoclonal Anti-T-Cell Antibody and Complement for the Prevention of Graft-Versus-Host Disease. A Prospective, Randomized, Double-Blind Trial. Annals of Internal Medicine 1986; 105:20-26.
13. Ash, R., Casper, J., Chitumbar, C., et al. Successful allogeneic transplantation of T cell depleted bone marrow from closely HLA matched unrelated donors. New England Journal of Medicine 1990; 322:485-494.
14. Butturini, A., Bortin, M.M., Seeger, R.C., Gale, R.P. In Cellular Immunotherapy of Cancer 1987, ed. J. Truitt, M. M. Bortin, and R.P. Gale, pp.371-390. New York: Alan R. Liss.

15. Martin, P.J., et al. Graft Failure in Patients Receiving T-cell-depleted HLA-identical Allogeneic Marrow Transplants. Bone Marrow Transplant 1988; 3:445-456.

16. Gaines BA, Yolonda L, Colson C, Kaufman L, Ildstad ST. Facilitating Cells Enable Engraftment of Purified Fetal Liver Stem Cells in Allogeneic Recipients. Exp Hematol 1996; 24:902-913.

17. Martin, P.J. and Kernan, N.A. T-Cell Depletion for GVHD Prevention in Humans. In Graft-vs-host disease 1997, 2nd ed., ed. Ferrara, Deeg, and Burakoff. pp. 615-637. New York: Marcel Dekker.

18. Truitt, R.L., Johnson, B.D., McCabe, C.M., and Weiler, M.B. Graft versus Leukemia. In Graft-vs-Host Disease, 2nd ed., ed. Ferrara, Deeg, and Burakoff. pp. 385-424. New York: Marcel Dekker.

19. Martin, P.J., Hansen, J.A., Storb, R. and Thomas, E.D.. Human Marrow Transplantation: An Immunological Perspective. Advances in Immunology 1987; 40: 379-438.

20. Reisner, Y., Kapoor, N., Kirkpatrick, D., Pollack, M.S., Dupont, B., Good, R.A., O'Reilly, R.J. Transplantation for acute leukaemia with HLA-A and B nonidentical parental marrow cells fractionated with soybean agglutinin and sheep red blood cells. Lancet 1981; 2:327-331.

21. Hale, G., Cobbold, S., Waldmann, H. T cell depletion with CAMPATH-1 in allogeneic bone marrow transplantation. Transplantation 1988; 45:753-759.

22. Noga, S.J. Graft Engineering: The Evolution of Hematopoietic Transplantation. Journal of Hematotherapy 1992; 1:3-17.

23. Noga, S. J., Donnenberg, A. D., Schwartz, C. L., Strauss, L. C., Civin, C. I., and Santos, G. W. Development of a Simplified Counterflow Centrifugation-Elutriation Procedure for Depletion of Lymphocytes from Human Bone Marrow. Transplantation 1986; 41(2):220-229.

24. Noga, S. J. Elutriation: New Technology for Separation of Blood and Bone Marrow. Lab Medicine. 19(4): 234-239.

25. Kauffman, M.G., Noga, S.J., Kelly, T.J., and Donnenberg, A.D. Isolation of Cell Cycle Fractions by Counterflow Centrifugal Elutriation. Analytical Biochemistry. 1990; 191:41-46.

26. Wagner, J.E., Donnenberg, A.D., Noga, S.J., Cremo, C.A., Gao, I.K., Yin, H.J., Vogelsang, G.B., Rowley, S.D., Saral, R., Santos, G.W. Lymphocyte Depletion of Donor Bone Marrow by Counterflow Centrifugal Elutriation: Results of a Phase I Clinical Trial. Blood 1988; 72(4):1168-1176.

27. Wagner, J.E., Santos, G.W., Noga, S.J., Rowley, S.D., Davis, J., Vogelsang, G.B., Farmer, E.R., Zehnbauer, B.A., Saral R., and Donnenberg, A.D. Bone Marrow Graft Engineering by Counterflow Centrifugal Elutriation: Results of a Phase I-II Clinical Trial. Blood 1990; 75(6):1370-1377.

28. Noga, S.J., Wagner, J.E., Rowley, S.D., Davis, J.M., Vogelsang, G.B., Hess, A.D., Saral, R., Santos, G.W, Donnenberg, A.D. Using Elutriation to Engineer Bone Marrow Allografts. Prog Clin Biol Res 1990; 333:345-361.
29. Noga, S.J., Wagner, J.E., Santos, G.W., and Donnenberg, A.D. Allograft Lymphocyte-Dose Modification with Counterflow Centrifugal Elutriation (CCE): Effects on Chronic GVHD and Survival in a Case/Control Study. In 33rd Annual ASH Meeting 1991, Denver.
30. Noga, S.J., Vogelsang, G.B., and Santos, G.W.. Allograft Lymphocyte Dose Modification (LDM) Prevents GVHD Without Compromising GVL Following BMT for Acute Leukemia. In 34th Annual ASH Meeting, 1992. Annaheim.
31. Wagner, J.E., Zahurak, M., Piantadosi, S., et. al. Bone marrow transplantation of chronic myelogenous leukemia in chronic phase: Evaluation of risks and benefits. Journal of Clinical Oncology 1992; 10:779-789.
32. Flinn, I., Orentas, R., Noga, S.J., Marcellus, D., Vogelsang, G.B., Jones, R.J., and Ambinder, R.F. Low Risk of Epstein-Barr Virus (EBV)-Associated Post-Transplant Lymphoproliferative Disease (PTLD) in Patients Receiving Elutriated Allogeneic Marrow Transplants may Reflect Depletion of EBV Infected Lymphocytes from the Graft. Blood 1995; 86(10):626a.
33. Schattenberg A, De Witte T, Salden M, et al. Mixed hematopoietic chimerism after allogeneic transplantation with lymphocyte-depleted bone marrow is not associated with a higher incidence of relapse. Blood 1989; 73:1367-1372.
34. Wagner, J.E., Donnenberg, A.D., Noga, S.J., Rowley, S.D., and Santos, G.W. The Role of Post-Transplant Cyclosporine A (CsA) Immunosuppressive Therapy on Engraftment of Lymphocyte Depleted Bone Marrow. In 30th Annual ASH Meeting 1988. San Antonio.
35. Jones, R.J., Wagner, J.E., Celano, P., Zicha, M.S. and Sharkis, S.J.. Separation of pluripotent haematopoietic stem cells from spleen colony-forming cells (CFU-S). Nature 1990; 347:188-189.
36. Noga, S.J., Davis, J.M., Schepers, K., Eby, L., and Berenson, R.J. The Clinical Use of Elutriation and Positive Stem Cell Selecton Columns To Engineer the Lymphocyte and Stem Cell Composition of the Allograft. Prog. Clin. & Biol. Res 1994; 392:317-324.
37. Reisner, Y., Martelli, M.F., and Lustig, E. Stem Cell Dose Increase Offers New Possibilities for BMT Across Major Histo-compatibility Barriers in Lethally and Sublethally Irradiated Recipients. Blood 1994; 84:346a.
38. DeWitte, T., Hoogenhout, J., De Pauw, B., Joldrinet, R., Janssen, J., Wessels, J., Van Daal, W., Justinx, T. and Haanen, C.. Depletion of Donor Lymphocytes by Counterflow Centrifugation Successfully Prevents Acute Graft-Vs-Host Disease in Matched Allogeneic Marrow Transplantation. Blood 1986; 67:1302.

39. Berenson, R.J., Shpall, E.J., Auditore-Hargreaves, K., Heimfeld, S., Jacobs, C., Krieger, M.S. Transplantation of CD34$^+$ Hematopoietic Progenitor Cells. Cancer Investigation 1996; 14(6):589-596.

40. Civin, C.I., Trishmann, T., Kadan, N.S., Davis, J. Noga, S., Cohen, K., Duffy, B., Groenewegen, I., Wiley, J., Law, P., Hardwick, A., Oldham, F., and Gee, A. Purified CD34-Positive Cells Reconstitute Hematopoiesis. Journal of Clinical Oncology 1996; (8):2224-2233.

41. Noga, S.J. and Civin, C.I. Positive Stem Cell Selection of Hematopoietic Grafts for Transplantation. In Graft-vs-Host Disease 1996; 2nd ed., ed. J. Ferrara, H. Deeg, and S. Burakoff, pp. 717-731. New York: Marcel Dekker.

42. Noga, S.J., Seber, A., Davis, J.M., Berenson, R.J., Vogelsang, G.B., Braine, H.G., Hess, A.D., Marcellus, D., Miller, C.A., Sharkis, S.J., Goodman, S.N., Santos, G.W., and Jones, R.J. CD34 Augmentation Improves Allogeneic T Cell Depleted Bone Marrow Engraftment. Journal Hematotherapy 1998; 7(2):151-157.

43. Noga, S.J., Vogelsang, G.B., Seber, A., Davis, J.M., Schepers, K., Hess, A.D., and Jones, R.J. CD34$^+$ Stem Cell Augmentation of Allogeneic, Elutriated Marrow Grafts improves Engraftment but Cyclosporine A (CSA) is Still Required to Reduce GVHD and Morbidity. Transplant Proceedings 1997; 29(1-2):728-732.

44. O'Donnell PV, Jones RJ, Vogelsang GB, Seber A, Ambinder RF, Flinn I, Miller CA, Marcellus DC, Griffin C, Abrams R, Braine HG, Grever M, Hess AD, Piantadosi S, Noga SJ. CD34$^+$ Stem Cell Augmentation of Elutriated, Allogeneic Bone Marrow Grafts: Results of a Phase II Clinical Trial of Engraftment and Graft-Versus-Host Disease Prophylaxis in High Risk Hematologic Malignancies. BMT 1998; 22(10): 947-955.

45. Noga, S.J., Berenson, R.J., Davis, J.M., Hess, A.D., Braine, H.G., Vogelsang, G.B., Miller, C.A., Jones, R.J. CD34$^+$ Stem Cell Augmentation of T Cell Depleted Allografts Reduces Engraftment Time, GVHD, and Length of Hospitalization. British Journal of Hematology 1994; 87:41a.

46. Noga, S., Miller, C, Berenson, R. Braine, H., Sproul, J., Jones, R. Combined Use of CD34$^+$ Stem Cell Augmentation and Elutriation Reduces the Morbidity and Cost of Allogeneic Bone Marrow Transplantation. American Society of Clinical Oncology 1994; 13:309a.

47. Henslee-Downey PJ, Abhyankar SH, Parrish RS et al. Use of Partially Mismatched Related Donors Extends Access to Allogeneic Marrow Transplant. Blood 1997; 89:3864-3872.

48. Beatty PG, Hansen JA, Thomas ED, et al. Marrow transplantation from unrelated donors for treatment of hematologic malignancies: effect of mismatching for one HLA locus. Blood 1993; 81:249-253.

49. Noga SJ. To TCD or not to TCD? Presented at the BMT in Children Symposium, June 1998, Palm Beach, Fl.

50. Reisner, Y., Martelli, M.F., and Lusting, E. Stem cell dose increase offers new possibilities for BMT across major histocompatibility barriers in lethally and sublethally irradiated recipients. Blood 1994; 84:346a.

51. Friedrich W, Muller S, Schreiner T, et al. The Combined Use of Positively Selected, T-Cell Depleted Blood and Bone Marrow Stem Cells in HLA Non-Identical Bone Marrow Transplantation in Childhood Leukemia. Experimental Hematology. 1995; 23:854a.

52. Yeager, A.M., Holland, H.K., Mogul, M.J., Forte, K., Lauer, M., Boyer, M.W., Turner, C.W., Vega, R.A., Beatty, P.G., Jacobs, C.A., Benyunes, M.C., and Wingard, J.R. Transplantation of Positively Selected CD34$^+$ Cells from Haploidentical Parental Donors for Relapsed Acute Leukemia in Children. Blood 1995; 86(10):291a.

53. Bacigalupo, A., Mordini, N., Pitto, A., Piaggio, G., and Podesta, M. CD34$^+$ Selected Stem Cell Transplants in Patients with Advanced Leukemia from 3 Loci Mismatched Family Donors. Blood 1995; 86(10):937a.

54. Korbling M, Przepiorka D, Engel H, et al. Allogeneic Blood Stem Cell Transplantation (Allo-PBSCT) in 9 Patients with Refractory Leukemia and Lymphoma: Potential Advantage of Blood over Marrow Allografts. Blood 1994; 84:396.

55. Link H, Arseniev L, Bahre O, et al. Transplantation of Allogeneic Peripheral Blood and Bone Marrow CD34$^+$ Cells after Immunoselection. Experimental Hematology 1995; 23:855a.

56. Bensinger WI, Buckner CD, Shannon-Dorcy K, Rowley S, Appelbaum FR, Benyunes M, Clift R, Martin P, Demirer T, Storb R, LeeM, Schiller G: Transplantation of Allogeneic CD34$^+$ Peripheral Blood Stem Cells in Patients with Advanced Hematologic Malignancy. Blood 1996; 88:4132-4138.

57. Strober S. T cells, GVHD, and Allogeneic Peripheral Blood Progenitor Cell Transplantation. Proceedings 5th International Symposium on Recent Advances in Hematopoietic Stem Cell Transplantation – Clinical Progress, New Technology and Gene Therapy: 119-120, San Diego, CA, 1997.

58. Kusnierz-Glaz CR, Still BJ, Amano M, Zukor JD, Negrin RS, Blume KG, Strober S. G-CSF-induced co-mobilization of CD4$^-$CD8$^-$ T cells and Hematopoietic Progenitor Cells (CD34$^+$) in the Blood of Normal Donors. Blood 1998; 89(7): 2586-2595.

59. Takaue Y, Kawano Y, Watanabe T. Autologous and Allogeneic Transplantation with Blood CD34$^+$ cells: a Pediatric Experience. In: Hematopoietic Stem Cell Therapy. Champlin R, Palsson B, Ho AD (eds), Cambridge University Press, London, in press, 1998.

60. Yeager AM, Amylon M, Wagner J. Allogeneic Stem Cell Transplantation from HLA-Haploidentical Relatives as Treatment for Children with Hematologic Malignancy: a Phase I/II Study Using Mobilized Peripheral Blood Progenitor Cells (PBSCs) that have Undergone CD34 Selection Followed by CD2 Depletion. Blood 1997; 90 (suppl 1):217a.

15

MONOCLONAL ANTIBODY AND RECEPTOR ANTAGONIST THERAPY FOR GVHD

James L.M. Ferrara, M.D.
University of Michigan Cancer Center, Ann Arbor, MI 48109
Ernst Holler, M.D.
Regensberg University Hospital, Regensburg, Germany, D93042
Bruce Blazar, M.D.
University of Minnesota, Minneapolis, MN 55455

INFLAMMATORY CYTOKINES IN GVHD: PATHOPHYSIOLOGY

Recent experimental evidence suggests that dysregulation of complex cytokine networks occurring in three sequential steps is responsible for many of the systemic manifestations of acute graft versus host disease (GVHD) (Figure 1). The first step of GVHD pathophysiology begins with the transplant conditioning regimen, which in clinical BMT includes total body irradiation (TBI) and/or chemotherapy. The conditioning is an important variable in the pathogenesis of acute GVHD because it damages and activates host tissues, including intestinal mucosa, liver and skin. Activated host cells then secrete inflammatory cytokines, e.g. tumor necrosis factor (TNF-α) and IL-1. The presence of inflammatory cytokines during this phase may upregulate adhesion molecules and MHC antigens by mature donor T cells in the second step of acute GVHD. This inflammatory context helps to explain the observation that enhanced risk of GVHD after clinical BMT is associated with certain intensive conditioning regimens that cause extensive injury to epithelial and endothelial surfaces and the subsequent release of inflammatory cytokines.

During the second step of acute GVHD, donor T cells proliferate and secrete IL-2 and IFN-γ (Th1 cytokines) in response to host alloantigens. During autologous BMT, donor and recipient are the same, and thus no allospecific T cell activation occurs. Th1 cytokines play a central role in the expansion of donor T cells and the activation of other effector cells such as large granular lymphocytes (LGLs) and natural killer (NK) cells. LGLs, NK cells and monocyte/macrophages appear to be prominent in the effector arm of GVHD and may contribute to the pathological damage, i.e. induce the changes of GVH *disease* following the T cell mediated GVH *reaction*. The initial hypothesis that the cytolytic function of lymphocytes directly causes the majority of tissue damage and necrosis has been modified and may be more appropriately restricted to specific target organs, e.g. the liver.

Figure 1. GVHD Pathophysiology

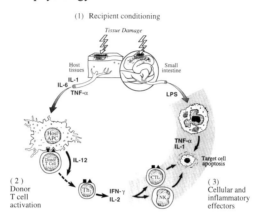

During the step three of acute GVHD physiology, increased secretion of the inflammatory cytokines TNF-α and IL-1 mononuclear phagocytes – which had been primed with Th1 cytokines during step two, occurs after triggering by a secondary stimulus which may be provided by lipopolysaccharide (LPS or endotoxin). LPS can leak through the intestinal mucosa damaged by the conditioning regimen and subsequently stimulate gut-associated lymphocytes and macrophages. LPS reaching skin tissues may also stimulate kertinocytes, dermal fibroblasts and macrophages to produce similar cytokines in the dermis and programmed cell death pathway. TNF-α mediated apoptosis may be particularly important in acute GVHD of the intestine. In addition to these preinflammatory cytokines, excess nitric oxide produced by activated macrophages may contribute to the deleterious effects on GVHD target tissues, particularly immunosuppression. Induction of inflammatory cytokines may thus synergize with the lytic component of GVHD provided by CTL and NK cells, resulting in the amplification of local tissue injury and further promotion of an inflammatory response which ultimately leads to the observed target tissue destruction in the BMT host. Blockage of these cytokines, either directly or indirectly, thus becomes an attractive therapeutic strategy.

The proteins, tumor necrosis factor alpha (TNF-α) and interleukin-1 (IL-1), are secreted during inflammatory processes of natural or "innate" immunity to infectious microbes or other foreign proteins. The cellular sources of TNF-α and IL-1 are often, but not always, mononuclear cells, and an abundance of cell types are known to produce them. These proteins are also produced during processes of acquired immunity, thus enhancing natural immunity; they often have synergistic, pleiotropic, and occasional redundant effects on target cells, activating lymphocytes as well as performing certain effector functions. TNF-α was originally described as a protein produced after activation of macrophages following lipopolysaccharide (LPS) stimulation and which induced hemorrhagic necrosis of transplantable murine sarcomas (1). TNF-α is now known to be a critical proinflammatory cytokine capable of mediating the deleterious effects of severe infectious complications such as septic shock (2,3). It is central to proinflammatory responses that result in a wide variety of systemic effects, including fever, acute phase responses, hematopoietic growth factor production, activation of endothelial cells and the destruction of epithelial cells and kertinocytes (4-6). These direct effects are accompanied by increased expression of a variety of molecules critical to immune responses such as intercellular adhesion molecules (ICAMs) and HLA class I antigens on epithelial and endothelial cells (5,6). Furthermore, a costimulatory role for TNF-α in activation of cytotoxic T cells has been reported (7).

IL-1 shares multiple proinflammatory properties with TNF-α (2), making both monokines candidates for involvement in the pathophysiology of BMT related complications. IL-1 is a polypeptide with two isoforms, IL-1α and IL-1β. IL-1 was first described as "endogeneous pyrogen" and was later shown to be a lymphocyte stimulating factor. Endotoxin is the most important known stimulus for IL-1 production, and approximately 5 molecules per lymphocyte is sufficient to stimulate IL-1 mRNA transcription. Recent studies suggest that cells undergoing apoptosis or programmed cell death produce IL-1 more efficiently (8) and IL-1 appears to be important in the regulation of apoptosis. Over-expression of IL-1 converting enzyme (ICE) induces apoptosis in cell lines (9) and ICE-deficient mice are resistant to apoptosis through the Fas pathway (10,199). IL-1 and TNF-α appear to be linked in this pathway because the Fas antigen (CD95) is a cell-surface protein with high homology to the TNF-α receptor (12,13).

Endotoxin is a principal inducer of inflammatory cytokines, and stimulation of TNF-α and IL-1 by endotoxin is the most likely explanation for the well-known role of bacterial microflora in development of GVHD. Sensitivity to endotoxin and its ability to trigger release of TNF-α are greatly enhanced in mice with GVHD, and this priming is predominantly due to the costimulatory role of IFNγ in the setting of BMT is the result of activation of donor Th1 cells, which occurs subsequent to the recognition of alloantigens. A second mechanism of IFNγ induction involves viral infections such as cytomegalovirus (15,16), a pathway that is of great potential significance in the context of BMT. Reproducible increases of IFNγ serum levels have also been noted during pre-transplant conditioning by Niederwieser et al (16). There is also increasing evidence for induction of inflammatory cytokines by cytotoxic drugs and ionizing irradiation. Induction of TNF-α mRNA had been demonstrated in cultures of human sarcoma cells (17) and in myeloid cell lines as well as normal monocytes/macrophages (18,19). In these systems, doses as low as 2 Gy induce TNF-α mRNA after 1 hour and reached a maximum after 3 hours. Clinically, increases of serum TNF-α and soluble TNF-receptor p55 (sTNF-R p55) have been observed following total body irradiation (TBI) with fractions of 4 Gy in patients prepared for allogeneic BMT (20). Both TNF-α and Interleukin 6 (IL-6) are released after a single TBI dose of 10 Gy (21). In an experimental SCID model, pretransplant conditioning induced systemic TNF-α within four hours of TBI. IL-1α levels increased slightly later, peaking at 72 hours (22). Systemic cytokine release was accompanied by increased expression of both TNF-α, and, subsequently, IL-6 in colonic tissue. These results have been independently confirmed in other experimental models, where IL-1α mRNA was induced 100-fold in the spleens of mice one week after receiving either syngeneic or allogeneic BMT; IL-1α production then returned to normal in syngeneic (but not allogeneic) BMT recipients (23). Although experimental data on cytokine induction by cytotoxic drugs that are used for pretransplant conditioning are rare, significant induction seems likely. While only minimal amounts of systemic and tissue expression of TNF-α and IL-1α were detected in mice conditioned by bulsulphan/cyclophosphamide regimens, large increases in TNF-α serum levels have been seen in patients receiving CVB (Cyclophosphamide, Etoposide, BCNU) conditioning prior to autologous BMT, suggestive that at least this combination chemotherapy can cause TNF-α release (see below). Cyclophosphamide alone is known to trigger TNF-α release from normal mononuclear cells in vitro (24).

Parallel to the heterogeneity of mechanisms resulting in the release of inflammatory cytokines, a vast number of cellular sources may be involved in this process. Donor monocytes and, to a lesser extent, donor CD4[+] T cells can produce TNF-α. Host macrophages are also candidate sources of TNF-α (25). Organs such as the lung and the liver (with significant populations of alveolar macrophages and Kupffer cells, respectively) are likely to be important producers of systemic cytokines. The concept of macrophage-derived production of cytokines might also help to explain the causal relationship between pretransplant risk factors and post-transplant complications, because macrophages have a half-life of about 2 to 3 months and are only slowly replaced by donor monocytes (26,27). In patients with chronic myeloid leukemia (CML), tissue macrophages may be a source of cytokine dysregulation throughout the period of acute GVHD. Other cells capable of TNF-α production are NK cells and keratinocytes (28). Mast cells have also recently been recognized as potent reservoirs of performed TNF-α, which can be released rapidly during the process of degranulation; these cells are thus ideal candidates for initiation of an inflammatory cascade without prior de novo synthesis of cytokines (29,30).

Mixed lymphocyte cultures are thought to represent in vitro models of host-vs. - graft and graft-vs.-host reactions, but MLC reactivity does not generally correlate with the incidence and severity of GVHD (J. Hansen, personal communication). Nevertheless, in many centers MLCs are used in the selection of suitable donors in allogeneic BMT. In a study of HLA-disparate MLCs, Dickinson used MLC supernatants to induce GVHD histology in skin explant assays (31). In these experiments, histological severity of GVHD was significantly associated with the amount of TNF-α and IFNγ (31). Thus, in a simplified model of GVHD in vitro, TNF-α is not merely an index of cellular activation but is also a direct mediator of target organ pathology.

Convincing data regarding a direct pathophysiological role of TNF-α were first presented by Piguet in 1987 (33). In a P → F1 model of MHC-incompatible BMT, lethally irradiated mice were injected with bone marrow and lymph node T cells. The observed skin and gut lesions of acute GVHD as well as weight loss (a systemic indicator of GVHD) were significantly prevented by weekly administration (day +7 to day +35) of a polyclonal antibody that neutralized TNF-α (33,34). Since that time, several investigators have confirmed Piguet's observations (30,35-37). In different models of acute GVHD, administration of TNF-α antibodies starting either after BMT or from day +7 have reduced the mortality from GVHD and its associated signs, including immunosuppression and mast cell degranulation. In most of these studies, antibodies neutralizing TNF-α were less effective than the use of a T cell-depleted bone marrow in preventing GVHD (30, 33, 35-37). In one study, the protective effects of anti TNF-antibodies seemed to be restricted to acute GVHD (30). It should be noted that in some studies, expression of TNF-α was less pronounced than the expression of IL-1 or IFNγ, demonstrating that TNF-α is but one important cytokine among several that are dysregulated (38, 39).

Convincing data regarding a direct role for IL-1 in GVHD were published by Abyankhar et al (23). Using a well-described mouse model of GVHD to minor histocompatibility antigens in a BMT model, mRNA for IL-1, IL-2, and TNF-α were evaluated after transplant by a semi-quantitative RT-PCR technique. In the spleen, IL-1α levels were increased almost two orders of magnitude the first week after transplant in both the spleen and the skin. One month after transplant, when GVHD was clinically apparent, IL-1α mRNA levels were 600-fold higher. Administration of IL-1 receptor antagonist from day +10 to day +20 after transplant significantly increased survival from approximately 20% to 80%. Thus, IL-1α appears to be a critical effector molecule in this experimental model of acute GVHD.

The observation of systemic inflammatory cytokine release during pretransplant conditioning and its correlation with poor outcome following BMT in clinical studies (see below) suggest that release of inflammatory cytokines before the transplant might increase activation of donor T cells, perhaps by upregulating HLA and adhesion molecules on epithelial and endothelial targets (5, 6). To explore the pathophysiological relevance of this pathway in an experimental model, a P $\rightarrow$ F1 mouse system was investigated giving only two injections of a polyclonal neutralizing TNF-α antibody prior to irradiation BMT. Using a low dose of donor T cells for induction of GVHD, this approach was as effective in prevention of mortality and weight loss. The role of conditioning-related release of TNF-α in the induction of GVHD was elegantly confirmed in a study by Xun and his colleagues (22). In this study, lethal, acute GVHD was prevented by prolonging the interval between TBI and BMT for at least four days, i.e., to a time when conditioning-related TNF-α levels had declined. Injection of the soluble rhuTNFR:Fc, an engineered TNF-α-antagonist made by linking two soluble TNF-receptors (p80) with the Fc portion of human IgG1, resulted in a comparable protection from GVHD without any interval between TBI and BMT. It should be noted, however, that neither of these approaches completely eliminated acute GVHD, nor did the use of a less aggressive conditioning regimen with busulfan and cytoxan.

The importance of timing between the conditioning regimen and the injection of donor cells has been confirmed by several independent laboratories, including an analysis of a murine model of GVHD using cyclophosphamide alone (40). The role of pretransplant conditioning, especially ionizing irradiation, in the induction of GVHD is also supported by the clinical observation of intensified GVHD lesions in irradiated areas (41). This mechanism has been confirmed by experimental studies where GVHD histology occurred primarily in murine skin that had been irradiated and transplanted prior to the induction of GVHD in the recipients (42).

Chronic GVHD has been observed in experimental models where acute GVHD is prevented with anti-TNF-α, suggesting that early release of TNF-α and conditioning-related tissue damage accelerate and amplify acute GVHD but are not relevant to the induction of chronic GVHD. This dichotomy implies that

336

prophylactic neutralization of inflammatory cytokines will not be able to induce tolerance to host antigens, a fact only one study has documented TNF-α expression in a murine model of chronic GVHD (38). In this report, TNF-α mRNA expression was not increased, IFNγ was suppressed, and IL-4 was over-expressed in splenocytes, suggesting a shift towards a Th2 profile in chronic GVHD. These results would suggest that the proinflammatory cascade (IFNγ -> TNF-α) does not operate during the pathophysiology of chronic GVHD, but further studies are needed.

A review of the published data on systemic TNF-α levels during the first three months following BMT clearly demonstrates that TNF-α serum levels are increased in patients not only developing acute GVHD, but those experiencing acute endothelial complications such as VOD or capillary leakage syndrome (43-45). This association of elevated TNF-α levels with a variety of pathological conditions, as well as its wide range of normal values, has so far precluded its use as an independent diagnostic parameter for acute GVHD. We have shown that a close correlation exists between acute GVHD and elevated sTNFR p55 levels (46) (Table 1). The shedding of soluble receptors subsequent to induction of TNF-α has been reported for a variety of clinical conditions; in the future, sTNFR levels might prove to be a more suitable and sensitive approach for clinical monitoring, because soluble receptors are more stable than native cytokines and circulate in normal individuals with significant (nanogram) levels, which may facilitate the detection of minor shifts in their concentrations.

A second and more precise approach to predictive assays may be the analysis of cytokine production by peripheral blood mononuclear cells (PBMC). Quantitative data can be obtained by evaluation of cytokine expression using either immunodetection of intracytoplasmatic cytokine protein (47) or PCR analysis of cytokine mRNA (23, 45). Such techniques have shown increased expression of both TNF-α and IL-1 in patients with GVHD. It should be noted that PBMC analysis presumes that peripheral circulating cells are relevant to the pathophysiology of acute GVHD; other critical cell populations, such as tissue macrophages or endothelial cells, may be major producers of relevant cytokines but may be inaccessible to analysis. Detailed correlations of serum or PBMC cytokines levels with tissue cytokine expression are therefore needed.

One of the most important findings in studies regarding the systemic release of TNF-α is the strong correlation between the time of first elevated levels of TNF-α and the occurrence of transplant-related complications (TRC) (48). In an update of studies in Munich, 222 patients receiving either allogeneic related donor (n= 161), unrelated donor (n= 34) or autologous BMT (n= 35) have been analyzed for daily serum TNF-α levels starting from admission until day +10 after BMT. Patients receiving HLA-identical sibling donor BMT are divided into 4 subgroups: 1) patients with increased TNF-α serum levels prior to treatment and without any clinical symptoms of "chronic" cytokine release (as previously described) (49); 2) patients with low levels prior to chemotherapy and an acute increase during pretransplant conditioning; 3) patients with acute release observed between the day +1 and day +10 following BMT; and 4) patients without any pathological TNF-α serum levels prior to day +10 after BMT. Patients with de novo release of TNF-α (group 2) have an extremely poor prognosis due to occurrence of severe treatment related complications (TRC) including acute GVHD. Their outcome is significantly worse when release of TNF-α occurs during pretransplant conditioning, indicating that host-derived cytokine release is important to the induction of GVHD.

Table 1. Maximal release of TNF-α soluble TNF-receptor p55 (sTNFR p55) in sequential serum samples obtained between day 0 and day +100 following BMT (Mean± SEM, pg/ml). TNFα was determined by ELISA. Patients were grouped according to the type of BMT and occurrence or absence of complications. Maximal levels between groups were compared by Wilcoxon tests; both TNFα and sTNFR were significantly elevated in patients with GVHD grade II (p<0.01). TNFα levels in frozen control samples (n=20) were 28 ± 36 pg/ml, sTNFR p55 levels 3000 ± 300pg/ml. TNFα levels in fresh control samples (n=30) were 48 ± 20pg/ml.

BMT Type	Autologous	Allogeneic			
complication	__	a GVHD grade 0-I	aGVHD grade II	aGVHD grade III/IV	VOD/ Capillary Leak
TNFα (cryo)	30 (46) n=4	50 (11) n=21	97 (36) n=8	326 (152) n=17	726 (360) n=6
TNFα (fresh)	111 (28) n=14	181 (48) n=13	365 (80) n=11	477 (103) n=14	554 (161) n=13
sTNFR p55	5,500 (1,800) n=5	4,100 (1,200) n=9	8,500 (2,400) n=12	14,300 (5,700) n=11	26,400 (10,800) n=6

A still puzzling observation is the extremely low incidence of TRC in patients with "chronic" release of TNF-α (group 1). Increased serum levels in these patients correlate with increased spontaneous production of TNF-α by PBMC in culture. Unique features of this subgroup are its low incidence of GVHD and the absence of disease correlations to stage, age or previous infectious complications, implying existence of some intrinsic or even genetically fixed mechanisms responsible for the increased production of TNF-α. Analyses of polymorphisms within the TNF-α gene are presently being performed to investigate this hypothesis. In thalassemia patients, a subgroup with high TNF-α levels prior to BMT has also been observed; although there was some correlation of TNF-α level with liver fibrosis, there is a stronger association with HLA-DQw1, suggesting a mechanism of genetically fixed cytokine dysregulation (51). In spite of the small numbers of patients with spontaneous TNF-α release, further evaluation of this group may lead to important insights regarding mechanisms of cytokine mediated damage. For example, chronic TNF-α secretion may lead to desensitization to TNF-α, or other cytokines may be simultaneously induced in this network that have protective effects. Recently, Tan and colleagues have identified a novel factor produced by Th1 T cell clones that protects NOD mice from the development of diabetes (52). In addition, polymorphisms of the TNF-α gene and promoter region have been found to correlate with increased TNF-α production in heart transplant recipients (53). Further insights into regulation of cytokine networks and their impact on disease could lead to therapeutic interventions and provide an alternative approach to the prevention of TRC in the future.

Correlation of conditioning-related release of TNF-α and BMT outcome has now been observed in a Swedish study (54).

Experimental findings from several laboratories confirm murine studies reported by Xun (22) and Lehnert (40). Although the murine models have shown an almost exclusive role for TBI in the induction of excess TNF-α, comparison of conditioning regimens in patients in Munich have not yet shown a significantly higher incidence of TNF-α release in those receiving TBI-CY regimens (23% TNF-α release during conditioning, 24% between day +1 and day +10) compared to BUCY regimens (16% TNF-α release during conditioning, 15% between day +1 and +10). These data already suggest occurrence of some cytokine release during non-TBI-containing regimens, but a more detailed analysis allowing identification of responsible cytotoxic agents is not yet available. Recently, this issue was clarified by analyzing circadin kinetcs of TNF-anti-TNF-complexes in patients receiving monoclonal anti-TNF-α throughout conditioning (55). In these patients, binding of TNF-α to circulating antibody facilitated detection of TNF-α production during both TBI/CY and BU/CY conditioning regimens. In TBI/CY-treated patients, every single dose of TBI (as well as every dose of CY) was followed by an increase of TNF-anti-TNF-complexes; in BU/CY-treated patients, only CY induced significant peaks. In contrast, oral application of BU had no effect on levels of these complexes. These data clearly indicated TNF-α is induced by both TBI and CY in vivo, confirming that cytokine release is not restricted to TBI in humans. As already discussed, the concept of chemotherapy induced cytokine release is further supported by analysis of patients receiving autologous BMT following CVB-conditioning, where 8/35 patients showed significant release of TNF-α during the course of conditioning. Even in autologous BMT, transplant related mortality was increased (37.5% versus7.4% in patients with or without TNF-α release, respectively) which was mainly due to pulmonary complications.

Some clinical risk factors predisposing to acute release of TNF-α during the course of conditioning have been identified (36). Increases of TNF-α levels were significantly (p<0.001) correlated with a diagnosis of CML or myelodysplastic syndrome. Fever or skin exanthems during conditioning were strongly associated (p<0.001) with TNF-α release; in addition, failure of gastrointestinal decontamination, as indicated by the presence of pathological stool specimens on the day of BMT was also associated with acute release of TNF-α (p<0.05). Interestingly, these risk factors mirror the concept of three of the major mechanisms involved in host-associated cytokine dysregulation: pretransplant conditioning itself, underlying disease, and translocation of bacteria from a damaged intestinal mucosa.

CLINICAL USE OF ANTAGONISTS OF INFLAMMATORY CYTOKINES

Corticosteroid

When discussing the use of specific cytokine antagonists for the treatment and prevention of acute GVHD, it should be remembered that corticosteroids, which are still the treatment of choice in first line treatment of acute GVHD exhibit potent and broad cytokine antagonism. There is increasing evidence that corticosteroids act via suppression of cytokine gene activation rather than by cytoxicity (56). Antibodies directed against cytokines or T cells or IL-2 receptor have been helpful in corticosteroid resistant acute GVHD. In a French trial (58), BC7, a complete murine IgG1 Mab, was given to 19 patients with grade III or IV acute GVHD over a period of 8-12 days in addition to baseline immunosuppression that included cyclosporine and corticosteroids. Eight patients achieved a very good partial response (42.1%) and further six patients had a partial response (31.5%) while five patients (26.3%) had no response. Skin (61%) and gut (72%) lesions responded better than liver lesions (38.5%). In 9/11 evaluable responding patients acute GVHD recurred after cessation of BC7 treatment; two patients became long-term survivors.

A German trial used Mab 195F(ab)$_2$-fragment of a murine IgG3 antibody with a high capacity for neutralization of human TNF-α in five patients with advanced acute GVHD (59). Again, symptoms of GVHD improved quite rapidly in 4 of these 5 patients with a skin response in 4/4 and a liver and gut response in 3/4 (60). As observed with Mab BC7, signs of GVHD recurred after cessation of treatment Mabs were safe and did not result in an increased incidence of infections or hematopoietic side effects. These were the first clinical studies to demonstrate the involvement of TNF-α not only as an indicator, but also as an effector molecule of acute GVHD in skin and gut lesions and, to a lesser extent, in liver lesions. However, due to rapid recurrence of GVHD symptoms in the majority of patients, they also clearly indicated that established GVHD will not resolve with short-term treatment of anti-TNF-α alone.

Table 2. Combined treatment of refractory acute GVHD with OKT3 (5mg/d) and TNF-antagonists (7 day course).

Treatment regimen	fever > 39°C after 1st dose OKT3	dyspnea after 1st dose of OKT3	CR/PR of acute GVHD at day +14	4 month survival
OKT3 + Pred.	8 / 8	6 / 8	5 / 8	3 / 8
OKT3 + PTX	4 / 7	2 / 7	6 / 7	3 / 7
OKT3 + Mab195	2 / 7	1 / 7	6 / 7	4/7

Pred.=prednisolone 4mg/kg/day; PTX=pentoxifylline 2100mg/day + low dose prednisolone (<3mg/kg); Mab195F=monoclonal antibody, which neutralizes TNFα (d1-3:3x1mg/kg, d4-7: 1x1mg/kg) + low dose prednisolone (<3mg/kg)

Combined treatment of refractory acute GVHD using a seven day course of daily injections of Mab 195F and OKT3® (n=7), OKT3® and pentoxifylline (PTX) (in a daily continuous infusion (n=7)), or OKT3® and high-dose corticosteroids (n=8) has also been investigated. Combination of OKT3® with Mab195F not only resulted in improvement of acute responses and intermediate survival but also proved to be very effective with regard to prevention of the cytokine release syndrome associated with the first dose of OKT3® (Table 2). Alternative approaches, such as combining anti-TNF-α Mab BC7 with anti-CD2 Mab followed by maintenance treatment with IL-2 receptor Mab, are currently underway in other centers.

In an attempt to use TNF-α antagonists in an earlier period of acute GVHD, a multicenter phase II trial was initiated combining a 7 day course of Mab195F with high dose corticosteroids for primary treatment of acute GVHD grade II or more. In an interim analysis of 33 patients treated thus far in our center, the response rate at day +30 was 75% in patients following HLA identical sibling donor BMT, indicating that neutralization of TNF-α may not be sufficient to treat the more intense forms of acute GVHD. Though the final analysis is pending, we observed no increase in infectious complications and no inteference with hematopoietic recovery.

Based on studies on systemic release of TNF-α and the beneficial effects of early neutralization of TNF-α in murine models, a phase I/II trial of Mab 195F given throughout the period of pretransplant conditioning (in addition to standard immunosuppression with cyclosporine and methotrexate) was initiated in 1991. This study included high risk patients receiving related donor BMT defined by an age above 40 years and a diagnosis of CML or myelodysplastic syndrome. Mab 195F was given in 3 dose levels. In all patients treatment was started prior to the first dose of TBI or cytotoxic drugs and stopped at midnight on the day before BMT. While the low dose proved inefficient with regard to prevention of GVHD, the high dose group was stopped due to observation of 2 late graft failures occurring more than 3 months after BMT without complete prevention of GVHD (for details see (55)). Due to beneficial effects seen in the first 4 patients receiving the intermediate dose, this dose was chosen according to the study protocol for evaluation in further 10 patients. Results of this study group were compared with a historical control group of age and disease matched patients. As the study group and historical controls were imbalanced with regard to the conditioning regimens used and a recent study from Seattle suggests delayed onset and a reduced incidence of acute GVHD in patients receiving BU/CY conditioning regimens (61), results of the Mab 195F prophylaxis study were analyzed separately. Patients receiving Mab195F prophylaxis showed no increase of infectious complications during aplastic phase or in the first 100 days following BMT and no delay of hematopoietic engraftment. Chimerism, as detected by isoenzyme typing and cytogenetic analysis of bone marrow in CML patients, was complete at day +30 in 17/18 patients of the historical control and in 12/14 patients receiving Mab195F prophylaxis. In addition, onset of acute GVHD was delayed, with a trend toward total reduction in overall incidence. Importantly, there was a reduction of severe GVHD (grade III/IV) and a four month survival rate of 79% in the Mab195F groups versus 67% in the historical control group. These phase II data demonstrate that neutralization of TNF-α in the period of pretransplant conditioning can be safely applied in the setting of human allogeneic BMT and await confirmation in a randomized trial, which is currently underway.

Pentoxifylline

Pentoxifylline (PTX), a well-established drug formerly used for its feasible rheologic effects in patients with arteriosclerosis, recently generated considerable interest for its suppression of TNF-α transcription via its phosphodiesterase activity. This effect could be clearly demonstrated in animals and human volunteers receiving LPS injections as well as in several studies on prevention of the cytokine release syndrome following the first dose of anti-CD3 Mabs (for review see (63)). Based on these effects and on the first reports on favorable effects of PTX in patients with amphotericin nephrotoxicity in the setting of BMT, a phase I/II study with oral PTX given for the whole period of allogeneic BMT was performed by Bianco et al (62) and suggested reduction of regimen-related toxicity as well as of acute GVHD when compared with historical controls. Since that report, several studies (63) were unable to repeat these beneficial observations. These negative results in subsequent trials are problematic, as TNF-α-suppressing activities of PTX have been clearly documented in a variety of experimental conditions. However, TNF-α levels were not evaluated in these trials. The most likely explanation for the negative results observed in randomized PTX trials is that clinically achievable PTX levels are too low to suppress TNF-α release; this effect has been directly documented in a recent small study where patients receiving PTX prophylaxis and suffering from acute GVHD still had significant levels of TNF-α in their serum (64). It is also possible that PTX has other deleterious effects that counterbalance the beneficial reduction in TNF-α secretion. Investigation of new phosphodiesterase-inhibitors or related drugs that inhibit transcription of TNF-α still seems an attractive approach for prevention of TNF-α release in the setting of allogeneic BMT and deserves more detailed analysis of bioavailability and efficacy with respect to experimental and clinical endpoints.

Interleukin 1 Receptor Antagonist (IL-1ra)

A third member of the interleukin family, interleukin-1 receptor antagonist (IL-1ra), is an important, specific inhibitor of IL-1 activity. IL-1ra was isolated from human mononuclear cells and its cDNA was sequenced in 1990 (65). IL-1ra is a 17kD polypeptide (with a glycosylated form of 25 kD) that has a 26% homology to IL-1β and a 19% homology to IL-1α. IL-1ra, which contains a leader sequence and a signal peptide, is secreted from cells and acts as a pure antagonist with no agonist activity (66). The biologic activity of IL-1 is therefore extremely tightly regulated, with the same cell producing both agonists and antagonists. Purified IL-1ra competes with both IL-1α and IL-β to bind IL-1 receptors with approximately the same affinity as either isoform. IL-1ra blocks IL-1 activity both *in vitro* and *in vivo*; thymocyte proliferation, endothelial and neutrophil adhesion, and cytokine synthesis are all inhibited, but *in vitro* 100-fold excesses of IL-1ra are required to produce such inhibition neutralized to achieve optimal effect. In that case, broader cytokine antagonists would be preferable, and it might be difficult to prove superiority of any single antagonist as compared to corticosteroids. Involvement of TNF-α in various phases of BMT suggests that prolonged neutralization is needed to optimize protection from cytokine-mediated damage. Chronic administration of potent TNF-α antagonists, such as Mabs, raises concerns regarding interference with antimicrobial defense. Neutralization of TNF-α in models of chronic bacterial infection such as peritonitis has been reported to increase mortality (72), presumably due to the need for TNF-α in focusing the inflammatory response and subsequently preventing bacterial spread and diffuse inflammation. A similar mechanism may pertain to the containment of viral infections, stressing the need to define optimal windows for neutralization of TNF-α in BMT.

Cytokine Shields

Recent evidence suggests that newly identified cytokines have unexpected activities and may act in certain circumstances as cytokine "shields." One such cytokine shield against experimental acute GVHD is IL-11. Administration of IL-11 from day −2 to day +14 after BMT prevented lethal graft-versus-host disease (GVHD) in a murine BMT model (B6 ->B6D2F1) across MHC and minor antigen barriers (73). IL-11 administration polarized the donor T cell cytokine responses to host antigen after BMT with a 50% reduction in IFNγ and IL-2 secretion and a 10-fold increase in IL-4. This polarization of T cell responses was associated with reduced IFNγ serum levels and decreased IL-12 production in mixed lymphocyte cultures (MLC). In addition, IL-11 prevented small bowel damage and reduced serum endotoxin levels by 80%. Treatment

344

with IL-11 also reduced TNF-α serum levels and suppressed TNF-α secretion by macrophages to LPS stimulation in vitro. IL-11 thus decreased GVHD morbidity and mortality by three mechanisms: (a) polarization of donor T cells; (b) protection of the small bowel; and (c) suppression of inflammatory cytokines such as TNF-α. Brief treatment with IL-11 may represent a novel strategy to prevent T cell-mediated inflammatory processes such as GVHD.

Neutralization of inflammatory cytokines as an alternative approach to prevent or treat early GVHD should be considered in the context of effective GHVD prevention by T cell depletion. The problem of an increased relapse rate observed after T cell depletion might be approached by subsequent reinfusion of donor T cells in a period where patients have recovered from conditioning-related damage as suggested by Waldmann (74). However, the period where the presence of donor T cells is required to control residual disease is still poorly defined. Recent work in murine GVL models suggests that there is a limited window of time in which T cells are required to produce an anti-tumor effect (75). Reducing non-specific inflammation induced by pretransplant conditioning but preserving donor T cell maturation in an early post-transplant period as it is achieved by prophylactic neutralization of TNF-α or related cytokines might prove an attractive alternative approach to temporal dissociation of GVHD and GVL effects. Such an approach appears to be supported by murine studies (22) as well as by results of the phase I/II trial on prophylactic neutralization of TNF-α, because the incidence and severity of acute GVHD are reduced without modulation of chronic GVHD.

Other transplant complications

A second and as yet poorly analyzed issue is the pathophysiological role of TNF-α in other acute transplant-related complications that contribute to early mortality following BMT. There is clinical evidence that systemic release of TNF-α is associated with the occurrence of veno-occlusive disease (VOD) (60,76). A possible contribution of liver macrophages, i.e. Kupffer cells, to pathophysiology of VOD seems likely because they are the largest macrophage compartment of the body and the first macrophages in the line of defense against endotoxin and other microbial products translocated from a damaged gastrointestinal mucosa. Prostaglandins have been reported to interfere with Kupffer cell activation and cytokine production, which may explain the beneficial effects of prophylactic PGE2 infusion on occurrence and severity of VOD (77). Such effects may be partially explained by local cytokine production, although we have been unable to observe modulation of TNF-α levels in patients receiving PGE2 prophylaxis (E. Holler, unpublished data). Similar pathways of cytokine-mediated pathophysiology appear to underlie interstitial pneumonitis or idiopathic pneumonia syndrome (78) and late pulmonary complications such as fibrosis. Again, Piguet has reported a necrotizing alveolitis associated with experimental GVHD, which is characterized by massive expression of TNF-α mRNA within the lung (79) and which is reversed by anti-TNF-α Mabs. In a more recent study, neutralizing anti-TNF-α antibodies strongly suppressed development of CMV-mediated pneumonitis (16). In addition, radiation induced damage of the lung, which contributes significantly to pulmonary complications in clinical BMT, is characterized by enhanced expression of fibrogenic cytokines such as TGFβ (80) which in turn is strongly induced by TNF-α. Thus, further investigation of TNF-antagonists for prevention or even early treatment of interstitial pneumonitis is clearly justified.

OVERVIEW OF T CELL COSTIMULATION BLOCKADE TO INDUCE TOLERANCE

As described above, donor T cells initiate GVHD in response to host alloantigens. The activation of T cells to alloantigen is mediated by a cascade of cell-surface and intracellular signals that are initiated via binding of the TCR/CD3 complex. (Figure 2). Even with high-affinity TCR-MHC/peptide interactions, additional T cell signals are required to drive T cell activation and expansion. Studies by Jenkins and Schwartz (81) showed that antigen-specific responses of Th1 clones were regulated by inducible cell-surface molecules present on antigen presenting cells (APC). Exposure to antigen on APC in the presence of paraformaldehyde prevented the expression of these costimulatory molecules on the T cell clone and led to a state of non-responsiveness termed anergy. Anergy develops in T cells that are specific for the antigen present during the time period of inadequate costimulation, and thus an attractive strategy would be to induce specific anergy of transplanted donor T cells to host alloantigens either *ex vivo* or *in vivo*. Such anergy would preserve the functional capacity of the remaining T cells to respond to infectious agents or residual leukemia cells or to provide cytokines for promotion of donor alloengraftment.

Costimulatory molecules include members of the immunoglobin (Ig) supergene family (e.g. CD28:B7), tumor necrosis factor (TNF)/nerve growth factor (NGF) receptor families [e.g. CD40 ligand (CD40L) (CD154):CD40, 4-1BB (CD137): 4-1BB ligand; OX40 (CD134): OX40 ligand], and adhesion molecules (e.g. LFA-1: ICAM-1, CD2:CD48). Ligation of the appropriate receptor on activated T cells by one or more of these proteins may directly provide positive signals or may modify the expression of other costimulatory determinants on the T cell surface or APC. In contrast to these positive signals are negative signals which downregulate immune responses primarily by inducing cell death (e.g. Fas (CD95): Fas L), and that compete for the same substrates as the positive regulators (e.g. CTLA-4 (CD152)), or that directly transduce negative regulatory signals (e.g. IL-10). The net balance of positive and negative regulators of T cell activation determines whether donor alloreactive T cells can reach the critical threshold stage of activation necessary to expand and cause systemic GVHD; thus both positive and negative regulatory pathways can be targeted to prevent the development of disease.

Figure 2.

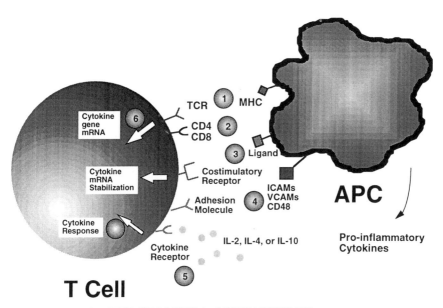

BLOCKADE OF THE CD28/CTLA-4:B7 PATHWAY

In vivo Blockade

In regard to blocking positive costimulatory signals, the best studied interaction involves that of CD28/CTLA-4 on T cells with B7 ligands (CD80;CD86) on APC. CD28 is constitutively expressed on all murine T cells (82) and its natural ligands, B7-1 (CD86), are predominantly found on activated APC (85-91). There is direct evidence to show that interruption of CD28/CTLA-4:B7 interactions impairs immune responses *in vivo*. Such studies were initially performed with CTLA-4-Ig, a protein consisting of the extracellular domain of CTLA-4 with high-affinity for its ligand B7 which was fused to the Cγ1 Legs moiety of Ig (83), and adapted for either human or murine systems. CTLA-4-Ig binds with high avidity to both CD80 and CD86 and effectively prevents the binding of CD28 to either ligand, precluding CD28 mediated positive signaling of the T cell. The administration of CTLA-4-Ig to rodents suppresses sheep red blood cell responses (84), prevents rejection of xenogeneic islet cells (85) and cardiac allografts (86), and reduces immune responses to self antigens such as myelin basic protein (87) and islet cell antigens (88).

CD80 and CD86 are both upregulated during GVH responses in the spleen, liver and colon in a B6→B10.BR murine BMT system. Unfortunately, infusion of high doses of CTLA4-Ig ≤ (250 mcg) every other day from day −1 for periods as long as 1 month post BMT protects only a small proportion of recipients from GVHD lethality and these surviving mice had evidence of GVHD (89). Actuarial survival of CTLA-4-Ig treated mice were significantly prolonged in several experiments, although the mortality rates varied between 37-100%. No survival advantage was conferred in preliminary studies in which mCTLA-4-Ig (murine) was compared to hCTLA-4-Ig human infusions (89), in contrast to the results of Wallace et al (90) which demonstrated a higher degree of protection from GVHD lethality with the mCTLA-4-Ig protein. In both of these studies, donor type lymphohematopoietic reconstitution was not impaired by CTLA-4-Ig treatment. To determine whether CTLA-4-Ig might be more effective against GVHD development in strain combinations in which disease was more dependent on $CD4^+$ as compared to $CD8^+$ T cells, the results of the B6 → B10.BR system were compared to the mHA-disparate CBA/J ($H2^k$)→B10.BR system (91). In both GVHD systems, hCTLA-4-Ig infusion was biologically active in prolonging survival, but did not prevent mortality. These results also suggested that CTLA-4-Ig protection was not related to any particular T cell subset.

The majority of hCTLA-4-Ig treated recipients in these experiments did not have detectable levels of circulating hCTLA-4-Ig as measured seven days after discontinuation of the injections (89). The CD28:B7 blockade approach was therefore changed from fusion proteins to anti-CD80 and CD86 Mab which can persist longer *in vitro* and can distinguish the individual contributions of the B7 ligands. Sublethally irradiated bm1 or bm12 recipients of T cell subset-purified MHC class I- or class II-disparate B6 $CD8^+$ and $CD4^+$ lymph node (LN) T cells and combined infusion of anti-CD80 and anti-CD86 Mab given in doses ≤ 250mcg i.p. for 3-4 weeks post-transplant had survival rates of 94% and 100%, respectively; by contrasts no control animals survived (92). Although both CD80 and CD86 bind to CD28 and CTLA-4, these two ligands have distinct functions and are expressed at different periods of time after induction (93-96). Most APC require stimuli for the induction of CD80 and CD86 expression, and CD86 is induced more rapidly than CD80 (97, 98). Both these antigens are expressed on activated T cells (87, 101-103). Interestingly, treatment with either Mab alone was only partially effective for GVHD mediated by CD4$^+$ T cells, and completely ineffective when GVHD was mediated by CD8$^+$ T cells (92).

To understand how CD28:B7 blockade affects donor T cells early post-BMT, thoracic duct lymphocytes (TDL) were analyzed 4-6 days post-BMT, a time when TDL are highly enriched for alloreactive donor T cells (104). Combined anti-CD80 and anti-CD86 Mab infusion in B6-SCID recipients of purified MHC class II-disparate bm12 CD4$^+$ LN T cells completely prevented lethal GVHD (92). Treated recipients had up to a 100-fold reduction in donor TDL T cells in comparison to irrelevant Mab-treated controls indicating that a major effect of anti-B7 Mab is to inhibit T cell expansion. Hakim et al (105) also observed inhibition of donor T cell expansion in non-irradiated F1 recipients or parental donor grafts that had received hCTLA-4-Ig infusions.

Interestingly, anti-B7 Mab-treated donor TDL T cells responses to host antigens were intact as measured by limiting dilution in the presence of exogenous IL-2 (92). It was clear that anti-B7 treatment did not delete alloreactive donor T cells, and this result suggested that anergy that had been induced *in vivo*, was reversible in the presence of IL-2 *in vitro*. Flow cytometric analysis of CD4$^+$ TDL cells, obtained 3 weeks post-transfer from anti-B7 Mab-treated B6-SCID recipients of CD4$^+$ bm12 lymph node T cells, indicated that a smaller portion of cells expressed CD80 than CD86, the reverse of that observed for irrelevant Mab-treated controls (92). These data suggested that anti-B7 Mab affected the upregulation of the late activation antigen, CD80, on donor T cells. To determine if CD80 expression on donor CD4$^+$ T cells was important in the causation of GVHD, experiments were performed in which CD4$^+$ LN T cells from 129/Svems (H2^b) CD80-deleted (knockout) mice were infused into sublethally irradiated MHC class II-disparate bm12 recipients. Approximately 25% of recipients of CD80-knockout T cells survived for the 80-day observation period, in contrast to the uniform lethality observed by day 21 post-transfer in recipients of wild-type T cells (92). Thus, the upregulation of CD80 on donor T cells may be critical to the induction of severe, lethal GVHD.

Ex vivo blockade of the CD28:B7 pathway

An alternative to the regulation of donor T cell responses *in vivo* after BMT is to tolerize donor T cells to recipient alloantigens by CD28:B7 blockade prior to infusion. Such an approach would have several advantages, including: 1) elimination of recipient exposure to reagent/materials with side-effects *in vivo*;

2) assurance of receptor blockade *ex vivo*; 3) economy of material due to the shorter tolerization period; 4) improved hematopoietic recovery and immune reconstitution from the lack of interference from tolerizing agents *in vivo*; 5) improved quality control of tolerance induction *ex vivo*; and 6) enhanced specificity of tolerance induction to host alloantigens rather than leukemia or viral antigens (which may reach critical antigenic threshold levels *in vivo*). With respect to leukemic antigens, preliminary studies have indicated that the blockade of CD28:B7 interaction *in vivo* with anti-B7 Mab can inhibit GVL effects from developing late post-BMT, while the forced expression of B7 ligands on leukemia cells can stimulate a GVL effect to acute myeloid leukemia even early post-BMT (106,107). Proof of principle anergy induction of donor T cells to alloantigen-bearing stimulators was provided by Tan et al. (108) who showed that human peripheral blood mononuclear cells (PBMC) can be rendered specifically non-responsive to alloantigen when cultured in the presence of hCTLA-4-Ig. Using a similar approach, B6 donor splenocytes from a 3-4 day culture with host-stimulators were exposed to saturating concentrations of hCTLA-4-IG in the presence of T cell depleted B10.BR splenocyte stimulators (109). Although these cells exhibited hyporesponsiveness *in vitro* and had significantly lower cell recovery than control cultures, they did not consistently prolong actuarial survival when infused into recipients.

Because the strength of TCR signal can also be influenced by adhesogenic interactions (particularly that of LFA-1), a combined approach of *ex vivo* CD28:B7 and LFA-1:ICAM co-blockade was investigated. The *ex vivo* incubation of bulk B6→ B10.BR splenocyte MLR cultures with anti-LFA-1 Mab reduced the MLR response to 14-27% of those observed in sham incubated controls (109). When combined with hCTLA-4-Ig, the addition of anti-LFA-1 Mab reduced the MLR response to 0-11% of controls. Yet, despite these impressive reductions in MLR responses, no protection from GVHD lethality was observed when these cultured cells were infused *in vivo* (109).

Since cardiac allograft survival improved if recipients were first primed to alloantigen for two days prior to CTLA-4-Ig infusion (110), the culture system used above was modified so that B6→B10.BR splenocyte MLR cultures were established three days prior to incubation for three hours with hCTLA-4-Ig and/or anti-LFA-1 Mab (109). B10.BR recipients of these primed, B6 cells were also treated *in vivo* with both hCTLA-4-Ig and anti-LFA-1 Mab for 1 month after BMT and experienced 90-100% survival for ≥ 110 days, in contrast to ≤ 30% in controls that received primed cells not exposed to *ex vivo* or *in vivo* treatments. Although recipients had some evidence of clinical GVHD, there was a clear advantage to the use of primed cells together with combined *ex vivo* and *in vivo* treatments with both hCTLA-4-Ig and anti-LFA-1 Mab. The importance of LFA-1:ICAM co-blockade in this approach was further supported by other studies demonstrating that either LFA-1:ICAM-1 blockade (111) or the use of ICAM-1 gene knockout (ko) recipients could induce a state of hyporesponsiveness associated with reduced organ graft rejection (112).

Additional modifications of the *ex vivo* approach may lead to further improvements. First, substitution of anti-CD80 and anti-CD86 Mab for hCTLA-4-Ig may be effective, based upon the more effective results obtained by Gribben et al (113). Second, extension of the MLR culture system by five to seven days should be attempted, based upon anergy induction experiments performed by Roncarolo and colleagues (114) who showed that the induction of alloantigen-specific nonresponsiveness in human $CD4^+$ T cells in an MLR culture was optimum after 10 days of incubation. Third restriction of the alloantigen response to $CD4^+$ T cells in an isolated MHC class II disparity may be necessary since the best evidence of anergy induction in mice and humans involves that T cell subset. These and other modifications will require testing to determine whether it is possible to generate alloantigen-hyporesponsiveness donor T cells that have a markedly reduced capacity to mediate GVHD when infused *in vivo*.

BLOCKADE OF THE CD40L:CD40 PATHWAY

In vivo Blockade

CD40 is a 50 kDa glycoprotein member of the NGFR/TNF receptor family and is expressed on B cells, professional APC, endothelial cells, and some epithelial cells (115-118). CD40L, a type II integral membrane glycoprotein, is the T cell counter-receptor for CD40 and is transiently expressed on antigen-activated $CD4^+$ cells (119-124). CD40L also transduces a signal to CD40-expressing B cells to upregulate molecules involved in T cell costimulation, such as CD80 and CD86 (125-127). Although both CD28-dependent and –independent pathways are involved in the induction of CD40L expression on activated T cells (128), the kinetics and density of CD40L expression are increased by CD28:B7-mediated costimulation (129). T cells can be rendered tolerant when exposed to antigen in a situation where B cells are incapable of receiving a CD40 signal (130,131). Blockade of CD40L:CD40 interaction in rodents has been shown to inhibit humoral and cellular inflammatory responses in a variety of models, including collagen-induced allografts (134). The *in vivo* administration of anti-CD40L Mab has been shown to inhibit the GVH reaction of parental splenocytes transplanted into non-irradiated F1 recipients (135). These findings have been extended in the B6→B10.BR BMT system where anti-CD40L Mab treatment (200mcg daily from day 1 to 5, then 2x per week until day 29) resulted in a 60% actuarial survival rate at day 95   vs. 0% in controls (136). To determine whether $CD8^+$ or $CD4^+$ T cells were differentially affected by anti-CD40L Mab, sublethally irradiated bm1 or bm12 recipients were given highly purified $CD8^+$ or $CD4^+$ B6 lymph node T cells, respectively (136). Anti-CD40L Mab had 56% long-term (day 140) survival, in contrast to 0% in controls.

To determine if host B cell regulation of donor T cell function was critical to the effect of anti-CD40L Mab, B6-SCID mice were used as recipients of bm12 $CD4^+$ lymph node T cells (136). Anti-CD40L Mab infusion protected a similar proportion of wild-type and SCID recipients, indicating that anti-CD40L Mab did not mediate its protective effects through interrupting T-B cognate interaction. To understand how CD40L:CD40 blockade affected donor T cells early post-BMT, donor $CD4^+$ TDL T cells from the bm12→ B6-SCID strain combination were analyzed (136). Yields from Mab-treated mice were reduced by > 2.5-fold and anti-host proliferative responses were inhibited by > 2.5-fold, although *in vivo* priming was not completely eliminated by anti-CD40L Mab. To determine whether anti-CD40L Mab inhibited the generation of proinflammatory or immunomodulatory cytokines (e.g. IFNγ, nitric oxide, etc.) mRNA in situ hybridization was performed on TDL or splenocytes obtained at periodic intervals post-transfer (136). All cells from Mab-treated recipients expressing IL-2, IL-12, and IFNγmRNA were markedly diminished at all times compared to controls, indicating that Th1-associated GVHD responses were susceptible to CD40L:CD40 blockade. In the BALB/c→ B6 BM rejection system, anti-CD40L Mab also inhibited graft rejection so that sublethally irradiated recipients of pan-T-cell-depleted BM grafts had significantly higher levels of donor engraftment two months after BMT compared to controls (90% vs. 60%) (136). Together with the GVHD results, these data support the concept that the blockade of CD40L:CD40 interactions may provide highly beneficial effects on the outcome of allogeneic BMT.

Ex vivo blockade

Recent experiments have demonstrated that blockade of CD40L *ex vivo* can render donor $CD4^+$ cells tolerant to host alloantigens (137). Using the B6→bm12 BMT systems, donor B6 $CD4^+$ T cells were incubated for a period of 10 days in MLR cultures with irradiated bm12 host stimulates in the presence of anti-CD40L Mab. Injections of tolerized $CD4^+$ cells into bm12 recipients caused 0% mortality, whereas injection of 33-fold fewer caused 97% mortality within 25 days of transfer. Injections of IL-2 *in vivo* were not able to break tolerance and T cells preserved vigorous responses to antigens not present in the tolerizing culture. Thus *ex vivo* tolerization may have significant therapeutic potential for allogeneic BMT.

OTHER MEMBERS OF THE NGF/TNF RECEPTOR FAMILY AS TARGETS FOR MODULATION

Of the remaining NGFR/TNF receptor family members which provide T cell costimulation, published data are available only as to the *in vivo* blockade of theOX40:OX40L interaction for GVHD prevention. OX40 is rapidly upregulated (peak expression 24 h) on activated $CD4^+$ and $CD8^+$ T cells (138). The counter-receptor for OX40 is OX40L, a type-II membrane protein which is expressed on activated B cells, endothelial cells, and activated T cells (138-140). Binding of OX40L to OX40 on activated T cells stimulates IL-4 production and increases the adhesion to vascular endothelium (138). The cross-linking of OX40L on B cells stimulates B cell proliferation, differentiation and isotype switching (138-140). OX40 is also expressed on T cells involved in autoimmune process, such as EAE and rheumatoid arthritis (141). OX40 appears to be upregulated in T cells during GVHD generation in rats (142), mice (143), and humans (141). Recent data indicate that 40-50% of $CD4^+$ and $CD8^+$ TDL isolated on day 6 post-BMT in the B6→B10.BR GVHD system express OX40 (B.R. Blazar, unpublished data). Anti-OX40 Mab infusion appears to block a Th2-mediated chronic GVH response in (DBA/2 x C57BL/6) F1 recipients of DBA/2 splenocytes and to skew the response to a Th1-type acute GVH response (143). These data suggest that OX 40 is expressed on T cells involved in regulating GVHD and that anti-OX40 Mab can alter the course of GVH toward a Th1 response. Ongoing studies are directed toward understanding how anti-OX40 Mab affects donor T cells in GVHD systems mediated by $CD8^+$ as well as $CD4^+$ T cells. Future studies will investigate targeting of other members of the NGFR/TNF receptor family known to be capable of providing T cell costimulation, such as 4-1BB:4-1BBL (144, 145).

Costimulatory signals, including CD28, CTLA-4 and CD40, also can regulate the expression of cell survival proteins, such as bcl_{xL} and IL-2 (144-146). In the absence of costimulation, T cells undergo programmed cell death (147). Fas (APO-1, CD95), a 48kD transmembrane glycoprotein that is structurally related to TNF-α, was originally described as a cell-surface molecule that regulates apoptotic death (148,149). Fas also can provide a costimulatory signal for cellular activation and proliferation to freshly isolated T cells. Activation-induced cell death of T cells can be mediated by Fas, a member of the NGF/TNF receptor family (12). Fas ligand is a 40 kD-type II transmembrane protein member of the TNF family that is expressed on activated lymphocytes (150,151). Ligation of Fas by anti-Fas Mab (152) or by binding to Fas ligand (151-153) induces apoptosis (154,155). Binding Fas ligand to Fas-expressing target cells represents an important mechanism of CTL killing (156). Because the Fas antigen which induces apoptosis is expressed on effector cells such as activated lymphocytes and GVH target cells such as the liver, lung, and thymus (157), investigators have explored the possibility that interruption of the Fas:FasL pathway will inhibit GVHD-induced injury. Recent studies in which FasL-deficient donor T cells are infused into irradiated (158,159) or non-irradiated (160) allogeneic recipients have shown that mortality from acute GVHD is delayed compared to recipients of wild-type cells. An intact Fas:FasL pathway was required for the generation of hepatic inflammation (159), alopecia (159), and B cell hypoplasia (161) but not cachexia associated with GVHD. These data indicate that approaches which preclude the ligation of the Fas receptor on host target tissues are also likely to possess therapeutic potential to reduce the toxicity of allogeneic BMT. Many of these blockades may represent non-cross reactive strategies, particularly in combination with cytokine modulations, and clinical trials should soon be initiated to determine whether these strong pre-clinical data will translate into novel approaches to improve allogeneic BMT for our patients.

Table 3. Summary of the results of the phase II trial using the anti-TNFα Mab195F (3 x 1mg/kg) during pretransplant conditioning as an additive prophylaxis. Patients were separately analyzed according to the type of pretransplant conditioning.

	overall incidence of GVHD grade II		median time to onset of GVHD II (d)		overall incidence of GVHD grade III/IV	
	TBI	BU	TBI	BU	TBI	BU
anti-TNF-alpha	2/3	5/11	26	50	0/3	2/11
historical control	9/9	7/9	14	35	6/9	4/ 9

TBI=total body irradiation (4Gy/day x 3-4 days) followed by cyclophosphamide, BU= oral busulphan (4mg/kg/day x 4 days) followed by cyclophosphamide. The overall incidence of GVHD grade II observed until d 100 was not statistically different between groups, onset of aGVHD was delayed (p< .05 for TBI, <.10 for BU) in anti-TNFα patients. This trended toward reduced incidence of severe GVHD (grade III/IV) in patients receiving TNFα during TBI conditioning (p<.10).

Table 4. IL-1ra treatment for steroid-resistant GVHD.

Age	GVHD Proph.	GVHD Therapy	IL-->1ra Dose (mg/kg)	GVHD Stage			Overall Grade
				Skin	Gut	Liver	
40	CSA/PRED	Cyc., Pred.	3,200	0-->0	4-->1	NE	2-->1
41	None	Cyc., MePr	1,600	2-->0	4-->0	3-->3	3-->2
47	3	MePr	3,200	3-->4	NE	3-->4	3-->4
37	1	MePr	800	0-->0	4-->0	0-->0	3-->0
4	1	MePr	6	3-->3	3-->0	0-->0	3-->2
3	1	MePr	6	3-->4	3-->2	2-->3	3-->4
34	1	MePr	400	3-->0	0-->0	3-->0	3-->0
33	1	MePr	800	4-->2	0-->0	2-->NE	2-->1
39	1	MePr	800	2-->1	0-->0	2-->1	2-->1
31	2	MePr	1,600	3-->3	2-->0	3-->4	4-->4
34	2	MePr	1,600	3-->1	1-->0	0-->3	2-->2
42	2	MePr	1,600	3-->4	4-->4	2-->3	4-->4
20	3	MePr	3,200	1-->2	1-->1	1-->4	2-->3
40	3	MePr	3,200	0-->0	3-->1	1-->NE	2-->1
50	4	MePr	3,200	3-->2	0-->NE	2-->NE	2-->NE
29	3	MePr	3,200	4-->1	0-->0	0-->1	3-->1
5	3	MePr	12	2-->0	4-->0	2-->3	3-->2
			Response (%)	8/14 (57%)	9/11 (82%)	2/11 (18%)	10/16 (63%)

Median age (range): 34 years (3-50). Median time to IL-1ra (range): 33 days (3-128) Abbreviations: MePr = methylprednisolone; CSA/PRED = cyclosporine/prednisone; Cyc. = cyclosporine, Pred. = prednisone; NE = unevaluable. Prophylactic regimens used: 1) = cyclosporine 1.5mg/kg twice a day, methotrexate 10mg/m^2 days 1, 8,15,22, and 28; 2) = cyclosporine 1.5mg/kg twice a day, methotrexate 10mg/m^2 days 1,8,15,22, and 28, plus methylprednisolone 3mg/kg/day beginning on day 7; 3) = cyclosporine 1.5mg/kg twice a day, methotrexate 15mg/m^2 on day 1 and then 10mg/m^2 on days 3,6, and 11, plus methylprednisolone 3mg/kg/day beginning on day 7; 4) = cyclosporine 1.5mg/kg twice a day, methotrexate 15mg/m^2 on day 1 and then 10mg/m^2 on days 3,6, and 11.

REFERENCES

1. Carswell EA, Old LJ, Kassel RL, et al. An endotoxin-induced serum factor that causes necrosis of tumors. Proc Natl Acad Sci. USA. 1975;72:3666-3670.
2. Fiers W. Tumor necrosis factor. Characterization at the molecular, cellular and *in vivo* level. FEBS Letters. 1991;285:199-212.
3. Tracey KJ, Vlassara H, Cerami A. Cachetctin/tumor necrosis factor. Lancet 1989;1:1122-1126.
4. Deem RL, Shanahan F, Targan SR. Triggered human mucosal T cells release tumor necrosis factor alpha and interferon gamma which kill human colonic epithelial cells. Clin Exp Immonol. 1991;83:79-84.
5. Pober JS. Effects of tumor necrosis factor and related cytokines on vascular endothelial cells. In: Tumor necrosis factor and related cytokines. 1987:170-184.
6. Johnson DR, Pober JS. Tumor necrosis factor regulation of major histocompatibility complex gene expression. Immunol Res. 1991;10:141-155.
7. Robinet E, Branelle D, Termitjtelen AM, et al. Evidence for tumor necrosis factor – a involvement in the optimal induction of class I allospecific T cells. J Immunol. 1990;144:4555-4561.
8. Hogquist KA, Nett MA, E.R. U, Chaplin DD. Interleukin-1 is processed and released during apoptosis. Proc Natl Acad Sci. USA. 1991;88:8485.
9. Yuan J, Shaham S, Ledoux S, et al. The C. elegans cell death gene ced-3 encodes a protein similar to mammalian interleukin-1 beta converting enzyme. Cell 1993;75:641-652,
10. Kuida K, Lippke JA, Ku G, et al. Altered cytokines export and apoptosis in mice deficient in interleukin-1B converting enzyme. Science 1995;267:2000-2003.
11. Miura M, Zhu H, Rotello R, et al. Induction of apoptosis in fibroblasts by IL-1 beta converting enzyme, a mammalian homolog of the C. elegans cell death gene ced-3. Cell 1993;75:653-660.
12. Itoh N, Yonehara S, Ishii A, et al. The polypeptide encoded by the cDNA for human cell surface antigen Fas can mediate apoptosis. Cell 1991;66:233-243.
13. Ju ST, Panka DJ, Cui H, et al. Fas (CD95)/Fas L interactions required for programmed cell death after T cell activation. Nature 1995;373:444-448.
14. Nestel FP, Price KS, Seemayer TA, et al. Macrophage priming and lipopolysaccharide-triggered release of tumor necrosis factor alpha during graft-versus-host disease. J Exp Med 1992;175:405-413.

15. Niederwieser D, Herold M, Woloszuczuk W, et al. Endogenous IFN-gamma during human bone marrow transplantation. Transplantation 1990;50:620-625.
16. Haagmans BL, Stals FS, van der Meide PH, Bruggeman CA, et al. Tumor necrosis factor alpha promotes replication and pathogenicity of rat cytomegalovirus. J Virol 1994;68:2297-2304.
17. Hallahan DE, Spriggs DR, Beckett MA, Kufe DW, et al. Increased tumor necrosis factor-a mRNA after cellular exposure to ionizing radiation. Proc Natl Acad Sci USA 1989;86:10104-10107.
18. Sherman ML, Datta R, Hallahan DE, et al. Regulation of tumor necrosis factor gene expression by ionizing radiation in human myeloid leukemia cells and peripheral blood monocytes. J Clin Invest 1991;87:1794-1797.
19. Iwamoto KS, McBride WH. Production of 13-hydroxyoctadecadienoic acid and tumor necrosis factor-a by murine peritoneal macrophages in response to irradiation. Radiat Res 1994;139:103-108.
20. Hoffman RA, Langrehr JM, Simmons RL. The role of inducible nitric oxide synthetase during graft-versus-host disease. Transplant Proc 1992;24:2856.
21. Girinsky TA, Pallardy M, Comoy E, et al. Peripheral blood corticotropin-releasing factor, adrenocorticotropic hormone and cytokine (interleukin beta, interleukin 6, tumor necrosis factor alpha) levels after high- and low-dose total-body irradiation in humans. Radiat Res 1994;139:360-363.
22. Xun CQ, Thompson JS, Jennings CD, et al. Effect of total body irradiation, busulfan-cyclophosphamicde, or cyclophosphamide conditioning on inflammatory cytokine release and development of acute and chronic graft-versus-host disease in H-2 incompatible transplanted SCID mice. Blood 1994;83:2360-2367.
23. Abhyankar S, Gilliland DG, Ferrara JLM. Interleukin-1 is a critical effector molecule during cytokine dysregulation in graft-versus-host disease to minor histocompatibility antigens. Transplantation 1993;56:1518-1523.
24. Hoffman B, Hintermeier-Knabe R, Holler E, et al. Evidence of induction of TNF-alpha by irradiation and cytotoxic therapy preceeding bone marrow transplantation- *in vivo* and *in vitro* studies. Networks 1992;3:257.
25. Brugger W, Reinhardt D, Galanos C, et al. Inhibition of *in-vitro* differentiation of human monocytes to macrophages by lipopolysaccharides (LPS); Phenotypic and functional analysis. Intern Immunol 1991:3:221-227.
26. Thomas ED, Ramberg RE, Sale GE, et al. Direct evidence for a bone marrow origin of the alveolar macrophage in man. Science 1976;192:1016-1018.

27. Perreault C, Pelletier M,. Belanger R, et al. Persistence of host Langerhans cells following allogeneic bone marrow transplantation: Possible relationship with acute graft-versus-host disease. Br J Haemotol 1985:60:253-260.
28. Barker JN, Mitra RS, Griffith CEM, et al. Keratinocytes as initiators of inflammation. Lancet 1991;337:211-214.
29. Walsh LJ, Trincheri F, Waldorf HA, Whitaker D, et al. Human dermal mast cells contain and release tumor necrosis factor alpha which induces enothelial leukocyte adhesion molecule-1. Proc Natl Acad Sci USA 1991;88:4420-4424.
30. Murphy GF, Sueki H, Teuscher C, Whitaker D, Korngold R. Role of mast cells in early epithelial target cell injury in experimental acute graft-versus-host disease. J Invest Dermatol 1994;102:451-461.
31. Dickinson AM, Sviland L, Dunn J, et al. Demonstration of direct involvement of cytokines in graft-versus-host disease reactions in an *in vitro* skin explant model. Bone Marrow Transplant 1991;7:209-216.
32. Dickinson AM, Sviland L, Jackson G, et al. Monoclonal anti-TNF-alpha suppresses graft-versus-host diesease. J Exp Med 1987;166:1280-1289.
33. Piguet PF, Grau GE, Allet B, et al. Tumor necrosis factor/cachetin is an effector of skin and gut lesions of the acute phase of graft-versus-host disease. J Exp Med 1987;166:1280-1289.
34. Piguet PF, Grau GE, Vasseli P. Tumor necrosis factor and immunopathology. Immunol Res 1991;10:122-140.
35. Shalaby MR, Fendly B, Sheehan KC, et al. Prevention of the graft-versus-host reaction in newborn mice by antibodies to tumor necrosis factor-alpha. Transplantation 1989;47:1057-1061.
36. Holler E, Thierfelder S, Nehrends U, et al. Anti-TNF-alpha and pentoxifylline for prophylaxis of a GVHD in murine allogeneic bone marrow transplantation. Oncology 1992;15:31-35.
37. Wall DA, Sheehan KC. The role of tumor necrosis factor-alpha and interferon gamma in graft-versus-host disease and related immunodeficiency. Transplantation 1994;57:273-279.
38. Allen RD, Staley TA, Sidman CL. Differential cytokine expression in acute and chronic murine graft-versus-host disease. Eur J Immunol 1993;23:333-337.
39. Ferrara JL, Abhyankar S, Gilliland DG. Cytokine storm of graft-versus-host disease: a critical effector role for interleukin-1. Transplant Proc 1993;25:1216-1217.
40. Lehnert S, WBR Amplification of the graft-versus-host reaction by cyclophosphamide: Dependence on timing of drug administration. Bone Marrow Transplant 1994;13:473-477.

41. Zwaan FE, Janson J, Noordijk EM. Graft-versus-host disease limited to area of irradiated skin. Lancet 1980;1:1081-1082.
42. Desbarats J, Seemayer TA, Lapp WS. Irradiation of the skin and systemic graft-versus host disease synergize to produce cutaneous lesions. Am J Pathol 1994;144:883-888.
43. Holler E, Kold HJ, Moller A, et al. Increased serum levels of tumor necrosis factor alpha precede major complications of bone marrow transplantation. Blood 1990;75:1011-1016.
44. Tanaka J, Imamura M, Kasai M, et al. Rapid analysis of tumor necrosis factor-alpha mRNA expression during veno-occlusive disease of the liver after allogeneic bone marrow transplantation. Transplantation 1993;55:430-432.
45. Tanaka J, Imamura M, Kasai M, et al. Cytokine gene expression in peripheral blood mononuclear cells during graft-versus-host disease after allogeneic bone marrow transplantation. B J Haematol 1993;85:558-565.
46. Holler E, Kolb HJ, Hintermeier-Knabe R, et al. Involvement of cytokines in graft-versus-host disease and graft-versus-leukemia activity. In: Bergmann L, Mitrou PS, eds. Cytokines in Cancer Therapy. Basel;Karger 1994:318-329.
47. Rowbottom AW, Norton J, Riches PG, et al. Cytokine gene expression in skin and lymphoid organs in graft-versus-host disease. J Clin Pathol 1993;46:341-345.
48. Holler E, Kolb HJ, Hintermeier-Knabe R, et al. The role of tumor necrosis factor alpha in acute graft-versus-host disease and complications following allogeneic bone marrow transplantation. Transplant Proc 1993;25:1234-1236.
49. Holler E, Hinetermeier-Knabe R, KolbHJ, et al. Low incidence of transplant related complications in patients with chronic release of TNF-alpha before admission to bone marrow transplantation- a clinical correlate of cytokine desensitization. Pathobiology 1991;59:171-175.
50. Holler E, Ferrara JLM. Antagonists of Inflammatory Cytokines: Prophylactic and Therapeutic Applications. In: Ferrara JLM, Deeg HJ, Burakoff SJ, ed. Graft-versus-Host Disease. 2nd ed. New York; Marcel Dekker, Inc. 1997;667-692.
51. Meliconi R, Uguccioni M, Lalli E, et al. Increased serum concentrations of tumor necrosis factor in beta-thalassaemia: Effect of bone marrow transplantation. J Clin Pathol 1992;45:61-65.
52. Akhar I, Gold JP, Pan LY, et al. CD4$^+$ B islet cell-reactive T cell clones that suppress autoimmune diabetes in nonobese diabetic mice. J Exp Med 1995;182:87-97.

53. Turner DM, Grant SCD, Lamb WR, et al. A genetic marker of high TNF-a production in heart transplant recipients. Transplantation 1995;60:1113-1117.

54. Remberger M, Ringden O, Markling L. TNFα levels are increased during bone marrow transplantation conditioning in patients who develop acute GVHD. Bone Marrow Transplant 1995;15:99-104.

55. Holler E, Kolb HJ, Hintermeier-Knabe R, et al. Modulation of acute graft-versus-host disease after allogeneic bone marrow transplantation by tumor necrosis factor alpha (TNFα) release in the course of pretransplant conditioning: Role of conditioning regimens and prophylactic application of a monoclonal antibody neutralizing human TNF-alpha (MAK 195F). Blood 1995;86:890-899.

56. Almawi WY, Lipman ML, Stevens AC, et al. Abrogation of glucocorticosteroid-mediated inhibition of T cell proliferation by the synergistic action of IL-1, IL-6 and IFNgamma. J Immunol 1991;146:3523-3527.

57. Holler E, Kolb HJ, Wilmanns W. Treatment of GVHD-TNF-antibodies and related antagonists. Bone Marrow Transplant. 1993;3:29-31.

58. Herve P, Flesch M, Tiberghien P, et al. Phase I-II trial of a monoclonal anti-tumor necrosis factor alpha antibody for the treatment of refractory severe acute graft-versus-host disease. Blood 1992;81:3362-3368.

59. Moller A, Emling F, Blohm D, et al. Monoclonal antibodies to human tumour necrosis factor alpha: In vitro and in vivo application. Cytokine 1990;2:162-169.

60. Holler E, Kolb HJ, Hintermeier-Knabe R, et al. Systemic release of tumor necrosis factor alpha in human allogeneic bone marrow transplantation: Clinical risk factors, prognostic significance and therapeutic approaches. In: Link, Freund, Schmidt, Welte, eds. Cytokines in Hemapoeisis, Oncology and AIDS II. Berlin-Heidelberg: Springer, 1992:435-442. Vol II.

61. Clift RA, Buckner CD, Thomas WI, et al. Marrow transplantation for chronic myeloid leukemia: a randomized study comparing cyclophosmphamide and total body irradiation with busulfan and cyclophosphamide. Blood 1994;84:2036-2043.

62. Bianco JJ, Appelbaum FR, Guiffre A, et al. Phase I-II trial of pentoxifylline for the prevention of transplant-related toxicities following bone marrow transplantation. Blood 1991;78:1205-1211.

63. Kahls P, Lechner K, Stockschlader M, et al. Pentoxifylline did not prevent transplant-related toxicity in 31 consecutive allogeneic bone marrow transplant recipients. Blood 1992;80:2683.

64. Malich U, Tischler HJ, Petersen D, et al. Pentoxifylline and levels of tumor necrosis factor alpha after bone marrow transplantation. In: "19th Annual Meeting of the EBMT":, ed. Garmisch-Partenkirchen, MMV-Verlag, Munchen. 1993:807.

65. Eisenberg SP, Evans RJ, Arend WP, et al. Primary structure and functional expression from complementary DNA of a human interleukin-1 receptor antagonist. Nature 1990:343:341-346.

66. Arend WP. Interleukin-1 receptor antagonist. Adv Immunol. 1993:54:167-227.

67. Granowitz EV, Clark BD, Mancilla J, et al. Interleukin-1 receptor antagonist competitively inhibits the binding of interleukin-1 to the type II interleukin-1 receptor. J Biol Chem 1991;266:14147-14150.

68. Arend WP, Welgus HG, Thompson RC, et al. Biological properties of recombinant human monocyte-derived interleukin-1 receptor antagonist. J Clin Invest 1990;85:16941697.

69. Haskill S, Martin G, Van Le L, et al. CDNA cloning of an intracellular form of the human interleukin-1 receptor antagonist associated with epithelium. Proc Natl Acad Sci USA 1990;88:3681-3685.

70. Aukrust P, Froland S, Liabakk NB, et al. Release of cytokines, soluble cytokine receptors, and interleukin-1 receptor antagonist after intravenous immunoglobin administration *in vivo*. Blood 1994;84:2136-2143.

71. Antin JH, Weinstein HJ, Guinan EC, et al. Recombinant human interleukin-1 receptor antagonist in the treatment of steroid-resistant graft-versus-host disease. Blood 1994;84:1342-1348.

72. Echtenacher B, Falk W, Maennel DN, et al. Requirement of endogeneous tumor necrosis factor/cachetin for recovery from experimental peritonitis. J Immunol 1990;145:3762-3766.

73. Hill GR, Cooke KR, Teshima T, et al. Interleukin-11 promotes T cell polarization and prevents acute graft-versus-host disease after allogeneic bone marrow transplantation. J Clin Invest 1998;102:115-123.

74. Waldmann H, Cobbold S, Hale G. What can be done to prevent graft-verus-host disease? Curr Opin Immunol 1994;6:777-783.

75. Truitt R, Johnson B, McCabe C. Graft Versus Leukemia. In: Graft-vs-Host Disease 2nd ed. Ferrara, Deeg, Burkaoff: New York: Marcel Dekker, Inc., 1997:385-424.

76. Bearman SI. The syndrome of hapatic veno-occlusive disease after marrow transplantation. Blood 1995;85:3005-3020.

77. Glickman E, Jolivet I, Scrobohaci ML, et al. Use of protaglandin E1 for prevention of liver veno-occlusive disease in leukemic patients with allogeneic bone marrow transplantation. Brit J Haematol 1990;74:277-281.

78. Cooke KR, Kobzik L, Martin TR, et al. An experimental model of idiopathic pneumonia syndrome after bone marrow transplantation. I. The roles of minor H antigens and endotoxin. Blood 1996;8:3230-3239.

79. Piguet PF, Grau GE, Collart MA, Vassalli P, et al. Pneumopathies of the graft-versus-host reaction. Alveolitis associated with an increased level of tumor necrosis factor MRNA and chronic interstitial pneumonitis. Lab Invest 1989;61:37-45.

80. Rubin P, Finkelstein J, Shapiro D. Molecular biology mechanisms in radiation induction of pulmonary injury syndromes: Interrelationship between the alveolar macrophage and the septal fibroblast. Int J Radiat Oncol Biol Phys 1992;24:93-101.

81. Jenkins MK, Schwartz RH. Antigen presentation by chemically modified splenocytes induces antigen specific T cell unresponsiveness *in vitro* and *in vivo*. J Exp Med 1987; 165:302-319.

82. Gross JA, Callas E, Allison JP. Identification and distribution of the costimulatory receptor CD28 in the mouse. J Immunol 1992;149:380-388.

83. Linsley PS, Brady W, Urnes M, et al. CTLA-4 is a second receptor for the B cell activation antigen B7. J Exp Med 1991;174:561-569.

84. Linsley PS, Wallace PM, Johnson J, et al. Immunosuppression in vivo by a soluble form of the CTLA-4 T cell activation molecule. Science 1992;257:792-795.

85. Lenschow DJ, Zeng Y, Thistlethwaite JR, et al. Long-term survival of xenogeneic pancreatic islet grafts induced by CTLA-4Ig. Science 1992;257:789-792.

86. Turka LA, Linsley PS, H.L., et al. T cell activation by the CD28 ligand B7 is required for cardiac allograft rejection in vivo. Proc Natl Acad Sci USA 1992;89:11102-11105.

87. Miller SD, Vanderlugt CL, Lenschow DJ, et al. Blockade of CD28/B7-1 interaction prevents epitope spreading and clinical relapses of murine EAE. Immunity 1995;3:739-745.

88. Lenschow DJ, Ho SC, Sattar H, et al. Differential effects of anti-B7-1 and anti-B7-2 monoclonal antibody treatment on the development of diabetes in the nonobese diabetic mouse. J Exp Med 1995;181:1145-1155.

89. Blazar BR, Taylor PA, Linsley PS, et al. In vivo blockade of CD28/CTLA4:B7/BB1 interaction with CTLA4-Ig reduces lethal murine graft-versus host disease across the major histocompatibility complex barrier in mice. Blood 1994;83:3815-3825.

90. Wallace PM, Johnson JS, MacMaster JF, et al. CTLA-4Ig treatment ameliorates the lethality of murine graft-versus-host disease across major histocompatibility complex barriers. Transplantation 1994;58:602-610.

91. Blazar BR, P.A. T, Gray GS, Vallera DA. The role of T cell subsets in regulating the in vivo efficacy of CTLA4-Ig in preventing graft-versus-host disease in recipients of fully MHC or minor histocompatibility (miH) only disparate donor inocula. Transplantaion 1994;58L1422-1426.

92. Blazar BR, Sharpe AH, Taylor PA, et al. Infusion of anti-B7.1 (CD80) and anti-B7.2 (CD86) monoclonal antibodies inhibit murine graft-versus-host disease lethality in part via direct effects on CD4[+] and CD8[+] T cells. J Immunol 1996;157:3250-3259.

93. Lenschow DJ, Sperling AI, Cooke MP, et al. Differential up-regulation of the B7-1 and B7-2 costimulatory molecules after Ig receptor engagement by antigen. J Immunol 1994;153:1990-1997.

94. Linsley PS, Greene J, Brady W, et al. Human B7-1 (CD80) and B7-2 (CD86) bind with similar avidities but distinct kinetics to CD28 and CTLA4 receptors. Immunity 1994;1:793-801.

95. Kuchroo VK, Das MP, Brown JA, et al. B7-1 and B7-2 costimulatory molecules activate differentially the Th1/Th2 developmental pathways:application to autoimmune disease therapy. Cell 1995;80:707-718.

96. Freeman GJ, Boussiotis VA, Anumanthan A, et al. B7-1 and B7-2 do not deliver identical costimulatory signals, since B7-2 but not B7-1 preferentially costimulates the initial production of IL-4. Immunity 1995;2:523-532.

97. Lenschow DJ. Expression and functional significance of an additional ligand for CTLA-4. Proc Natl Acad Sci USA 1993;90:11054-11058.

98. Hathcock KS, Laszlo G, Pucillo C, et al. Comparative analysis of B7-1 and B7-2 costimulatory ligands: expression and function. J Exp Med 1994;180:631-640.

99. Azuma M, Yssel H, Phillips JH, et al. Functional expression of B7/BB1 on activated T lymphocytes. J Exp Med 1993;25:207-211.

100. Das MRP, Zamvil SS, Borriello F, et al. Reciprocal expression of co-stimulatory molecules, B7-1 and B7-2, on murine T cells following activation. Eur J Immunol 1995;25:207-211.

101. Hirokawa M, Kitabayashi A, Kuroki J, et al. Signal transduction by B7/BB1 induces protein tyrosine phosphorylation and synergizes with signalling through T cell receptor/CD3. Immunol 1995;86:155-161.

102. Sansom DM, Hall ND. B7/BB1, the ligand for CD28 is expressed on repeatedly activated T cells in vitro. Eur J Immunol 1993;23:295-298.

103. Racke MK, Scott DE, Quigley L, et al. Distinct role for B7-1 (CD80) and B7-2 (CD86) in the initiation of experimental encephalomyelitis. J Clin Invest 1995;96:2195-2203.

104. Sprent J, von Boehmer H. Activation of T lymphocytes to M locus determinants in vivo. I. Quantitation of T cell proliferation and migration into thoracic duct lymph. Eur J Immunol 1976;6:352-358.
105. Hakim FT, Cepeda R, Gray GS, et al. Acute graft-versus-host reaction can be aborted by blockade of costimulatory molecules. J Immunol 1995;155:1757-1766.
106. Blazar BR, Boyer MW, Taylor PA, et al. The role of CD28:B7 in the persistent graft-vs-leukemia (GVL) effect of delayed post-BMT splenocyte infusions in mice. Blood 1995;86:115.
107. Boyer MW, Vallera DA, Taylor PA, et al. The role of B7 costimulation by murine acute myeloid leukemia in the generation and function of a CD8[+] T cell line with potent *in vivo* graft-versus-leukemia properties. Blood 1997;89(9):3477-3485.
108. Tan P, Anasetti C, Hansen JA, et al. Induction of alloantigen-specific hyporesponsiveness in human T lymphocytes by blocking interaction of CD28 with its natural ligand B7/BB1. J Exp Med 1993;177:165-173.
109. Blazar BR, Taylor PA, Panoskaltis-Mortari A, et al. Co-blockade of the LFA1:1CAM and CD28/CTLA4:B7 pathways is a highly effective means of preventing acute lethal graft-versus-host disease induced by fully major histocompatibility complex-disparate donor grafts. Blood 1995;85:2607-2618.
110. Lin H, Bolling SF, Linsley PS, et al. Long term acceptance of major histocompatibility complex mismatched cardiac allografts induced by CTLA-4Ig plus donor-specific transfusion. J Exp Med 1993;178:1801-1806.
111. Isobe M, Yagita H, Okumura K, et al. Specific acceptance of cardiac allograft after treatment with antibodies to ICAM-1 and LFA-1. Nature 1992;255:1125-1127.
112. Sligh JE, Ballantyne CM, Rich SS, et al. Inflammatory and immune responses are impaired in mice deficient in intercellular adhesion molecule-1. Proc Natl Acad Sci USA 1993;90:8529-8533.
113. Gribben JG, Guinan EC, Boussiotis VA, et al. Complete blockade of B7 family-mediated costimulation is necessary to induce human alloantigen-specific anergy: a method to ameliorate graft-versus-host disease and extend the donor pool. Blood 1996;87:4887-4893.
114. Groux H, Bigler M, deVries JE, et al. Interleukin-10 induces a long-term antigen-specific anergic state in human CD4[+] T cells. J Exp Med 1996;184:19-29.
115. Clark EA, Ledbetter JA. Activation of human B cells mediated through two distinct cell surface differentiation antigens, Bp35 and Bp50. Proc Natl Acad Sci USA 1986;72:4494-4498.

116. Hart DNJ, McKenzie JL. Isolation and characterization of human tonsil dendritic cells display a unique antigenic phenotype. J Exp Med 1988;168:157-170.

117. Schriever F, Freedman AS, Freeman G, et al. Isolated human follicular dendritic cells display a unique antigenic phenotype. J Exp Med 1989; 169(6): 2043-2058.

118. Galy AHM, Spits H. CD40 is functionally expressed on human thymic epithelium. J Immunol 1992;149:775-782.

119. Hollenbaugh D, Grosmaire LS, Kullas CD, et al. The human T cell antigen p39, a member of the TNF gene family, is a ligand for the CD40 receptor: expression of a soluble form of gp39 with B cell co-stimulatory activity. EMBO J 1992;11:4313-4321.

120. Armitage RJ, Fanslow WC, Strockbine L, et al. Molecular and biological characterization of a murine ligand for CD40. Nature 1992;357:80-82.

121. Noelle RJ, Roy M, Sheperd DM, et al. A 39 kDa protein on activated helper T cells bind CD40 and transduces the signal for cognate activation of B cells. Proc Natl Acad Sci USA 1992;89:6550-6554.

122. Lederman S, Yellin MJ, Inghirami G, et al. Molecular interactions mediating T-B lymphocyte collaboration in human lymphoid follicles; roles of T cell B cell-activating molecule (5c8 antigen) and CD40 in contact-dependent help. J Immunol 1992;149:3817-3826.

123. Hermann P, Van-Kooten C, Gaillard C, et al. CD40 ligand postive CD8[+] T cell clones allow B cell growth and differentiation. Eur J Immunol 1995;25:2927-2977.

124. Grammer AC, Bergman MC, Miura Y, et al. The CD 40 ligand expressed by human B cells costimulates B cell responses. J Immunol 1995;154:4996-5010.

125. Ranheim EA, Kipps TJ. Activated T cells induced expression of B7/BBI on normal or leukemic B cells through a CD40-dependent signal. J Exp Med 1993;177:925-935.

126. Kennedy MK, Mohler KM, Shanebeck KD, et al. Induction of B cell costimulatory function by recombinant murine CD40. Eur J Immunol 1994;24:116-123.

127. Klaus SJ, Pinchuk LM, Ochs HD, et al. Costimulation through CD28 enhances T cell dependent B cell activation via CD40-CD40L interaction. J Immunol 1994;152:5643-5652.

128. Ding L, Green JM, Thompson CG, et al. B7/CD28-dependent and – independent induction of CD40 ligand expression. J Immunol 1995;155:5124-5132.

129. Jaiswal AL, Dubey C, Swain SL, et al. Regulation of CD40 ligand expression on naïve CD4 T cells – a role for TCR but not costimulatory signals. Int Immunol 1996;8:275-285.

130. Buhlmann JE, Foy TM, Aruffo A, et al. In the absence of a CD40 signal, B cells are tolerogenic. Immunity 1995;2:645-653.

131. Hollander GA, Castigli E, Kulbacki R, et al. Induction of alloantigen-specific tolerance by B cells from CD40 deficient mice. Proc Natl Acad Sci USA 1996;1996:4994-4998.

132. Durie FH, Fava RA, Foy TM, et al. Prevention of collagen-induced arthritis with an antibody to gp39, the ligand for CD40. Science 1993;261:1328-1330.

133. Gerritse K, Laman JD, Noelle RJ, et al. CD40-CD40 ligand interactions in experimental allergic encephalomyelitis and multiple sclerosis. Proc Natl Acad Sci USA 1996;93:2499-2504.

134. Parker DC, Greiner DL, Phillips NE, et al. Survival of mouse pancreatic islet allografts in recipients treated with allogeneic small lymphocytes and antibody CD40 ligand. Proc Natl Acad Sci USA 1995;92:9560-9564.

135. Durie FH, Aruffo A, Ledbetter J, et al. Antibody to the ligand of CD40, gp39, blocks the occurrence of the acute and chronic forms of graft-vs-host disease. J Clin Invest 1994;94:1333-1338.

136. Blazar BR, Taylor P, Panoskaltsis-Mortari A, et al. Blockade of CD40 Ligand-CD40 Interaction Impairs CD4$^+$ T Cell Mediated Alloreactivity by Inhibiting Mature Donor T Cell Expansion and Function after Bone Marrow Transplantation. J Immunol 1997;158:29-39.

137. Blazar BR, Taylor PA, Noelle RJ, et al. CD4$^+$ T cells tolerized ex vivo to host alloantigen by anti-CD40 ligand (CD40L:CD154) antibody lose their graft-versus-host disease lethality capacity but retain nominal antigen responses. J Clin Invest 1998;102:473-482.

138. Imura A, Hori T, Imada K, et al. The human OX40/gp34 system directly mediates adhesion of activated T cells to vascular endothelial cells. J Exp Med 1996;1996:2185-2195.

139. Baum PR, Gayle RBr, Ramsdell F, et al. Molecular characterization of murine and human OX40/OX40 ligand systems: identification of a human OX40 ligand as the HTLV-1 regulated protein gp34. EMBO J 1994;13:3992-4001.

140. Stuber E, Storber W. The T-cell-B-cell interaction via OX40-Ox40L is necessary for the T-cell-dependent humoral immune response. J Exp Med 1996;183:979-989.

141. Weinburg AD, Bourdette DN, Sullivan TJ, et al. Selective depletion of myelin-reactive T cells with the anti-OX40 antibody ameliorates autoimmune encephalomyelitis. Nat Med 1996;2:183-189.

142. Tittle T, Steinkeler C, Weinberg A, et al. Identification of the T cells causing acute GvHD. FASEB J 1996;10:1435.

143. Durie FH. Conversion of chronic graft-versus-host disease to that of the acute phenotype using in vivo administration of an antibody to OX40. FASEB J 1996;10:1435.

144. Pollok KE, Kim YJ, Zhou Z, et al. Inducible T cell antigen 4-IBB. Analysis of expression and function. J Immunol 1993;150(3): 771-781.

145. DeBenedette MA, Chie NR, Pollok KE, et al. Role of 4-IBB ligand in costimulation of T lymphocyte growth and its upregulation on M12 B lymphomas by cAMP. J Exp Med 1995;181:985-992.

146. Boise LH, Minn AJ, Noel PJ, et al. CD28 costimulation can promote T cell survival by enhancing the expression of Bcl-xL. Immunity 1995;3:87-98.

147. Van Parijs L, Ibraghimov A, Abbas AK. The roles of costimulation and Fas in T cell apoptosis and peripheral tolerance. Immunity 1996;4:321-328.

148. Yonehara S, Ishii A, Yonehara M. A cell-killing monoclonal antibody (anti-Fas) to a cell surface antigen co-downregulated with the receptor of tumor necrosis factor. J Exp Med 1989;163:1747-1756.

149. Trauth BC, Klas C, Peters AM, et al. Monoclonal antibody-mediated tumor regression by induction of apoptosis. Science 1989;245:301-305.

150. Suda T, Takahashi T, Golstein P, et al. Molecular cloning and expression of the Fas ligand, a novel member of the tumor necrosis factor family. Cell 1993;75:1169-1178.

151. Suda T, Nagata S. Purification and characterization of the Fas-ligand that induces apoptosis. J Exp Med 1994;179:873-879.

152. Ogasawara J, Watanabe-Fu Kunaga R, Adachi M, et al. Lethal effect of the anti-Fas antibody in mice [published erratum appears in Nature 1993;365:568]. Nature 1993;364:806-809.

153. Suda T, Tanaka M, Miwa K, et al. Apoptosis of mouse naïve T cells induced by recombinant soluble fas ligand and activation-induced resistance to fas ligand. J Immunol 1996;157:3918-3924.

154. Watanabe-Fukunaga R, Brannan CI, Copeland NC, et al. Lympho-proliferation disorder in mice explained by defects in Fas antigen that mediates apoptosis. Nature 1992;356:314-317.

155. Takahashi T, Tanaka M, Brannan CI, et al. Generalized lymphoproliferative disease in mice, caused by a point mutation in the Fas ligand. Cell 1994;76:969-976.

156. Rouvier E, Luciani MF, Goldstein P. Fas involvement in Ca(2+)-independent T cell mediated cytotoxicity. J Exp Med 1993;177:195-200.

157. Watanabe-Fukunaga R, Braman CI, Itoh N, et al. The cDNA structure, expression and chromosomal assignment of the mouse Fas antigen. J Immunol 1992;148:1274-1279.

158. Braum MY, Lowin B, French L, et al. Cytotoxic T cells deficient in both functional fas ligand and perforin show residual cytolytic activity yet lose their capacity to induce lethal acute graft-versus-host disease. J Exp Med 1996;183:657-661.
159. Baker MB, Altman NH, Podack ER, et al. The role of cell-mediated cytotoxicity in acute GVHD after MHC-matched allogeneic bone marrow transplantation in mice. J Exp Med 1996;183:2645-2656.
160. Via C, Nguyen P, Shustov A, et al. A major role for the Fas pathway in acute graft-versus-host disease. J Immunol 1996;157:5387-5393.
161. Baker MB, Riley RL, Podack ER, et al. GVHD-associated lymphoid hypoplasia and B cell dysfunction is dependent upon donor T cell-mediated Fas-ligand function, but not perforin function. Proc Natl Acad Sci USA 1997;94:1366-1371.

16

ADOPTIVE IMMUNOTHERAPY FOR LEUKEMIA: DONOR LYMPHOCYTES TRANSDUCED WITH THE HERPES SIMPLEX THYMIDINE KINASE GENE

Charles J. Link Jr., M.D.[1]* Ann Traynor, M.D.[2];
Tatiana Seregina, Ph.D.[1], and Richard K Burt, M.D.[2]

[1]Human Gene Therapy Research Institute, Des Moines, IA 50309
[2]Northwestern University School of Medicine, Chicago, IL 60611;

Acknowledgments: This work (CJL and RKB) is supported in part by a grant from the Leukemia Society of America.

INTRODUCTION

Compared to autologous BMT, an allogeneic transplant can cure hematopoietic malignancies by transfer of donor cells that exert an anti-neoplastic effect called Graft-versus-Leukemia (GVL) (1). This GVL effect is so potent that some patients who relapse after allogeneic bone marrow transplantation can be reinduced into remission by donor lymphocyte infusions (DLI) (2,3). As with an allogeneic transplant, the main side effect of DLI is graft versus host disease (GVHD). The safety of this therapy might be improved by engineering the donor cells to permit their destruction if significant GVHD occurs. To this end, a number of clinical investigators are evaluating a strategy of infusing allogeneic lymphocytes which have been genetically modified by insertion of a latent suicide gene (4-8).

Mechanisms of GVL

GVL is an immune response of the donor cells against the recipient's leukemia. The targets for this immune reaction remain undefined although the close association with the GVHD process suggests that common mechanisms may operate. However, GVL may occur without GVHD. Lymphocyte reactivity between HLA-identical siblings is due to differences in minor histocompatibility antigens which are peptides presented on the cell surface by major histocompatibility complex (MHC) molecules. Two important characteristics of minor antigens are their tissue-restricted distribution and differences in ability to elicit an immune response. Several possible mechanisms could explain the differences between GVL and GVHD. T cell recognition of minor antigens that are present on both leukemic cells and normal recipient tissues could result in both GVL and GVHD. Quantitative differences in the presentation of these antigens by leukemic and normal cells could also create variability in the GVHD-GVL association. Some minor antigens have a tissue-restricted distribution. A normal myeloid antigen that remains present on the leukemia cells could elicit an anti-myeloid effect causing GVL without GVHD. Recognition leukemia-specific antigens could also produce GVL without GVHD.

Both CD8⁺ and CD4⁺ cells are thought to participate in GVL. CD8⁺ and CD4⁺ T cells can be cytotoxic using either the perforin mechanism that causes direct cell lysis or the Fas mechanism that results in apoptosis through receptor-ligand interaction. CD4⁺ T cells could enhance the GVL reaction by secreting cytokines such as IL-2 that help CD8⁺ T cells to clonally expand or other cytokines such as TNFα or IFNγ that could mediate a direct cytotoxic effect or recruit other secondary effector cells. Natural killer (NK) cells are also thought to play a role in the GVL by mediating cytotoxicity in a MHC-unrestricted fashion.

The minor antigens on leukemic cells responsible for GVL are in large part unknown. Even if leukemic specific minor antigens are known, the generation and propagation of leukemic specific lymphocytes is technically difficult. In addition, the subset of lymphocytes necessary to induce and maintain GVL is unknown. To circumvent these obstacles we are infusing lymphocytes which contain a latent suicide gene in case significant GVHD should occur.

SUICIDE STRATEGY

The herpes simplex thymidine kinase (HStk) gene is a negative selectable marker or "suicide" gene. HStk sensitizes the transduced cells to ganciclovir (GCV), an anti-Herpes drug (20). GCV is a substrate for phosphorylation by herpes thymidine kinase resulting in a monophosphate (MP) form of the drug within HStk transduced cells. Endogenous cellular phosphorylases convert GCV-MP to GCV-triphosphate (GCV-TP) which incorporates into DNA and inhibits DNA polymerase. The result is cell death for the HStk expressing cells. Since the human thymidine kinase enzyme, which is present in all human cells, has very low affinity for GCV, little systemic toxicity occurs.

An interesting *in vitro* and *in vivo* observation noted with HStk is that only a portion of tumor cells need to be transduced with this gene to effect complete tumor destruction. This has been termed "metabolic cooperation" or "bystander effect" (1, 9). The bystander effect arises at least in part by transfer of GCV-MP to neighboring cells via gap junctions from an HStk infected cell. Gap junctions are absent on lymphocytes and there is no evidence of a bystander effect from HStk transduced lymphocytes.

Viruses are a natural method of transferring genetic material into cells. If the viral backbone is genetically modified, it can function as a vehicle or vector to transfer new and even non-human genes into human cells. Retroviral vectors are currently the method of choice for the transfer and long term, stable expression of exogenous DNA into human lymphocytes (10, 11). Moloney murine leukemia virus-based vectors have been designed to be replication incompetent and to minimize the possibility of recombinant regeneration of a replication-competent virus (10, 11). Our initial protocol uses a HStk containing Moloney murine retrovirus to transduce donor lymphocytes prior to infusion. Since the efficiency of retroviral transduction is generally low, our retroviral construct also contains a selectable marker to isolate transduced lymphocytes. The selectable marker in our current trial is the neo^r (neomycin phosphotransferase) gene which allows selection for gene transfer in the presence of the neomycin analog, G418.

Clinical Study using HStk gene modified lymphocytes

The schema of our HStk DLI protocol is shown in figure 1. Four patients with chronic myelogenous leukemia, three patients with acute myelogenous leukemia, and one patient with cutaneous T cell lymphoma have received HStk DLI. No adverse reactions associated with gene modified lymphocytes have been observed in any of the patients. Two patients died of complications associated with their disease before receiving cell infusions and two additional patients' cells could not be grown *ex vivo*. Screening for replication competent retroviral testing was negative in all patients who received HStk modified donor lymphocytes. After infusion, the range of HStk positive peripheral blood lymphocytes varied from 0 to 3.8%. One patient with AML had a transient cytogenetic response to gene modified lymphocyte infusions. Two other patients entered remission, including a patient with CTCL and another patient with AML.

None of the CML patients that were treated with adoptive lymphocytes at the doses used demonstrated evidence of remission induction. One patient developed chronic GVHD that failed PUVA, corticosteroids and cyclosporine therapy. Following ganciclovir treatment (twice daily for five days) significant regression of GVHD occurred.

Several European groups have also reported results from infusion of allogeneic HStk transduced lymphocytes. Dr. Bordignon and colleagues proposed the first clinical study using HStk gene modified lymphocytes as a method to modulate GVHD after allogeneic bone marrow transplantation(4, 5). The vector used in their protocol contained two transgenes, the HStk-neo fusion gene and the truncated intracellular domain of the low affinity nerve growth factor receptor (NGFR). The NGFR gene was used as a selectable marker to permit rapid cell surface selection by flow cytometry of transduced cells. In the Bordignon study, no toxicity or complication was observed that could be attributed to the gene transfer procedure itself. In seven of the eight patients genetically modified lymphocytes could be detected in circulation or in biopsy specimens after infusion. Two patients developed acute GVHD. One patient developed chronic GVHD. Biopsy of GVHD lesions revealed the presence of the HStk transgene by PCR. Transduced cells were present up to 12 months after infusion and transgenic cells retained their immunologic activity. Three patients had complete responses including one patient each with acute myelogenous leukemia and chronic myelogenous leukemia, respectively. Two patients with chronic myelogenous leukemia exhibited partial responses. In the two patients who developed acute GVHD, ganciclovir eliminated transduced cells and resulted in regression of hepatic and cutaneous GVHD.

Two patients developed specific immune responses against the HStk transduced cells that resulted in their destruction. A specific immune response was defined against the cell surface marker that had been used to select for the transduced cell, the truncated nerve growth factor receptor (NGFR). This occurrence was observed at eight and nine months respectively in two patients after BMT. Another patient was noted who developed chronic GVHD that subsequently showed partial in vivo resistance to ganciclovir. When the transduced cells were analyzed *ex vivo* after being removed from the patient, they continued to show ganciclovir sensitivity. This suggests that despite HStk gene expression, in vivo resistance may have been related to the cell cycle dependent nature of ganciclovir killing (3).

Tiberghien et. al, (6, 7) have reported preliminary results using T cells transduced with retroviral construct containing HStk and neomycin resistance genes. Three patients at high risk for GVHD received gene modified T-lymphocytes at the time of a T cell depleted allogeneic BMT. No acute toxicity was observed. Two patients who developed GVHD had complete resolution of symptoms after administration of ganciclovir (6).

SUMMARY

The overall goal of adoptive immunotherapy with genetically modified lymphocytes is to decrease the morbidity and mortality associated with allogeneic bone marrow transplantation. The initial data reviewed here suggest that the behavior of the allogeneic HStk transgenic cells can be modified after administration to patients. Further study is needed to identify the response rates and risks associated with this procedure. In particular, larger studies will be needed with appropriate randomization to determine if the response rate to genetically modified cells is equivalent to the response rates with unmodified cells. Wider application of these techniques in the initial setting of allogeneic transplantation will undoubtedly occur and such trials have been initiated at several institutions. Careful attention to vector, suicide gene, selectable marker, efficiency of transduction, and cell dose will be necessary when comparing different trials since these variables will probably affect transgenic cell survival and response rates.

Figure 1. Protocol Schematic
Allogeneic Bone Marrow Transplant Followed by Relapse
↓
Apheresis of Original Transplant Donor and
Transduction of Donor Lymphocytes
↓
Administration of Cytoreductive Therapy to Recipient if Clinically Indicated
↓
Reinfusion of Donor Lymphocytes. May be given as multiple infusions over 1 to 4 weeks.

Lymphocyte Dose to be Administered

Patient Population	CD3+ Lymphocytes / Kg Recipient Weight
HLA-identical Sibling	0.1-2.5×10^8
HLA-Mismatched Related or HLA-Unrelated Donor	0.01-1.0×10^8

↓
Weekly Grading of GVHD and Leukemia Response
↓
Development of Clinically Significant Graft Versus Host Disease.
Treat with Standard Therapy
(corticosteroids with or without cyclosporine)
↓
Infusion of Ganciclovir for Progressive or Unresponsive GVHD After 72 Hours
5 mg/kg b.i.d. IV for 5 to 21 days

REFERENCES

1. Horowitz MM, Gale RP, Sondel PM, Goldman JM, Kersey J, Kolb HJ, Rimm AA, Ringden O, Rozman C, Speck B, Truitt RL, Zwaan FE, Bortin MM. Graft-versus-leukemia reactions after bone marrow transplantation. Blood 1990; 75:555-562.
2. Kolb HJ, Mittermuller J, Clemm CH, Holler E, Ledderose G, Brehm M, Wilmanns W. Donor Leukocyte Transfusion for Treatment of Recurrent Chronic Myelogenous Leukemia in Marrow Transplant Recipients. Blood 1990; 76:2462-65.
3. Kolb HJ, Schattenberg A, Goldman JM, Hertenstein B, Jacobsen N, Arcese W, Ljungman P, Ferrant A, Verdonck L, Niederwieser D, van Rhee F, Mittermueller J, de Witte T, Holler E, Ansari H. Graft-versus-leukemia effect of donor lymphocyte transfusions in marrow grafted patients. Blood 1995; 86:2041-2050.
4. Bonini C, Ferrari G, Verzeletti S, Servida P, Zappone E, Ruggieri L, Ponzoni M, Rossini S, Mavilio F, Traversari C, Bordignon C. HSV-TK gene transfer into donor lymphocytes for control of allogeneic graft-versus-leukemia. Science 1997; 276:1719-1724.
5. Bordignon C, Bonini C, Verzeletti S, Nobili N, Maggioni D, Traversari C, Giavazzi R, Servida P, Zappone E, Benazzai E, Massimo B, Porta F, Ferrari G, Mavilio F, Rossini S, Blaese RM, Candotti F. Transfer of HSV-tk gene into donor peripheral blood lymphocytes for in vivo modulation of donor anti-tumor immunity after allogeneic bone marrow transplantation. Human Gene Ther 1995; 6:813-819.
6. Tiberghien P, Cahn JY, Milpied N, Ferrand C, Deconinck E, Brion A, Reynolds CW, Jacob W, Certoux JM, Chiang Y, Herve P. Administration of donor T cells expressing the Herpes-simplex thymidine kinase gene in conjunction with a T cell depleted allogeneic marrow graft. Blood 1996; 10 Suppl 1.
7. Tiberghien P, Reynolds CW, Keller J, Spence S, Deschaseaux M, Certoux J, Contassot E, Murphy WJ, Lyons R, Chiang Y, Herve P, Longo D, Ruscetti FW. Ganciclovir treatment of Herpes simplex thymidine kinase-transduced lymphocytes: An approach for specific in vivo donor T cell depletion after bone marrow transplantation. Blood 1994; 84:1333-1341.
8. Link CJ, Burt RK, Traynor AE, Drobyski WR. Adoptive immunotherapy for leukemia: Donor lymphocytes transduced with the herpes simplex thymidine kinase gene for remission induction. Human Gene Therapy, 1997; 8: 1287-99.
9. Bi WL, Parysek LM, Warnick R, and Stambrook PJ. In vitro evidence that metabolic cooperation is responsible for the bystander effect observed with HSV tk retroviral gene therapy. Hum. Gene Ther 1993; 4:725-731.

10. Miller AD. Retroviral vectors. Curr. Top. Microbiol. Immunol. 1992; 158:1-24.
11. Miller A D, Buttimore C. Redesign of retrovirus packaging cell lines to avoid recombination leading to helper virus production. Molec. Cell Biol 1986; 6:2895-2902.

17

CLINICAL APPLICATION OF HEMATOPOIETIC STEM CELL CULTURE AND EXPANSION

Stephen G. Emerson, M.D., Ph.D. and
Patricia D. Conrad, M.D.
University of Pennsylvania School of Medicine, Philadelphia, PA 19104 USA

The tremendous amplification inherent in hematopoietic development in vivo has long tantalized clinician scientists with the notion that this physiology could be harnessed for clinical application. In these scenarios, ex vivo culture of hematopoietic cells could be employed for the generation of myeloid and lymphoid cells of various maturities and degrees of modifications, ranging from amplified stem cells to transfusion doses of mature red blood cells and platelets. Over the past decade, advances in our understanding of hematopoietic physiology have allowed investigators to begin to address these issues, and clinical trials are beginning to explore these possibilities.

IS CLINICALLY RELEVANT HEMATOPOIETIC CELL EXPANSION REALISTIC OR ACHIEVABLE?

As hematopoietic cell expansion has proven to be a difficult task, many investigators have appropriately questioned the overall feasibility of the project. Can stem cell numbers ever be expanded without loss of self-renewal? Does stem cell proliferation always result in stem cell senescence? Studies from several systems indicate that stem cell renewal may be regulated by both microenvironmental and internal genetic factors. Early serial bone marrow transplantation studies in the mouse by Mauch and Hellman suggested that stem cells had a limited capacity for renewal(34,35). However, recent careful studies by Iscove indicate that the initial transplantation and repopulation confers a set limit on the number of stem cells that are produced in the recipient mouse. If one transplants sufficient numbers of hematopoietic cells from the 1° recipients, these will expand and produce equal numbers of transplantable stem cells in the 2° recipients, and this process can be carried out without apparent exhaustion. Thus, the BMT environment limits the number of stem cells produced in a given mouse, but individual stem cells are capable of many logs of self-renewal(36). Of note, the replicative ability of the stem cell pool may not be infinite, and may decline with development, either as a consequence of aging or simply the passage of time, as a consequence of decreased telomerase activity (37-41).

How environmental cues which stimulate stem cell renewal are communicated to stem cells is not well understood. Over the past fifteen years a series of soluble cytokines has been hypothesized to support stem cell expansion, including IL-1, IL-3, SCF, Flt-3 ligand, Il-11, TPO, and HGF/Scatter Factor. SCF and Flt-3 ligand clearly play roles in the maintenance of stem cell numbers in vivo, while SCF, Flt-3 and IL-11 appear to have the ability to modestly increase transplantable stem cell numbers in vitro(42-46). Similarly, specific cell surface geometries, including fibronectin domains and heparan sulfates, have been hypothesized to support and trigger stem cell renewal. However, in no case has any of these cytokines or adhesion substrates, alone or in combination, been convincingly shown to stimulate a major amplification of the competitive long-term repopulating stem cell pool.

CURRENT APPROACHES TO EX VIVO HEMATOPOIETIC EXPANSION

Incubation of selected CD34+ cells with combinations of high dose cytokines (HDC) has been widely studied. Haylock et al.(1) first found that CD34+ mobilized peripheral blood cells could be driven to proliferate in dilute culture in the presence of 10 ng/ml IL-1β, IL-3, IL-6, G-CSF, GM-CSF and SCF. Under these conditions, the CFU-GM pool expanded 20-60 fold over input over 14 days, and many more mature precursors were generated as well. These results have subsequently been reproduced by many other groups, including Srour et al.(2), Coutinho et al.(3), and Brugger et al.(4). Each of these expansion protocols shares the use of highly CD34+ selected cells, dilute culture conditions, and multiple high dose cytokines. Without each of these features, proliferation is very much reduced in these cultures. Similar results have been obtained with bone marrow and umbilical cord blood cells, with some interesting variations, as will be discussed below.

Most of the progenitor cell amplification in these cultures appears to be occurring by terminal differentiation of pre-progenitors and stem cells. Not only does the number of CD34+ cells themselves decline in these HDC cultures, but the number of more primitive long term culture initiating cells (LTCIC) declines as well (2,3,4,5). Thus these cultures are unlikely to support expansion of pluripotent stem cells, and may actually result in stem cell depleted cell preparations.

The alternative approach to *ex vivo* hematopoietic expansion has been *continuous perfusion based culture of unselected hematopoietic cell populations*

(CPC). Perfusion, often used in conjunction with CSFs, has been used to stimulate functional stromal cells to both support stem cell renewal and supply local proliferative and differentiative CSFs, including GM-CSF, IL-6 and SCF(6,7,8). Similar rapid medium exchange schedules on whole bone marrow led to prolonged, stable progenitor cell production in culture, indicative of stem cell self-renewal. This effect was achieved by a combination of stimulation of the stromal elements, and by removal of metabolic byproducts produced by the maturing myeloid cells(9,10).

Taking advantage of stromal cell stimulation and added cytokines, rapid medium exchange has recently been combined with the addition of selected doses of exogenous CSFs. Koller, Palsson et al.(11) found that incubation of bone marrow mononuclear cells under continuous perfusion and oxygenation in the presence of low doses of SCF, IL-3, GM-CSF and Epo resulted in a 10-20 fold expansion of total mononuclear cells and CFU-GM, along with a 4-8 fold expansion in LTCIC. Subsequent studies by Koller et al. have shown that both the presence of the stromal layer, the presence of non-CD34+ non-stromal accessory cells, and the medium exchange provided by perfusion each contribute to the maintenance and expansion of LTCIC in these systems(12). Zandstra et al. confirmed the effect of perfusion and cytokines in stimulating simultaneous LTCIC and progenitor cell expansion in stroma-replete bone marrow cells(13), demonstrating several fold expansion of LTCIC in stirred flask bioreactors. Taken together, these studies suggest that *ex vivo* expansion of the progenitor cell pool concomitant with maintenance and limited expansion of the LTCIC pool may be possible via a single step culture of fairly unmanipulated bone marrow.

Whether or not any of the currently employed human ex vivo hematopoietic culture techniques support the amplification of the most primitive human hematopoietic stem cell pool is not known. Clearly, techniques that foster the survival and net expansion of long-lived pluripotent stem cells will be essential for all allogeneic applications, and for at least some autologous stem cell support applications as well. Even in autologous, high dose chemotherapy support applications, since the number of stem cells that survive high dose preparative therapy will almost certainly vary widely among patients, it seems most prudent to attempt to provide hematopoietic infusions that themselves contain the requisite number of long-term repopulating stem cells.

SOURCES OF HEMATOPOIETIC CELLS FOR EXPANSION: BONE MARROW, PERIPHERAL BLOOD, UMBILICAL CORD BLOOD

Bone marrow, mobilized peripheral blood, and umbilical cord blood have all been successfully used as starting populations for *ex vivo* expansions. Each has its potential advantages, and each has its theoretical concerns as a clinical source. The advantage of *bone marrow* is that pluripotent stem cells are known to be present at the start of the culture, and all of the elements needed for their *in vivo* survival are likely to be present. In addition, in these studies the bone marrow cells have been put through little manipulation prior to culture, and in fact these cultures perform optimally when all bone marrow cellular elements are left in the starting cell population. Based upon numerical calculations, results of these studies project that an engrafting dose of hematopoietic stem and progenitor cells could be obtained with approximately 5×10^8 BMMC, which could be obtained from a small number of analytical scale bone marrow aspirates in the outpatient setting(11,12,14).

Mobilized peripheral blood CD34+ cells (MPB) show extremely high levels of progenitor and precursor cell expansion, with post-pre expansion progenitor cell ratios exceeding 50. The attractions of this approach are the availability of the starting material from circulating blood after patient mobilization with cytokines and/or chemotherapy, and the excellent track record of mobilized peripheral blood for very rapid hematopoietic reconstitution. A significant potential concern with cultured MPB CD34 cells is the long term durability of the grafts in highly myeloablated patients, since graft failure has been reported with the use of such cells as sole support(15). However, the combination of stromal based perfusion cultures with mobilized peripheral blood cells might provide an attractive alternative.

Umbilical cord blood cell (UCB) transplants could be directly augmented by ex vivo cultured cells. Based upon extensive in vitro studies(16,17,18,19,20), UCB was first utilized as a source of transplantable stem cells in 1990 by Gluckman et al. for a child with Fanconi's Anemia(21). Overall, the results of the >100 UCB transplants to date suggest that: 1)UCB stem cells exist and can engraft after infusion; 2)Engraftment kinetics are slower than for bone marrow or mobilized peripheral blood cells; and 3)Recipient graft-versus-host disease is no more severe, and perhaps milder, than with bone marrow donor cells(22). However, it is possible that the in vivo expansion potential of UCB cells is not infinite, nor easily influenced after reinfusion. While some larger children weighing as much as 70 Kg have successfully engrafted following UCB transplantation, a number of recipients weighing over 40 Kg have failed to engraft following UCB infusions from standard cord blood collections.

In the context of *ex vivo* expansion, studies by Lansdorp et al. (20) and Moore et al.(23) suggest that UCB may be cultured in high doses of soluble cytokines, without extensive loss of either phenotypically (CD34+) or functionally primitive cells. These results are quite distinct from those with bone marrow or peripheral blood hematopoietic cells cultured under the identical conditions by these investigators. Taken together, these studies suggest that *ex vivo* expansion of UCB could have tremendous impact on the applicability of UCB to diverse clinical settings, including the treatment of older children and adults.

HEMATOPOIETIC GROWTH FACTORS IN THE EX VIVO EXPANSION CULTURES

Ex vivo hematopoietic expansion cultures have been performed with a variety of combinations of cytokines, with little consensus emerging as to the optimal combination for clinical use. In general, high doses of proliferative cytokines appear to drive differentiation of primitive cells while simultaneously depleting the stem cell pool, while inhibitory cytokines (e.g. MIP-1α) both decrease the overall production of mature progenitors and precursors but favor primitive stem cell survival(1,2,3,4,5,24). Interestingly perfusion based stromal cultures result in the endogenous production of low levels of SCF, IL-6, Flt-3 ligand and undoubtedly other cytokines, perhaps favoring the survival of primitive hematopoietic cells while permitting some degree of amplification of the more mature progenitor and precursor pools (13,14,15).

Following this flurry of initial activity, more recent experiments have focused on those cytokines that murine transplantation experiments suggest have a role in true expansion of transplantable stem cells, as measured in competitive repopulation assays. These most notably include SCF, Flt-3 ligand, and perhaps IL-11. To date, however, no xenogeneic transplant experiments prove conclusively that the number of human competitive repopulating units are increased dramatically by these same cytokines, either alone or in combination.

Most recently, significant interest has been raised concerning the potential role of thrombopoietin (TPO) in stem cell expansion. Early reports suggested that TPO, particularly in combination with SCF and/or Flt-3 ligand, had the effect of producing stable in vitro hematopoietic cultures for several months, that could only be explained if the cultures were supporting several logs of primitive hematopoietic cell expansion (32). Follow up studies have indeed supported the notion that TPO amplifies multilineage differentiation of primitive hematopoietic cells. However, confirmatory reports of non-decaying hematopoietic cultures with ongoing production of progenitor cells over months of culture have not been forthcoming. Nonetheless, all of the available evidence suggests that a combination of TPO with SCF, possibly also including Flt-3 ligand, would be the current best approach to expanding primitive populations of human hematopoietic cells ex vivo.

INITIAL CLINICAL EXPERIENCE WITH *EX VIVO* EXPANDED HEMATOPOIETIC CELLS

Dexter and colleagues first returned cultured bone marrow to two patients in 1983(25,26), and Barnett, Eaves and colleagues have extensive experience in returning cultured bone marrow to patients with CML(27). Silver et al. first returned bone marrow mononuclear cells derived from 14 day perfusion cultures supplemented with IL-3, GM-CSF, Epo and SCF as adjuncts to autografts in 5 patients with Hodgkin's Disease and Non-Hodgkin's Lymphoma (28). Bender et al. studied 5 patients who received enriched CD34+ mobilized peripheral blood cells cultured the GM-CSF/IL-3 fusion protein PIXY321 for 12 days, the dose infused the day after reinfusion of the standard, non-cultured PBMC dose. In each of these studies, the investigators found no toxicities associated with the infusions (29).

Reports of *ex vivo* cultured CD34+ cells as sole autograft supports have now been publicly presented. Holyake et al. found that CD34+ PB cells cultured in IL-3, SCF, IL-6, IL-1β and Epo could rapidly reconstitute hematopoiesis following autografting preparation, but observed a worrisome incidence of subsequent graft failure(15). Brugger et al. published the results of very similar clinical trials, but only commented on early hematopoietic recovery(30). Of 6 patients who received ex vivo cultured cells alone 5 survived, with mean neutrophil recoveries to 500 and 1000 ANC occurring 2 days later than in patients receiving both native and cultured cells, while platelet recoveries were indistinguishable in the two small groups. Of substantial concern, however, no follow-up on these patients has been reported, so that the intermediate and long-term stability of these recoveries cannot be determined. Overall, while it is too early to know the durability of the hematopoietic recoveries in these patients, and while the chemotherapy regimen employed may not have been truly myeloablative, these results clearly support the notion that a fairly small number of enriched hematopoietic progenitor cells cultured *ex vivo* under these conditions will initiate hematologic reconstitution. If subsequent graft failure is indeed a problem with CD34+ selected expanded products, then stromal based cultures, or some other approach to maintaining primitive stem cells while expanding late progenitors and precursors, will need to be pursued instead. Similarly, sophisticated applications providing genetically modified stem cells will require persistence of modified long-term repopulating stem cells, which may itself require stromal based perfusion cultures (31) or similarly stem cell supportive approaches.

A clinical trial combining soluble cytokine expansion and perfusion-based expansion of UCB has recently been reported. In these studies, Kurtzberg and colleagues removed aliquots of UCB from thawed samples prior to reinfusion and cultured the aliquot in PIXY/Epo/Flt-3 ligand for 12 days. After the 12 day culture, these cells were reinfused into the patients, and their clinical course was followed. No demonstrable shortening of the neutrophil or platelet nadir was achieved in these patients, perhaps due to the cells being added on day 12, not day 0. Nonetheless, overall patient morbidity was low, and overall day 100 survival was substantially higher than in a recent group of comparably treated UCB transplant patients at the same center(33). Definitive evaluation of this approach awaits randomized clinical trials, which are now under design. In addition, case reports in abstract form have identified cases in which ex vivo expansion of UCB cells in perfusion bioreactors have allowed the sustained engraftment of large adults with relatively low UCB cell yields (47).

One of the major barriers to the full exploration of clinical trials is lack of cytokine availability, both by themselves and as supplements to stromal based cultures. To date, intellectual property issues have prevented the combination of the best candidate cytokines for study in clinical settings. Until such time as each of these cytokines is available for study in a pure, well-characterized formulation suitable for a FDA and IRB approved clinical trial, the optimal clinical results may indeed be elusive.

In summary, *ex vivo* stem and progenitor cell expansion has the potential for a wide variety of clinical applications (Table 1). The full range of applications will need to be determined by careful clinical trials assessing the efficacy of these cell products for short term nadir ablation and long term stem cell reconstitution, as well as more specialized cellular and genetic applications.

Table 1. Potential Clinical Application of Ex Vivo Expanded Hematopoietic Cells
A) Myelopoietic Support of Hematopoietically Compromised Host
    1) Autologous Bone Marrow Transplantation
    2) Allogeneic Bone Marrow Transplantation
    3) Non-Transplant Nadir Rescue
    4) Umbilical Cord Blood Transplantation

B) Ex vivo Education/Modification of Stem Cells and Derivative Cells
    1) T Cell Depletion of Stem Cell Grafts for Allogeneic Bone Marrow Transplantation
    2) T Cell Depleted Autologous Transplantation for Autoimmune Diseases
    3) Active Purging of Tumor Cells from Stem Cell Autografts in Vitro
    4) Adoptive Immunotherapy via T Cells Generated and Educated Ex Vivo
    5) Permanent Genetic Modification of Stem Cells

REFERENCES

1. Haylock, D.N., To, L.B., Dowse, T.L., Juttner, C.A., Simmons P.J.. *Ex vivo* expansion and maturation of peripheral blood CD34+ cells into the myeloid lineage. Blood 1992; 80:1405-1412.
2. Srour, E.G., Brandt, J.E., Briddell, R.A., Grigsby, S., Leemhuis, T., Hoffman, R. Long-term generation and expansion of human primitive hematopoietic progenitor cells *in vitro*. Blood 1993; 81:661-669.
3. Coutinho, L.H., Will, A., Radford, J., et al. Effects of recombinant human granulocyte colony-stimulating factor(CSF), human granulocyte macrophage-CSF, and gibbon interleukin-3 on hematopoiesis in human long-term bone marrow culture. Blood 1990; 75:21182129.
4. Brugger, W., Mocklin, W., Heimfeld, S., Berenson, R.J., Mertelsmann, Kanz L. *Ex vivo* expansion of enriched peripheral blood CD34+ progenitor cells by stem cell factor, interleukin 1β(IL-1β), Il-6, Il-3, interferon-γ and erythropoietin. Blood 1993; 81:2579-2584.
5. Henschler, R., Brugger, W., Luft, T., Frey, T., Mertelsmann, R., Kanz, L. Maintenance of transplantation potential in *ex vivo* expanded CD34+-selected human peripheral blood progenitor cells. Blood 1994; 84:2898-2903.
6. Caldwell, J., Locey, B., Palsson, B.O., Emerson, S.G.: The influence of culture perfusion conditions on normal human bone marrow stromal cell metabolism. J Cell Physiol 1991; 147:344-353.

7. Caldwell, J., Locey, B., Clarke, M.F., Emerson, S.G., Palsson, B.O.: The influence of culture conditions on genetically engineered NIH-3T3 cells. Biotech Prog 1991; 7:1-8.
8. Guba, S.C., Sartor, C.I., Gottschalk, L.R., Ye-Hu, J., Xiao, L.C., Mulligan, T., Emerson, S.G. Bone marrow stromal cells secrete IL-6 and GM-CSF in the absence of inflammatory stimuli: Demonstration by serum-free bioassay, ELISA, and reverse transcriptase polymerase chain reaction. Blood 1992; 80:1190-1198.
9. Schwartz, R., Palsson, B.O., Emerson, S.G.: Rapid medium and serum exchange increases the longevity and productivity of human bone marrow cultures. Proc Nat Acad Sci USA 1991; 88:6760-6764.
10. Schwartz, R., Emerson, S.G., Clarke, M.F., Palsson, B.O.: In vitro myelopoiesis stimulated by rapid medium exchange and supplementation with hematopoietic growth factors. Blood 1991; 78:3155-3161.
11. Koller, M.R., Emerson, S.G. Palsson, B.O. Large-Scale Expansion of Human Hematopoietic Stem and Progenitor Cells from Bone Marrow Mononuclear Cells in Continuous Perfusion Culture. Blood 1993; 82:378-384.
12. Koller, M.R., Palsson, M.A., Manchel, I., et al. Long-term culture-initiating cell expansion is dependent on frequent medium exchange combined with stromal and other accessory cell effects. Blood 1995; 86(5): 1784-1793.
13. Zandstra, P.W., Eaves, C.J., Cameron, C., and Piret, J.M. Cytokine depletion in long-term stirred suspension cultures of normal human marrow. J Hematoth 1995; 4:235.
14. Champlin, R., Mehra, R., Gajewski, J., Khouri, I., Geisler, D., Davis, M., Oba, K., Thomas, M., Armstrong, R.D., Douville, J., Weber, S., Silver, S., Muller, T., Deisseroth, A. Ex Vivo expanded progenitor cell transplantation in patients with breast cancer. Blood 1995; 86: Suppl 1166a.
15. Holyoake, T.L., Alcorn, M.J., Richmond, L., Pearson, C., Farrell, E., Kyle, B., Dunlop, D.J., Fitzsimons, E., Steward, W.P., Pragnell, I.B., Franklin, I.M. Phase I study to evaluate the safety of re-infusing CD34 cells expanded ex vivo as part or all of a PBPC transplant procedure. Blood 1995; 86: Suppl 1161a.
16. Broxmeyer, H.E., Douglas G.W., Hangoc G., Cooper, S., Bard, J., English, D., Arny, M., Thomas, L., Boyse, E.A. Human umbilical cord blood as a potential source of transplantable hematopoietic stem/progenitor cells. Proc Natl Acad Sci U.S.A. 1989; 86:3828-3823.
17. Broxmeyer, H.E., Hangoc, G., Cooper, S., Ribeiro, R.C., Graves, V., Yoder, N.M., Wagner, J., Vadhan-Raj, S., Benninger, L., Rubinstein, P. Growth characteristics and expansion of human umbilical cord blood and estimation of its potential for transplantation in adults. Proc Natl Acad Sci USA 1992; 89:4109-4113.

18. Fleischman, R.A., Mintz, B., Development of adult bone marrow stem cells in H-2-compatible and -incompatible mouse fetuses. J Exp Med 1984; 159:731-745.
19. Carow, C.E., Hangoc, G., Broxmeyer, H.E. Human multipotential progenitor cells (CFU-GEMM) have extensive replating capacity for secondary (CFU-GEMM): An effect enhanced by cord blood plasma. Blood 1993; 81:942-949.
20. Mayani, H., Lansdorp, P.M. Thy-1 expression is linked to functional properties of primitive hematopoietic progenitor cells from human umbilical cord blood. Blood 1994; 83:2410-2417.
21. Gluckman, E., Devergie, A., Bourdeau-Esperou, H., Theirry, D., Traineau, R., Auerbach, A., Broxmeyer, H.E. Transplantation of umbilical cord blood in Fanconi's anemia. Nouv Rev Fr Hematol 1990; 32:423-435.
22. Wagner, J.E., Kernan, N.A., Steinbuch, M., Broxmeyer, H.E., Gluckman, E. Allogeneic sibling umbilical-cord-blood transplantation in children with malignant and non-malignant disease. Lancet 1995; 346:214-219.
23. Moore, M.A.S., Hoskins, I. Ex vivo expansion of cord blood-derived stem cells and progenitors. Blood Cells 1994; 20:468-481.
24. Mayani, H, Little, M-T., Dragowska, W., Thornbury, G., Lansdorp, P.M. Differential effects of the hematopoietic inhibitors MIP-1α, TGF-β, and TNF-α on cytokine-induced proliferation of subpopulations of CD34+ cells purified from cord blood and fetal liver. Exp Hematol 1995; 23:422-427.
25. Spooncer, E., Dexter, T.M. Transplantation of long term cultured bone marrow cells. Transplantation 1984; 35:624-627.
26. Chang, J., Morgenstern, G., Deakin, D., Testa, N.G., Coutinho, L., Scharffe, J.H., Harrison, C., Dexter, T.H. Reconstitution of haemopoietic system with autologous marrow taken during relapse of acute myeloblastic leukaemia and grown in long-term culture. Lancet 1986; 294-295.
27. Barnett, M.J., Eaves, C.J., Phillips, G.L., Kalousek D.K., Klingemann, H.G., Lansdorp, P.M., Reece, D.E., Shepherd, J.D., Shaw, G.J., Eaves, A.C. Successful autografting in chronic myeloid leukaemia after maintenance of marrow in culture. Bone Marrow Transplantation 1989; 4:345-351.
28. Silver, S.M., Adams, P.T., Hutchinson, R.J., Douville, J.W., Paul, L.A., Clarke, M.F., Palsson, B.O., Emerson, S.G. Phase I evaluation of ex vivo expanded hematopoietic cells produced by perfusion culture in autologous bone marrow transplantation(ABMT). Blood Suppl 1993; 1 82:297a.
29. Bender, J.G., Zimmerman, T., Lee, W.J., Loudovaris, M.F., Qiao, X., Schilling, M.L., Smith, S.L., Unverzagt, K.L., Van Epps, D.E., Blake, M., Williams, D.E., Williams, S. Large scale selection and expansion of CD34+ cells in PIXY321: Phase I/II Clinical Studies. J Hematoth 1995; 4:237.

30. Brugger, W., Heimfeld, S., Berenson, R.J., Mertelsmann, R., Kanz, L. Reconstitution of hematopoiesis after high-dose chemotherapy by autologous progenitor cells generated *ex vivo*. N Engl J Med 1995; 333:283-287.

31. Eipers, P.G., Krause, J.C., Palsson, B.O., Emerson, S.G., Todd, R.F., Clarke, M.F. Retroviral infection of primitive hematopoietic cells in continuous perfusion culture. Blood 1995; 86:3754-3762;.

32. Pacibello, W., Sanavio, F., Garetto, L., Severino, A., Bergandi, D., Farrario, J., Faglioli, F., Berger, M., Aglietta, M. Extensive amplification and self-renewal of human primitive hematopoietic stem cells from cord blood. Blood 1997; 89:2644-2653;.

33. Jaroscak, J., P.L. Martin, B. Waters-Pick, R.D. Armstrong, T. Driscoll, R.P. Howrey, S. CastellinolJ. Douville, S. kBukrhop, K. Goltry, P. Rubinstein, A. Smith, J. Kurtzberg, J. A phase I trial of augmentation of unrelated umbilical cord blood transplantation with *ex vivo* expanded cells. Blood 1998; 92 Sup1: 523a.

34. Mauch P. Botnick LE. Hannon EC. Obbagy J. Hellman S. Decline in bone marrow proliferative capacity as a function of age. Blood. 1982; 60:245-252.

35. Mauch P. Hellman S. Loss of hematopoietic stem cell self-renewal after bone marrow transplantation. Blood. 1989; 74(2):872-875.

36. Iscove NN. Nawa K. Hematopoietic stem cells expand during serial transplantation in vivo without apparent exhaustion. Current Biology 1997; 7(10):805-808.

37. Lansdorp PM. Developmental changes in the function of hematopoietic stem cells. Experimental Hematology 1995; 23 (3):187-191.

38. Vaziri H. Dragowska W. Allsopp RC. Thomas TE. Harley CB. Lansdorp PM. Evidence for a mitotic clock in human hematopoietic stem cells: loss of telomeric DNA with age. Proceedings of the National Academy of Sciences of the United States of America 1994; 91(21):9857-9860.

39. Akiyama M. Hoshi Y. Sakurai S. Yamada H. Yamada O. Mizoguchi H. Changes of telomere length in children after hematopoietic stem cell transplantation. Bone Marrow Transplantation 1998; 21(2):167-171.

40. Wynn RF. Cross MA. Hatton C. Will AM. Lashford LS. Dexter TM. Testa NG. Accelerated telomere shortening in young recipients of allogeneic bone-marrow transplants. Lancet 1998; 351(9097):178-181.

41. Notaro R. Cimmino A. Tabarini D. Rotoli B. Luzzatto L. *In vivo* telomere dynamics of human hematopoietic stem cells. Proc Nat Acad Sci USA 1997; 94:13782-13785.

42. Bodine, D.M., Seidel, N.E., Zsebo, K.M, Orlic, D. In vivo administration of stem cell factor mice increases the absolute number of pluripotent stem cells. Blood 1993; 82:445-455.

43. Yonemura, Y., Ku, H., Lyman, S.D., Ogawa, M. In vitro expansion of hematopoietic progenitors and maintenance of stem cells: Comparison between flt3/flk2 ligand and kit ligand. Blood 1997; 89:1915-1921.
44. Nandurkar, H.H., Robb, L., Tarlinton, D., Barnett, L., Kontgen, F., Beglet C.G. Adult mice with targeted mutation of the interluekin-11 receptor display normal hematopoiesis. Blood 1997; 90:2148-2159.
45. Miller, C.L., Eaves, C.J. Expansion in vitro of adult murine hematopoietic stem cells with transplantable lympho-myeloid reconstituting ability. Proc Natl Acad Sci USA 1997; 94:13648-13651.
46. Macharehtschian K., Hardin, J.D., Moore, K.A., Boast, S., Goff, S.F., Lemischka, I, R. Targeted disruptoin of the fltk2/flt3 gene leads to deficiencies in primitive hematopoietic progenitors. Immunity 1995; 3:147-156.
47. Pecora, A.L., Stiff, P., Jennis, A., Goldberg, S., Rosenbluth, R., Price, P., Douvile, J., Armonstrong, R., Smith, A., Preti, R. Rapid and durable engraftment in two patients with high risk CML using unexpanded and expanded umbilical cord blood stem cells. 1999 ASBMT Meeting, Keystone, CO, Abstr. #62, p18.

18

NEW CYTOKINES AND THEIR CLINICAL APPLICATION

Ian K. McNiece, Ph.D.

Bone Marrow Transplant Unit, University of Colorado Health Sciences Center, Denver, CO 80262 USA

INTRODUCTION

The production of mature blood cells is controlled by a network of proteins called hematopoietic growth factors (HGFs). A number of HGFs were identified by their ability to stimulate colony formation in semi solid agar culture of normal bone marrow (1-2), and were called colony stimulating factors (3). It was shown that colonies of mature granulocytes were formed in the presence of granulocyte colony stimulating factor (G-CSF) (4), colonies of mature macrophages were formed in the presence of macrophage colony stimulating factor (M-CSF or CSF-1) (5) and mixed colonies of macrophages and granulocytes were formed in the presence of granulocyte-macrophage colony stimulating factor (GM-CSF) (6). Subsequently, some of the CSFs have been taken to clinical trials and are now used routinely in clinical treatments. G-CSF for example has been shown to stimulate recovery of neutrophils after chemotherapy and is used clinically to shorten the period of neutropenia after chemotherapy (7,8). Both G-CSF and GM-CSF are routinely used alone or in combination with chemotherapy to mobilize peripheral blood progenitor cells (PBPC) from the bone marrow to the peripheral circulation (9,10). The use of PBPC has replaced the use of bone marrow for cellular support following high dose chemotherapy, due to more rapid recovery in neutrophils and platelets resulting in a considerable decrease in overall costs of the transplant (11).

In the past 5 to 10 years a number of novel HGFs have been identified. These include Interleukin-11 (IL-11), Stem Cell Factor (SCF), Thrombopoietin (Tpo), and Flt-3 ligand (Flt-3L). At present a number of these novel HGFs are in clinical development and are in phase I studies or recently approved such as IL-11. In this chapter, the basic biology of these factors will be summarized and their clinical applications discussed.

An overview of the hematopoietic growth factors is presented in Table 1, listing the approved growth factors and the stage of clinical development of each factor.

Table 1: The Hematopoietic Growth Factors

Factor	Status	Clinical Indications
G-CSF	Approved	Neutropenia following chemotherapy, PBPC mobilization.
GM-CSF	Approved	Neutropenia following BMT, PBPC mobilization.
Epo	Approved	Anemia
IL-11	Approved	Thrombocytopenia following chemotherapy
SCF	PLA submitted[1]	Mobilization of PBPC in combination with G-CSF
FLT-3L	Phase I/II	Mobilization of PBPC

[1] Product licence application (PLA) submitted to the FDA

A number of other HGFs have been used in clinical studies but have not continued towards regulatory approval due to minimal clinical benefit or unacceptable toxicities. These include interleukin-1 (IL-1) which was evaluated for prevention of myelosuppression from chemotherapy (12), interleukin-3 (IL-3) which has been evaluated for hematopoietic recovery following chemotherapy and for mobilization of PBPC (13), and interleukin -6 (IL-6) which has been evaluated for recovery of platelets after chemotherapy (14). These HGFs demonstrate the complexity involved in taking HGFs to the clinic and ultimately to registration.

INTERLEUKIN-11 (IL-11)

IL-11 was first purified and cloned in 1990 from a nonhuman primate stromal cell line (15). The human IL-11 genomic sequence was subsequently cloned in 1992 (16). The protein has a molecular weight of approximately 19 kDa and binds to a multimeric receptor complex which contains an IL-11-specific alpha subunit and a 130 kDa beta subunit (gp130) (17). IL-11 is expressed in vivo in a wide range of tissue, including bone marrow fibroblasts, neurons of the central nervous system (CNS) and in developing spermatogonia of the testis (15,18,19).

In vitro, IL-11 has little stimulatory effect alone, but acts in synergy with other growth factors to stimulate colony formation of both primitive and committed progenitor cells (20). The primary hematopoietic activity of IL-11 is stimulation of megakaryocytopoiesis. In combination with IL-3, IL-11 enhances the growth of megakaryocyte colonies, resulting in increased numbers of colonies and an increase in the size of the colonies. IL-11 has been shown to stimulate both primitive (BFU-Mk) and committed (CFU-Mk) progenitor cells (21,22).

Treatment of normal mice and nonhuman primates with IL-11 results in marked stimulation of megakaryocytopoiesis. In nonhuman primates, IL-11 treatment results in an increase in circulating platelets by increasing the size and maturation rate of bone marrow megakaryocytes (23). IL-11 significantly increases peripheral WBC counts in mice following bone marrow transplant (BMT) or following sublethal irradiation in mice (24). A dose-dependent increase in platelet counts was also seen following BMT or sublethal irradiation (24).

Clinical Use of IL-11
RhIL-11 was evaluated in a randomized placebo-controlled study in patients with breast cancer receiving dose-intensive cyclophosphamide and doxorubicin (25). Women with advanced breast cancer, who received chemotherapy plus G-CSF, were randomized to blinded treatment with placebo or 50 µg/kg/d of rhIL-11 subcutaneously for 10 or 17 days after the first two chemotherapy cycles. Platelet transfusions were required in 22 of 37 (59%) in the placebo group versus 13 of 40 (32%) in the rhIL-11 treated group (P=.04). Treatment with rhIL-11 significantly reduced the total number of platelet transfusions required (P=.03) and the time to platelet recovery to more than 50,000 platelets/ul in the second cycle (P=.01). The majority of adverse events were reversible, mild to moderate in severity and likely related to fluid retention (25).

In November of 1997 the Food and Drug Administration (FDA) approved Neumega (Oprelvekin - rhIL-11) for the prevention of severe thrombocytopenia and the reduction of the need for platelet transfusion following myelosuppressive chemotherapy in patients with nonmyeloid malignancies who are at risk of severe thrombocytopenia. Oprelvekin, the active ingredient in Neumega, is produced in E.coli and the protein has a molecular weight of approximately 19 kDa and is non-glycosylated. The polypeptide is 177 amino acids in length and differs from the native IL-11 which has 178 amino acids including a proline at the amino-terminus of the protein.

STEM CELL FACTOR (SCF)

In 1990, several groups reported the isolation of a protein which was the ligand for the tyrosine kinase receptor, c-kit. SCF was identified by Zsebo and colleagues (26) by its ability to stimulate primitive progenitor cells in combination with other HGFs. SCF was shown to be identical to mast cell growth factor (MGF) (27), and kit ligand (KL) (28). There are two forms of SCF which result from alternate splicing of the DNA, resulting in a membrane bound form and a soluble form (29). The native soluble SCF exists as a dimeric glycoprotein with a molecular weight of approximately 45 kDa (26). The primary site of SCF production in the marrow is by stromal cells, including fibroblasts (27,29).

The in vitro properties of the recombinant rat and human SCF (rrSCF and rhSCF) suggest that it is a multipotent factor acting on cells of the myeloid, erythroid, mast and lymphoid lineages (30-34). In liquid culture of normal mouse bone marrow cells, rrSCF generates pure populations of mast cells (35), while in semi solid agar culture, rrSCF stimulates mixed colony formation of neutrophil, macrophage and megakaryocyte cells (30). Primitive erythroid progenitors (Burst Forming Unit-erythroid; BFU-e), in both human and mouse bone marrow, are stimulated by SCF in the presence of erythropoietin (Epo) (32-34,36). The addition of IL-3 to the combination of SCF plus Epo results in increased colony numbers equivalent to the sum of colonies formed with SCF plus Epo and IL-3 plus Epo. This suggests that the erythroid progenitors stimulated by SCF plus Epo are different to the erythroid progenitors stimulated by IL-3 plus Epo (32). IL-7 synergizes with rrSCF to stimulate pre-B cell colony formation in semi solid agar culture of normal mouse bone marrow cells (30,31). No effect on human pre B cell development has been detected for rhSCF and may be due to a limited role of rhIL-7 on early human B cell development. Williams and colleagues have examined the role of SCF in T cell development in thyroid lobe cultures. In these studies SCF was shown to synergize with IL-7 to stimulate increased proliferation of T cells (37). In agar culture of human bone marrow cells rhSCF synergizes with CSFs and erythropoietin to stimulate progenitor cells of the myeloid and erythroid lineages (32-34). SCF alone has limited if any effect on human megakaryocytopoiesis, however, both primitive and mature megakaryocyte progenitors (BFU-Mk and CFU-Mk) are stimulated by SCF in combination with other cytokines (38,39).

Highly purified mouse and human progenitors are stimulated by SCF in combination with other cytokines demonstrating a direct stimulatory effect of SCF on these cells (33,40,41). This is consistent with the detection of c-kit on cells with a primitive phenotype determined by antigen expression (42,43). In liquid culture of purified primitive mouse or human progenitor cells, SCF acts in combination with other cytokines to stimulate the amplification of progenitor cells (33,40,41). These studies have been performed at the single cell level and in the mouse, single cells generated up to 450 CFC (41). In all studies the amplification of progenitors led to more differentiated progeny, and in no studies presented to date has self renewal of primitive cells/progenitors been demonstrated as a result of stimulation by SCF. These properties demonstrate that SCF is a multilineage factor which may act directly upon a common lymphoid-myeloid stem cell.

Preclinical Studies of SCF

The in vivo biology of SCF has been studied in a number of animal models including rodents, dogs and nonhuman primates. In all species studied, SCF stimulates a broad range of biological responses within hematopoietic tissues. In mice, SCF has been shown to localize to the lungs and has been associated with mast cell degranulation (44). At doses of SCF of 100 µg/kg or greater, significant increases have been demonstrated for neutrophils, erythrocytes, mast cells, B and T lymphocytes and megakaryocytes (45). In addition, SCF has been shown to be an effective mobilization factor for peripheral blood progenitor cells (PBPC) (46,47).

Clinical Trials With SCF

Initial phase I studies were performed with SCF following chemotherapy in patients with advanced small-cell lung cancer (48) and patients with advanced carcinoma of the breast (49). At the doses of rhSCF tested (5 to 50 µg/kg/day), there was little if any effects on recovery of hematopoietic cells. However, a number of adverse events were reported in these studies including mild to moderate dermatologic reactions at the injection sites and multisymptom systemic anaphylactoid reactions (48-50). All of these reactions were transient and reversible. These clinical observations are consistent with the induction of mast cell hyperplasia as well as induction of mast cell activation and mediator release (50). Subsequently, a phase I/II study was performed to evaluate the effect of low doses of rhSCF (5 to 25 µg/kg/day) to synergize with rhG-CSF in PBPC mobilization. Breast cancer patients were mobilized with the combination of rhSCF plus rhG-CSF and compared to patients mobilized with rhG-CSF alone. The median number of CD34$^+$ cells collected was greater for patients receiving the combination of rhG-CSF and rhSCF, at doses greater than 10 µg/kg/day, compared to rhG-CSF alone (7.7 v 3.2 x 10^6/kg) (51). The time to hematopoietic engraftment and overall survival was similar for both treatment groups. Recently, a randomized phase III study of mobilization of rhSCF and rhG-CSF was performed in high-risk breast cancer patients. There were 175 evaluable patients without protocol violations. The aim of the study was to compare the number of aphereses required to collect a target of 5 x 10^6 CD34$^+$ cells/kg. By day 5 of leukapheresis, 67% of the rhSCF plus rhG-CSF patients had reached the target compared to 48% of those receiving rhG-CSF alone. This study demonstrated that the combination of rhG-CSF and rhSCF reduced the number of leukapheresis harvests required to collect 5 x 10^6 CD34$^+$ cells/kg compared to rhG-CSF alone (52). It is of concern that only 67% of the patients treated with the combination of rhSCF plus rhG-CSF reached the target of 5 x 10^6 CD34$^+$ cells/kg in this study. The package insert for the use of rhG-CSF states that the drug should be administered for 6 to 7 days with leukapheresis on days 5,6 and 7 with clinical support data demonstrating median ANC recovery of 9 to 11 days and median platelet recovery of 10 to 16 days. The challenge will be to identify those patients that will have lower leukapheresis yields with rhG-CSF alone and could benefit from the added treatment with rhSCF. The increased yields of CD34+ cells obtained with the combination of rhSCF plus rhG-CSF may become important in cell therapy procedures, such as tumor cell depletion, where significant losses of CD34+ cells occur. A product licencing application (PLA) was filed for rhSCF under the product name STEMGEN in 1996 and is currently under FDA review.

FLT-3 LIGAND (FLT-3L)

In 1991, two groups described the cloning of a novel murine tyrosine kinase receptor termed flt3 (53) and flk-2 (54) which was thought to be specific for hematopoietic stem cells and progenitor cells (54). Several years later, the human homolog of Flk2/Flt-3 was cloned from a CD34+ cell enriched library (termed STK-1(55)). The ligand for this receptor (FLT-3L) was subsequently identified by two groups. Lymann and colleagues cloned FLT-3L from a cDNA library made from a murine T-cell line which bound the soluble form of the flt-3 receptor (56). Hannum and colleagues purified FLT-3L from media conditioned by a murine stromal cell line by affinity chromatography using the mouse flt-3 receptor extracellular domain (57). Once the mouse FLT-3L cDNA had been isolated it was used to isolate cDNAs encoding the human gene (58). The product of the human FLT-3L gene is a type 1 transmembrane protein of 235 amino acids. A membrane bound form of FLT-3L is produced due to alternate splicing, resulting in the deletion of the proteolytic cleavage site (59).

The in vitro effects of FLT-3L overlap with SCF acting in combination with other growth factors to stimulate mature and primitive hematopoietic progenitor cells of the myeloid and lymphoid lineages (60). Both factors have limited if any effects alone on either primitive or mature progenitor cells. While SCF has a major stimulatory effect on mast cells, FLT-3L has no stimulatory effect on mast cells (61). The precise roles of FLT-3L and SCF in stimulation of lymphopoiesis still remains to be determined, however, the data from knockout mice suggest that FLT-3L may be more critical in early lymphoid development than SCF (60). In vivo, daily administration of FLT-3L in mice results in an increase in the number of lymphocytes, granulocytes and monocytes (62). Bone marrow cellularity is not affected by FLT-3L treatment. The effect on lymphoid cells occurs on more immature B cells associated with a decrease in both mature T and B cells (62). Similar to SCF, FLT-3L alone mobilizes progenitor cells into the peripheral blood of mice and synergizes with G-CSF and GM-CSF to give increased mobilization (63).

Clinical Use of FLT-3L
FLT-3L has been administered to normal healthy volunteers by subcutaneous injection at doses ranging from 10 to 100 μg/kg daily for 14 consecutive days (65). Injection site

reactions and enlarged lymph nodes were the only adverse reactions attributed to FLT-3L administration. After discontinuation of FLT-3L, all adverse events and laboratory changes resolved without sequelae. Increased circulating WBC levels and mobilization of CD34$^+$ cells, GM-CFC and BFU-E occurred for up to a week after the last dose. Circulating dendritic cells were also increased up to 30-fold by day 9 in FLT-3L treated individuals compared to placebo (66). The increase in dendritic cells was transient, with dendritic cells in the peripheral blood returning to normal levels within 7 days after cessation of treatment.

FLT-3L is manufactured by Immunex and the clinical grade soluble protein is termed Mobist. Mobist is being evaluated in phase I/II clinical trials in cancer patients for PBPC mobilization in combination with other growth factors and a phase II trial in patients with prostate cancer and non-Hodgkin's lymphoma to study its effects on tumor cell inhibition.

THROMBOPOIETIN (TPO)

For many years, investigators had been attempting unsuccessfully to isolate thrombopoietin. In 1986, Wendling and colleagues (67) described a transforming viral complex that induced a myeloproliferative syndrome in mice. Four years later the transforming gene v-mpl was identified and the cellular homologue of the viral gene, proto-oncogene c-mpl, was identified and shown to be specifically involved in megakaryocyte development (68,69). The ligand for c-mpl was subsequently isolated and cloned in 1994 by at least four independent groups and shown to have the properties consistent with thrombopoietin (Tpo) (70-73). Tpo has a molecular mass of 35 kDa and consists of a novel two-domain structure with an amino-terminal domain homologous to erythropoietin and a carboxy-terminal domain rich in serine, threonine and proline residues that contain several potential N-linked glycosylation sites (70,72). The primary sites of Tpo production are the liver and the kidneys, with production also occurring in the spleen and marrow (74). The Tpo molecule has problems with stability and therefore the group from Amgen Inc, truncated the molecule, retaining the Epo-like domain and splicing the glycosylation terminal. The truncated molecule was then conjugated to polyethylene glycol (PEG) to stabilize the molecule while retaining its biological activity. The pegylated molecule was termed rhPEG-MGDF (75).

The major effects of Tpo in vitro, are on megakaryocyte development. In bone marrow cultures, Tpo has been shown to stimulate both primitive (Mk-BFU) and mature (Mk-CFU) megakaryocyte precursor cells and to stimulate proplatelet and platelet formation (76-78). A number of studies have reported effects of Tpo on primitive hematopoietic precursor cells in combination with other growth factors. Tpo synergizes with SCF to stimulate Mk-CFU and is additive with IL-3 (76).

Many studies have evaluated the role of Tpo in vivo, particularly in mice and primates. In normal animals, Tpo induces a marked increase of platelet levels of 3 to 6 fold higher than base line levels (79,80). In animals, with irradiation and/or chemotherapy induced thrombocytopenia, treatment with Tpo results in more rapid recovery of platelet levels (76,81,82). However, in animals given marrow ablative therapy, treatment with Tpo has no effect on the nadir of thrombocytopenia but decreases the duration (81,82).

Clinical Use of Tpo
A number of clinical studies have been performed with Tpo. Patients with advanced solid tumors have been treated with Tpo following chemotherapy (83-85). In general, treatment with Tpo has had a minimal effect on thrombocytopenia, but has significantly enhanced the recovery of platelets to baseline levels. A study treating patients with lung cancer resulted in a platelet nadir of 180,000/ul in Tpo treated patients following chemotherapy compared to 111,000/ul in the placebo treated group, however the platelets returned to baseline by day 14 in the Tpo treated group vs 21 days in the placebo treated group (84).

Several studies have evaluated the use of Tpo in mobilization of PBPC. A study by Gajewski suggests that the addition of Tpo to G-CSF plus chemotherapy results in enhanced mobilization of PBPC.(85). This study however, did not include a control group mobilized with G-CSF plus chemotherapy, making this study difficult to evaluate.

Other studies have used Tpo with transplantation of either BM (87) or PBPC (88,89) to support high dose chemotherapy. There was no significant difference in the duration of severe thrombocytopenia following PBPC and treatment with Tpo, compared to placebo, however, following BM transplantation, patients treated with Tpo had accelerated time to platelet recovery associated with a 38% reduction in the severity of severe thrombocytopenia (87). The last area of clinical trials with Tpo is treatment of platelet donors to improve platelet apheresis yields. In 59 donors, an increased platelet yield was obtained with treatment with Tpo and infusion of the apheresis products, into cancer patients with chemotherapy-induced Grade IV thrombocytopenia, resulted in increased platelet increments (90).

THE EX VIVO ROLE OF HGF'S IN CELLULAR THERAPY

Ex Vivo Expansion of Progenitor Cells and Mature Cells
A number of studies have demonstrated the effects of multiple growth factor combinations on primitive progenitor cells and stem cells. The ability to stimulate primitive progenitor cells to generate committed progenitor cells and mature cells has been proposed as a method to eliminate neutropenia and thrombocytopenia following

high dose chemotherapy. A number of different cocktails of HGFs have been shown to stimulate the expansion of CD34$^+$ cells, however, these cocktails contain HGFs manufactured by different companies which has limited the access to clinical grade HGFs (91). The early clinical studies utilized combinations of SCF/IL-3/IL-6/IL-1/GM-CSF/Epo which were research grade factors (92). These studies showed little if any clinical benefit, however, they did demonstrate the safety of reinfusion of expanded cells (92). Alcorn and colleagues started with frozen bone marrow samples that were CD34 selected and expanded. Reinfusion of the expanded cells resulted in prolonged delays in engraftment and a back up product was given to a number of patients on this study (93). A major flaw in this study was the effect of selecting a frozen BM product which resulted in large losses of progenitor cells, such that the expanded product contained a similar progenitor cell number as the original starting BM. This complicates evaluation of the effect of the expanded cells. Other studies have used suboptimal HGF cocktails such as PIXY123 (GM-CSF/IL-3 fusion protein) plus G-CSF plus Epo resulting in low levels of expansion of progenitor cells (94).The cocktail of SCF plus G-CSF plus Tpo has been shown to stimulate a consistent expansion from PBPC and cord blood (CB) of 20 fold or more (95,96). This cocktail was tested in a primate study, where PBPC mobilized with G-CSF in normal baboons was CD34 selected, ex vivo expanded in the cocktail of SCF, G-CSF and MDGF for 10 days and the cells harvested (97). After washing, the expanded cells were reinfused into the baboons after lethal irradiation. The baboons treated with expanded cells and both G-CSF and MGDF after transplantation had greatly reduced neutropenia compared to baboons transplanted with unexpanded cells. Of 3 baboons, only one had a neutrophil count that dropped below 500 ANC/ul compared to control groups in which all 3 animals in 3 separate groups had nadirs below 200 ANC/ul in all animals. Baboons transplanted with expanded cells without treatment with G-CSF and MGDF post transplant had similar nadirs in neutrophils to animals transplanted with unexpanded cells demonstrating the need for growth factors following transplantation of expanded cells. Platelet nadirs were identical between all groups receiving either expanded or unexpanded cells with or without growth factors post transplant (97).

A recent study by Shpall and colleagues has utilized the cocktail of SCF, G-CSF and MGDF for the ex vivo expansion of umbilical cord blood (UCB) cells products for transplantation in the matched unrelated setting (98). This study has selected 40% of the frozen UCB product for expansion while 60% of the product is reinfused unmanipulated to ensure long term durable chimerism. The selected CD34$^+$ cells are cultured in a serum defined culture media containing SCF plus G-CSF plus Tpo at 100 ng/ml in teflon bags for 10 days. The cells are then harvested, washed and reinfused. The study has reported on the transplantation of 4 patients who were large adults with an average weight of approximately 70 kg who received less than 10^7 total cells per kg. All 4 patients engrafted neutrophils within 20 to 30 days, comparable to engraftment of unmanipulated UCB in smaller patients. Previous data from Gluckman and colleagues reported transplantation of unmanipulated CB in patients > 45kg showed that only 23% had engrafted neutrophils by day 60 (99). These data suggest a potential role of expanded UCB for transplantation of larger adult patients.

Gene Therapy

One of the main technologies for transduction of genes into hematopoietic cells is retroviral transduction. Retroviruses will not transfect quiescent cells and so HGFs are required to stimulate stem cells to enable efficient transduction. There is extensive evidence in murine models that retroviral vectors can introduce foreign genes at high efficiencies into stem cells resulting in long term persistent expression of the gene product in vivo (100-102). In these models, BM cells were harvested from mice and cultured with high titer viral supernatants in the presence of SCF plus IL-3 plus IL-6 (100). After 2 to 3 days of culture the cells were transplanted into irradiated mice and greater than 90% of the progenitor cells contained the viral gene at time periods in excess of 12 months of transplant (102).

Studies in humans have been less successful with low levels of transduction resulting from identical approaches with BM or PBPC products. Bodine and colleagues have demonstrated that human stem cells and primitive progenitor cells do not express the murine retroviral receptor (103). This suggests that the retrovirus cannot enter the stem cell and so low transduction efficiencies result. The mouse studies demonstrate the potential of retro viral gene transfer and it remains to be seen whether the technical barriers associated with transfer into human stem cells can be overcome. The role of HGFs in this setting will depend upon the vectors that allow for gene transduction and the need for activation of stem cells into cycle.

REFERENCES

1. Bradley TR, Metcalf D. The growth of mouse bone marrow cells in vitro. Aust J Exp Biol Med Sci 1966; 44:287-299.
2. Pluznick DH, Sachs L. The cloning of normal "mast" cells in tissue culture. J Cell Comp Physiol 1965; 66:319.
3. Metcalf D. Hemopoietic colonies. In: In vitro cloning of normal and leukemic cells. Berlin: Springer-Verlag, 1977.
4. Metcalf D, Nicola NA. Synthesis by mouse peritoneal cells of G-CSF, the differentiation inducer for myeloid leukemia cells: stimulation by endotoxin, M-CSF, and multi-CSF. Leuk Res 1985;9:35-50.
5. Warren MK, Ralph P. Macrophage growth factor CSF-1 stimulates human monocyte production of interferon, tumor necrosis factor, and colony stimulating activity. J Immunol 1986; 137:2281-2285.
6. Metcalf D, Burgess AW, Johnson GR, et al. In vitro actions on hemopoietic cells of recombinant murine GM-CSF purified after production in E. Coli: comparison

with purified native GM-CSF. J Cell Physiol 1986; 128:421-431.

7. Bronchud MH, Scarffe JH, Thatcher N, et al. Phase I/II study of recombinant human granulocyte colony stimulating factor in patients receiving intensive chemotherapy for small cell lung cancer. Br J Cancer 1987; 56(6):809-813.

8. Gabrilove JL, Jakubowski A, Fain K, et al. Phase I study of granulocyte colony-stimulating factor in patients with transitional cell carcinoma of the urothelium. J Clin Invets 1988; 82(4):1454-1461.

9. Sheridan WP, Begley CG, Juttner C, et al. Effect of peripheral-blood progenitor cells mobilized by filgrastim (G-CSF) on platelet recovery after high-dose chemotherapy. Lancet 1992; 339 (8794): 640-644.

10. Gianni AM, Siena S, Bregni M, et al. Granulocyte-macrophage colony-stimulating factor to harvest circulating haemopoietic stem cells for autotransplant. Lancet 1989; 2:580-585.

11. Peters WP, Rosner G. A bottom-line analysis of the financial impact of hematopoietic colony-stimulating factors and CSF-primed peripheral blood progenitor cells. Blood 1991; 78(suppl 1):14a.

12. Crown J, Jakubowski A, Kemeny N, et al. A phase I trial of recombinant human interleukin-1B alone and in combination with myelosuppressive doses of 5-fluorouracil in patients with gastrointestinal cancer. Blood 1990; 78:1420-1427.

13. Lindermann A, Ganser A, Seipelt G, et al. Biologic effects of recombinant interleukin-3 in vivo. J Clin Onc 1991; 9:2120-2127.

14. Veldhuis GJ, Willemse PH, Sleijfer DT, et al. Toxicity and efficacy of escalating doses of recombinant human interleukin-6 after chemotherapy in patients with breast cancer or non-small cell lung cancer. J Clin Oncol 1995; 13:2585-2593.

15. Paul S, Bennett F, Calvetti J, et al. Molecular cloning of a cDNA encoding interleukin 11, a stromal cell-derived lymphopoietic and hematopoietic cytokine. Proc Natl Acad Sci USA 1990; 87;7512-7516.

16. McKinley D, Wu Q, Yang-Feng T, et al. Genomic sequence and chromosomal location of human interleukin (IL)-11 gene. Genomics 1992; 13:814-819.

17. Yin T, Miyazawa K, Yang Y, et al. Interleukin (IL)-6 signal transducer, gp130, is involved in IL-11 mediated signal transduction. J Immunol 1993; 151:2555-2561.

18. Toyama K, Yoshida Y, Ohashi K, et al. Production of multiple growth factors by a newly established human thyroid carcinoma cell line. Jpn J Cancer Res 1992; 83:153-158.

19. Elias JA, Lentz V, Cummings PJ. Transforming growth factor-B regulation of IL-6 production by unstimulated and IL-1-stimulated human fibroblasts. J Immunol 1991; 146;3437-3443.

20. Leary A, Zeng HQ, Clark SC, Ogawa M. Growth factor requirements for survival in G_0 and entry into the cell cycle of primitive hemopoietic progenitors. Proc Natl Acad Sci USA 1992; 89:4013-4017.

21. Du XX, Williams DA. Effects of recombinant human interleukin-11 (IL-11) on

murine hematopoiesis in vitro. Blood 1993; 82:319a.

22. Bruno E, Briddell RA, Cooper RJ, Hoffman R. Effects of recombinant interleukin-11 on human megakaryocyte progenitor cells. Exp Hematol 1991; 19:378-381.

23. Bree A, Schlerman F, Timony G, et al. Pharmacokinetics and thrombopoietic effects of recombinant human interleukin-11 (rhIL-11) in nonhuman primates and rodents. Blood 1991;78:132a.

24. Du XX, Neben T, Goldman S, Williams DA. Effects of recombinant human interleukin-11 on hematopoietic reconstitution in transplant mice: acceleration of recovery of peripheral blood neutrophils and platelets. Blood 1993; 81:27-34.

25. Gordon MS, McCaskill-Stevens WJ, Battiato LA, et al. A phase I trial of recombinant human interleukin-11 (neumega rhIL-11 growth factor) in women with breast cancer receiving chemotherapy. Blood 1996; 87:3615-3624.

26. Zsebo KM, Wypych J, McNiece IK, et al. Identification, purification, and biological characterization of hematopoietic stem cell factor from Buffalo Rat Liver conditioned medium. Cell 1990; 63:195-201.

27. Anderson DM, Lyman SD, Baird A, et al. Molecular cloning of mast cell growth factor, a hematopoietin that is active in both membrane bound and soluble forms. Cell 1990; 63:235-243.

28. Huang E, Nocka K, Beier DR, et al. The hematopoietic growth factor KL is encoded by the Sl locus and is the ligand of the c-kit receptor, the gene product of the W locus. Cell 1990; 63:225-233.

29. Toksoz D, Zsebo KM, Smith KA, et al. Support of human hematopoiesis in long-term bone marrow cultures by murine stromal cells selectively expressing the membrane bound and secreted forms of the human homolog of the steel gene product, stem cell factor. Proc Natl Acad Sci USA 1992:89:7350-7354.

30. Martin FH, Suggs SV, Langley KE, et al. Primary structure and functional expression of rat and human stem cell factor DNAs. Cell 63:203-211, 1990.

31. McNiece IK, Langley KE, Zsebo KM. The role of stem cell factor in B cell differentiation: synergistic interaction with IL-7. J. Immunol. 146:3785-3790, 1991.

32. McNiece IK, Langley KE, Zsebo KM. Recombinant human stem cell factor synergizes with GM-CSF, G-CSF, IL-3 and Epo to stimulate human progenitor cells of the myeloid and erythroid lineages. Exp. Hematol. 19:226-231, 1991.

33. Bernstein ID, Andrews RG, Zsebo KM. Recombinant human stem cell factor enhances the formation of colonies by CD34[+] and CD34[+]lin- cells, and the generation of colony-forming cell progeny from CD34[+]lin- cells cultured with interleukin-3, granulocyte colony stimulating-factor or granulocyte-macrophage colony-stimulating factor. Blood 77:2316-2321, 1991.

34. Broxmeyer HE, Cooper S, Lu L, et al. Effect of murine mast cell growth factor (c-kit proto-oncogene ligand) on colony formation by human marrow hematopoietic progenitor cells. Blood 77:2142-2149, 1991.

35. Medlock E, Yung Y, McNiece I, et al. Role of stem cell factor (SCF) in the

stimulation of the mast cell lineage. Blood 76(10) suppl. 1:154 (abstr.), 1991.

36. Broxmeyer HE, Hangoc G, Cooper S, et al. Influence of murine mast cell growth factor (c-kit ligand) on colony formation by mouse marrow hematopoietic progenitor cells. Exp. Hematol. 19:143-146, 1991.

37. Namen AE, Widmer MB, Voice R, et al. A ligand for the c-kit proto-oncogene (MGF) stimulates lymphoid progenitor cells in vitro. Exp. Hematol. 19:749-754.

38. Briddell RA, Bruno E, Cooper RJ, et al. Effect of c-kit ligand on in vitro human megakaryocytopoiesis. Blood 78:2854-2859, 1991.

39. Avraham H, Vannier E, Cowley S, et al. Effects of the stem cell factor, c-kit ligand, on human megakaryocytic cells. Blood 79:365-371, 1992.

40. de Vries P, Brasel KA, Eisenman JR, et al. The effect of recombinant mast cell growth factor on purified hematopoietic stem cells. J. Exp. Med. 173:1205-1211, 1991.

41. Williams N, Bertoncello I, Kavnoudias H, Zsebo K, McNiece I. Recombinant rat stem cell factor stimulates the amplification and differentiation of fractionated mouse stem cell populations. Blood 79:58-64, 1992.

42. Briddell RA, Broudy VC, Bruno E, et al. Further phenotypic characterization and isolation of human hematopoietic progenitor cells using a monoclonal antibody to the c-kit receptor. Blood 79:3159-3167, 1992.

43. Ogawa M, Matsuzaki Y, Nishikawa S, et al. Expression and function of c-kit in hematopoietic progenitor cells. J. Exp. Med. 174:63-71, 1991.

44. Lynch DH, Jacobs C, DuPont D, et al. Pharmacokinetic parameters of recombinant mast cell growth factor (rMGF). Lymphokine Cytokine Res 1992;11:233-236.

45. Andrews RG, Knitter GH, Bartelmez SH, et al. Recombinant human stem cell factor, a c-kit ligand, stimulates hematopoiesis in nonhuman primates. Blood 1991; 78:1975-1980.

46. Andrews RG, Bensinger WI, Knitter GH, et al. The ligand for c-kit ligand, stem cell factor, stimulates the circulation of cells that engraft lethally irradiated baboons. Blood 1992; 80:2715-2720..

47. Briddell RA, Hartley CA, Smith KA, McNiece IK (1993). Recombinant rat stem cell factor synergizes with recombinant human granulocyte-colony stimulating factor in vivo in mice to mobilize peripheral blood progenitor cells which have enhanced repopulating ability. Blood 1993; 82:1720-1723.

48. Crawford J, Lau D, Erwin R, et al. A phase I trial of recombinant methionyl human stem cell factor (SCF) in patients (pts) with advanced non-small cell lung carcinoma (NSCLS). Proc Am Soc Clin Oncol 1993; 12:135a.

49. Demetri G, Costa J, Hayes D, et al. A phase I trial of recombinant methionyl human stem cell factor (SCF) in patients with advanced breast carcinoma pre- and post chemotherapy (chemo) with cyclophosphamide © and doxorubicin (A). Proc Am Soc Clin Oncol 1993; 12:142a.

50. Costa JJ, Demetri GD, Harrist TJ, et al. Recombinant human stem cell factor (kit ligand) promotes human mast cell and melanocyte hyperplasia and functional

activation in vivo. J Exp Med 1996; 183:2681-2686.

51. Glaspy JA, Shpall EJ, LeMaistre CF, et al. Peripheral blood progenitor cell mobilization using stem cell factor in combination with filgrastim in breast cancer patients. Blood 1997; 90:2939-2951.

52. Shpall EJ, Wheeler CA, Turner SA, et al. A randomized phase 3 study of PBPC mobilization by stem cell factor (SCF, STEMGEN) and filgrastim in patients with high-risk breast cancer. Blood 1997; 90(suppl 1):591a.

53. Rosnet O, Marchetto S, deLapeyriere O, et al. Murine Flt3, a gene encoding a novel tyrosine kinase receptor of the PDGFR/CSF1R family. Oncogene 1991; 6:1641-1650.

54. Matthews W, Jordan CT, Wiegand GW, et al. A receptor tyrosine kinase specific to haematopoietic stem and progenitor cell-enriched populations. Cell 1991; 65:1143-1152.

55. Small D, Levenstein M, Kim E, et al. STK-1, the human homolog of Flk-2/Flt-3, is selectively expressed in CD34$^+$ human bone marrow cells and is involved in the proliferation of early progenitor/stem cells. Proc Natl Acad Sci USA 1994; 91:459-463.

56. Lymann SD, James L, Vanden Bos T, et al. Molecular cloning of a ligand for the flt3/flk-2 tyrosine kinase receptor: a proliferative factor for primitive hematopoietic cells. Cell 1993; 75:1157-11.67.

57. Hannum C, Culpepper J, Campbell D, et al. Ligand for FLT3/FLK2 receptor tyrosine kinase regulates growth of haematopoietic stem cells and is encoded by variant RNAs. Nature 1994; 368:643-648.

58. Lyman SD, James L, Johnson L, et al. Cloning of the human homologue of the murine flt3 ligand: a growth factor for early hematopoietic progenitor cells. Blood 1994; 83:2795.

59. Lyman SD, James L, Escobar S, et al. Identification of soluble and membrane-bound isoforms of the murine flt3 ligand generated by alternative splicing of mRNAs. Oncogene 1995; 10:149-157.

60. Lyman SD, Jacobsen SE. c-kit ligand and flt3 ligand: stem/progenitor cells factors with overlapping yet distinct activities. Blood 1998; 91:1101-1134.

61. Hjertson M, Sundstrom C, Lyman SD, et al. Stem cell factor, but not flt3 ligand, induces differentiation and activation of human mast cells. Exp Hematol 1996; 24:748.-754.

62. Brasel K, McKenna HJ, Morrissey PJ, et al. Hematologic effects of flt3 ligand in vivo in mice. Blood 1996; 88:2004-2012.

63. Brasel K, McKenna HJ, Charrier K, et al. Flt3 ligand synergises with granulocyte-macrophage colony-stimulating factor or granulocyte colony-stimulating factor to mobilize hematopoietic progenitor cells into the peripheral blood of mice. Blood 1997; 90:3781-3788.

64. Molineux G, McCrea C, Yan XQ, McNiece I. Flt-3 ligand synergises with G-CSF to increase neutrophil numbers and to mobilize peripheral blood stem cells with

long-term repopulating potential. Blood 1997; 89:3998-4004

65. Lebsack ME, McKenna HJ, Hoek JA, et al. Safety of FLT3 ligand in healthy volunteers. Blood 1997; 90(suppl 1): 170a.

66. Maraskovsky E, Roux E, Teepe M, et al. Flt3 ligand increases peripheral blood dendritic cells in healthy volunteers. Blood 1997; 90 (suppl 1):581a.

67. Wendling F, Varlet P, Charon M, Tambourin P. MPLV: a retrovirus complex inducing an acute myeloproliferative leukemic disorder in adult mice. Virology 1986; 149:242-246.

68. Souyri M, Vigon I, Penciolelli JF, et al. A putative truncated cytokine receptor gene transduced by the myeloproliferative leukemia virus immortalizes hematopoietic progenitor cells. Cell 1990; 63: 1137-1147.

69. Vigon I, Mornon JP, Cocault L, et al. Molecular cloning and characterization of MPL, the human homolog of the v-mpl oncogene: identification of a member of the hematopoietic growth factor receptor superfamily. Proc Natl Acad Sci USA 1992; 89:5640-5644.

70. deSauvage FJ, Hass PE, Spencer SD, et al. Stimulation of megakaryocytopoiesis and thrombopoiesis by the c-mpl ligand. Nature 1994; 369: 533-8.

71. Hunt P, Li YS, Nichol JL, et al. Purification and biological characterization of plasma-derived megakaryocyte growth and development factor. Blood 1995; 86:540-547.

72. Lok S, Kaushansky K, Holly RD, et al. Cloning and expression of murine thrombopoietin cDNA and stimulation of platelet production in vivo. Nature 1994; 369:565-568.

73. Ogami K, Shimada Y, Sohma Y, et al. The sequence of a rat cDNA encoding thrombopoietin. Gene 1995; 158:309-310.

74. Foster DC, Sprecher CA, Grant FJ, et al. Human thrombopoietin: gene structure, cDNA sequence, expression, and chromosomal localization. Proc Natl Acad Sci USA 1994; 91:13023-13027.

75. Hokom MM, Lacey D, Kinstler OB, et al. Pegylated megakaryocyte growth and development factor abrogates the lethal thrombocytopenia associated with carboplatin and irradiation in mice. Blood 1995; 86:4486-4492.

76. Nichol JL, Hokom MM, Hornkohl A, et al. Megakaryocyte growth and development factor. Analysis of in vitro effects on human megakaryocytopoiesis and endogenous serum levels during chemotherapy-induced thrombocytopenia. J Clin Invest 1995; 95:2973-2978.

77. Choi ES, Nichol JL, Hokom MM, et al. Platelets generated in vitro from proplatelet-displaying human megakaryocytes are functional. Blood 1995; 85:402-413.

78. Choi ES, Hokom MM, Chen JL, et al. The role of megakaryocyte growth and development factor in terminal stages of thrombopoiesis. Br J Haemtol 1996; 95:227-233.

79. Kaushansky K, Lin N, Grossman A, et al. Thrombopoietin expands erythroid,

granulocyte-macrophage, and megakaryocyte progenitor cells in normal and myelosuppressed mice. Exp Hematol 1996; 24:265-269.

80. Farese AM, Hunt P, Boone T, MacVittie TJ. Recombinant human megakaryocyte growth and development factor stimulates thrombocytopoiesis in normal human primates. Blood 1995; 86:54-59.

81. Molineux G, Hartley C, McElroy P, et al. Megakaryocyte growth and development factor accelerates platelet recovery in peripheral blood progenitor cell transplant recipients. Blood 1996;88:366-376.

82. Harker LA, Marzec UM, Hunt P, et al. Dose-response effects of pegylated human megakaryocyte growth and development factor on platelet production and function in nonhuman primates. Blood 1996; 88:511-521.

83. Basser RL, Rasko JE, Clarke K, et al. Thrombopoietic effects of pegylated recombinant human megakaryocyte growth and development factor (PEG-rHuMGDF) in patients with advanced cancer. Lancet 1996; 348:1279-1281.

84. Begley G, Basser R, Clarke K, et al. Randomized, double-blind, placebo-controlled phase I trial of PEG-ylated megakaryocyte growth and development factor (PEG-rHuMGDF) administered to patients with advanced cancer before and after chemotherapy. Proc Annu Meet Am Soc Clin Oncol 1996; 15:719.

85. Vadhan-Raj S, Verschraegen C, McGarry L, et al. Recombinant human thrombopoietin (rhTPO) attenuates high-dose carboplatin (C)-induced thrombocytopenia in patients with gynecologic malignancies. Blood 1997; 89:580a.

86. Gajewski J, Korbling M, Donato M, et al. Recombinant human thrombopoietin (rhTPO) for mobilization of peripheral blood progenitor cells (PBPC) for autologous transplantation in breast cancer: Preliminary results of a phase I trial. Blood 1997; 89:221a.

87. Beveridge R, Schuster M, Waller E, et al. Randomized, double-blind, placebo-controlled trial of pegylated recombinant human megakaryocyte growth and development factor (PEG-rHuMGDF) in breast cancer patients (pts) following autologous bone marrow transplantation (ABMT). Blood 1997; 89:580a.

88. Bolwell B, Vredenburgh J, Overmoyer B, et al. Safety and biologic effect of pegylated recombinant human megakaryocyte growth and development factor (PEG-rHuMGDF) in breast cancer patients following autologous peripheral blood progenitor cell transplantation (PBPC). Blood 1997; 89:171a.

89. Glaspy J, Vredenburgh J, Demetri GD, et al. Effects of PEGylated recombinant human megakaryocyte growth and development factor (PEG-rHuMGDF) before high dose chemotherapy (HDC) with peripheral blood progenitor cell (PBPC) support. Blood 1997; 89:580a.

90. Kuter D, McCullough J, Romo J, et al. Treatment of platelet (PLT) donors with pegylated recombinant human megakaryocyte growth and development factor (PEG-rHuMGDF) increases circulating PLT counts (CTS) and PLT apheresis yields and increases platelet increments in recipients of PLT transfusions.

91. Haylock DN, To LB, Dowse TL, et al. Ex vivo expansion and maturation of peripheral blood CD34$^+$ cells into the myeloid lineage. Blood 1992; 80:1405-1412.
92. Brugger W, Mocklin W, Heimfeld S, et al. Ex vivo expansion of enriched peripheral blood CD34$^+$ progenitor cells by stem cell factor, interleukin-1B (IL-1B), IL-6, IL-3, Interferon--gamma, and erythropoietin. Blood 1993;81:2579-2584.
93. Alcorn MJ, Holyoake TL, Richmond L, et al. CD34-positive cells isolated from cryopreserved peripheral blood progenitor cells can be expanded ex vivo and used for transplantation with little or no toxicity. J Clin Oncol 1996; 14:1839-1847.
94. Williams SF, Lee WJ, Bender JG, et al. Selection and expansion of peripheral blood CD34$^+$ cells in autologous stem cell transplantation for breast cancer. Blood 1996; 87:1687-1691.
95. Stoney GB, Briddell RA, Kern BP, et al. Clinical scale ex vivo expansion of myeloid progenitor cells and megakaryocytes under GMP conditions. Exp. Hematol. 1996; 24(9):1043.
96. Briddell R, Kern BP, Zilm KL, et al. Purification of CD34$^+$ cells is essential for optimal ex vivo expansion of umbilical cord blood cells. J. Hematotherapy 1997; 6:145-150.
97. Andrews RG, Briddell RA, Gough M, McNiece IK. Expansion of G-CSF mobilized CD34$^+$ peripheral blood cells (PBC) for 10 days in G-CSF, MGDF and SCF prior to transplantation decreased post-transplant neutropenia in baboons. Blood 1997; 90:10(suppl 1), 92a.
98. Shpall EJ, Briddell R, Hami L, et al. Transplantation of leukemia patients receiving high dose chemotherapy with ex vivo expanded cord blood cells. ABMT meeting, Miami FL, April, 1998.
99. Gluckman E, Rocha V, Boyer-Chammard A et al. Outcome of cord-blood transplantation from related and unrelated donors. Eurocord Transplant Group and the European Blood and Marrow Transplantation Group. N Engl J Med 1997 Aug 7;337(6):373-81.
100. Bodine DM, McDonagh KT, Donahue RE, Nienhuis AW. Gene insertion into hematopoietic stem cells. Exp. Hematol 1992; 20:125-126.
101. Yan X-Q, Lacey D, Fletcher F, et al. Chronic exposure to retroviral vector encoded MGDF (mpl-ligand) induces lineage-specific growth and differentiation of megakaryocytes in mice. Blood 1995; 86(11):4025-4033.
102. Lusky BD, Zsebo KM, Williams DA. Pre-stimulation of murine bone marrow with steel factor increases retroviral-mediated gene transfer into long-lived hematopoietic stem cells. Blood 1991; 78(suppl. 1):256a.
103. Orlic D, Girard LJ, Jordan CT, et al. The level of mRNA encoding the amphotropic retrovirus receptor in mouse and human hematopoietic stem cells is low and correlates with the efficiency of retrovirus transduction. Proc Natl Acad Sci USA 1996; 93:11097-11102.

Index